Second

Dental Terminology

CHARLINE M. DOFKA, CDA, RDH, MS

THOMSON

DELMAR LEARNING   Australia Brazil Canada Mexico Singapore Spain United Kingdom United States

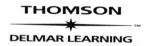

THOMSON

DELMAR LEARNING

Dental Terminology, Second Edition
by Charline M. Dofka, CDA, RDH, MS

Vice President, Health Care Business Unit:
William Brottmiller
Editorial Director:
Matthew Kane
Acquisitions Editor:
Kalen Conerly
Senior Product Manager:
Darcy M. Scelsi
Editorial Assistant:
Molly Belmont

Marketing Director:
Jennifer McAvey
Marketing Channel Manager:
Michelle McTyghe
Marketing Coordinator:
Andrea Eobstel
Technology Director:
Laurie Davis
Technology Project Manager:
Mary Colleen Liburdi

Production Director:
Carolyn Miller
Production Manager:
Barbara A. Bullock
Content Project Manager:
Anne Sherman

Library of Congress Cataloging-in-Publication Data

Dofka, Charline M.
   Dental terminology / Charline M. Dofka.—2nd ed.
      p. ; cm.
   ISBN 1-4180-1522-9
1. Dentistry—Terminology.
I. Title.
   [DNLM: 1. Dentistry—Programmed Instruction.
2. Dentistry—Terminology—English. WU 15 D653d 2007]
   RK28.D64 2007
   617.6001'4—dc22   2006032040

NOTICE TO THE READER

Contents

Preface

INTRODUCTION

Dental Terminology has been written in a user-friendly manner to help the new student or learner understand dental terms. Unlike the other dental dictionaries or reference books that provide words in a straight alphabetical sequence, this text presents terms related specifically to the science of dentistry, grouping them according to speciality or area of interest. The method of presentation employs a "sounds-like" pronunciation system and gives a definition that is more informative and used in relation to similar dental terms. Students will be able to relate the given word to its area of use and compare it to other terms associated with that speciality.

This book may serve as a reference resource for students or may be used in conjunction with a classroom text. The chapters are flexible and able to be adjusted to the specific area of interest. The material and review exercises may be used to reinforce current lessons or understanding in the classroom. On-the-job trainees and those with limited exposure to all dental fields will find this text helpful in understanding broad dental terminology.

ORGANIZATION AND FEATURES

The twenty chapters in this second edition of *Dental Terminology* cover the basic areas of interest or concentration. The first chapter provides a foundation. It explains the composition of dental terms by exploring prefix, root/combination, and suffix divisions, along with word composition. The remaining chapters introduce words relative to specific areas of dentistry. Each new word is printed in boldface, followed by a sounds-like pronunciation and technical definition, plus an example of common usage for most terms. Review exercises challenging the student to recall and apply this information are included with each chapter. Illustrations are scattered throughout the text to reinforce knowledge of many dental terms. An extensive glossary is provided for quick reference, and an appendix presents the word element.

NEW TO THIS EDITION

Chapter 1:

- Expanded explanation of prefixes and suffixes
- Additional exercises integrated within the chapter to reinforce learning

Chapter 2:

- Additional art to enhance understanding
- Expanded definitions for further clarification of some terms and concepts

Chapter 3:

- Expanded discussion related to periodontal membranes, gingival, cementum
- Expanded definitions related to odontology
- Addition of terms related to ridges found on teeth

Chapter 4:

- Added discussion related to places of employment for dental professionals
- Additional illustrations of instruments
- Additional descriptions of rotary instruments

Chapter 5:

- Addition of terms related to disease processes and classifications
- Additional content related to procedures to prevent disease and for proper sanitization

Chapter 6:

- New discussion of the sixth vital sign—pain
- Addition of some questions related to pain in the Chapter Review

Chapter 7:

- New section on procedure related to the initial examination

Chapter 8:

• New chapter on pain management

Chapter 9:

• Additional definitions on the latest technologies in radiography

Chapter 10:

• Added content on matrix placement

Chapter 11:

• New chapter on cosmetic dentistry

Chapter 12:

• Added discussion of implants

Chapter 13:

• Introduction of new tools and techniques

Chapter 14:

• Expanded procedure in maxiofacial surgery

Chapter 15:

• Additional content on methods of orthodontic correction

Chapter 17:

• New content on forensic tooth identification

ABOUT THE AUTHOR

Charline Manion Dofka graduated from West Liberty State College with a BS in Dental Hygiene and received an MS from the University of Dayton. She has taken postgraduate studies at Ohio State, West Virginia University, Kent State, and Ohio State University. Before becoming a dental assisting instructor and co-operative health occupations coordinator for thirty years, she was employed as a dental assistant/hygienist in oral surgery, orthodontic, and general practices.

Mrs. Dofka has recently retired from teaching, but maintains life membership in Iota Lambda Sigma a professional fraternity, DANB certification, registration as a dental hygienist. She is currently serving in consultation practice and advisory board capacity as well as working in volunteer activities.

FEEDBACK

The author hopes that *Dental Terminology* will aid the beginning student—or any interested person—in understanding and using dental terms. Comments, viewpoints, or input regarding this book or *Competency Skills for the Dental Assistant*, which she also has written, will be appreciated. The author may be contacted by E-mail at CharDent@aol.com.

REVIEWERS

Barbara Bennett, CDA, RDH, MS, Texas State Technical College, Harlingen, Texas

Robert Bennett, DMD, Texas State Technical College, Harlingen, Texas

Cindy Bradley, CDA, CDPMA, EFDA, Orlando Tech, Orlando, Florida

Patricia Frese, RDH, Med, Raymond Walters College, Cincinnati, Ohio

Terri Heintz, CDA, RDA, Des Moines Area Community College, Ankeny, Iowa

Kathryn Mosley, RDA, BS, MS, Silicon Valley College, Fremont, California

Denise Murphy, CDA, CDPMA, EFDA, Orlando Tech, Orlando, Florida

Juanita Robinson, CDA, EFDA, LDH, MSEd, Indiana University Northeast, Gary, Indiana

Kelly Svanda, CDA, Southeast Community College, Nehawka, Nebraska

Janet Wilburn, BS, CDA, Phoenix College, Phoenix, Arizona

HOW TO USE STUDYWARE™ TO ACCOMPANY DENTAL TERMINOLOGY, SECOND EDITION

The StudyWARE™ software helps you learn terms and concepts in *Dental Terminology, Second Edition*. As you study each chapter in the text, be sure to explore the activities in the corresponding chapter in the software. Use Study-WARE™ as your own private tutor to help you learn the material in *Dental Terminology, Second Edition*.

Getting started is easy. Install the software by inserting the CD-ROM into your computer's CD-ROM drive and following the on-screen instructions.

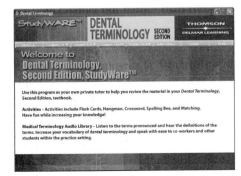

When you open the software, enter your first and last name so the software can store your quiz results. Then choose the chapter in which you are interested from the menu to take a quiz or explore one of the activities.

Menus

You can access the menus from wherever you are in the program. The menus include Quizzes, Activities, and Scores.

Activities. Have fun while increasing your knowledge! Activities include flashcards, spelling bee, hangman, crossword puzzles, and matching.

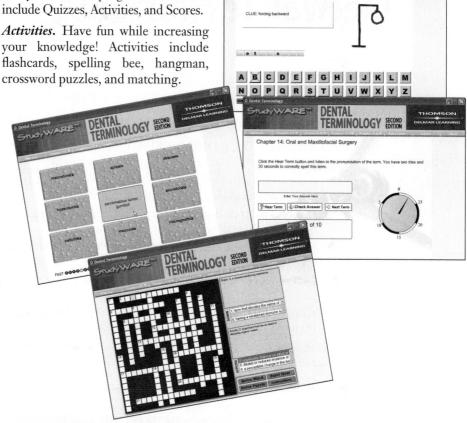

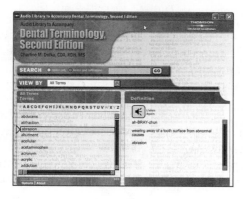

Audio Library. The StudyWARE™ Audio Library is a reference that includes audio pronunciations and definitions for more than 700 dental/medical terms! Use the audio library to practice pronunciation and review definitions. You can browse terms by chapter or search by key word. Listen to pronunciations of the terms you select, or listen to an entire list of terms.

CHAPTER 1

Introduction to Dental Terminology

OBJECTIVES

Upon conclusion of this chapter, the reader should be able to:

1. **Locate the dental word.** Words and abbreviations related to dentistry are printed in boldface when first mentioned in the text.

2. **Pronounce the dental word.** Words are divided by pronunciation groupings with indications for emphasis and pronunciation stress.

3. **Analyze the structure of the dental word.** Combination words are separated into meaningful parts to show word structure.

4. **Define the meaning of the dental word.** Definitions/meanings are presented for each listed term.

5. **Pluralize the dental word.** Words are changed from singular to plural by using the standard rules for changing word endings.

6. **Use the dental word.** Exercises in use of the words and terms are provided at the end of each chapter.

LOCATE THE DENTAL WORD

Dental words are arranged and listed alphabetically in dictionaries, reference works, or glossary listings. A few terms, such as AIDS (acquired immune deficiency syndrome) and HVE (high volume evacuator), are commonly listed in an abbreviated form made up of the first letters of several words. These acronyms (**ACK**-roh-nims) are listed along with other abbreviations representing a combination of word pieces or by initials that can indicate an occupation, a specialty, procedure, condition, or chemical. In filling prescriptions and writing labels the science of pharmacology uses many abbreviations, such as *b.i.d.* (twice a day). Radiology and dental charting procedures also use many acronyms and abbreviations.

Care must be taken when looking for or using acronyms or abbreviations to shorten words, as many abbreviations are not universal. For example, the abbreviation *imp* in general dentistry charting may indicate an impression, but an oral surgeon's office may use *imp* to designate an impaction. Some dental facilities develop a specific code or method of designating conditions and procedures. When in doubt about the spelling or meaning of an abbreviation or an acronym, it is best to spell out the word or look it up in a dictionary, glossary, or office manual.

Some examples of abbreviations or acronyms found in reference works are:

ALARA	as low as reasonably achievable
ANUG	acute necrotizing ulcerative gingivitis
CDA	Certified Dental Assistant
DDS/DMD	Doctor of Dental Surgery or Doctor of Dental Medicine
FFD	film focus distance or focal film distance
HIV	human immunodeficiency virus
HVE	high volume evacuation
MPD	maximum permissible dose
MSDS	Material Safety Data Sheet
PID	Position Indicating Device
PDR	*Physician's Desk Reference*
PPE	personal protection equipment
RDH	Registered Dental Hygienist
ZOE	zinc oxide eugenol

CAUTION: Some words are similar in sound and spelling but have different meanings. These **homonyms** (**HAHM**-oh-nims) may cause confusion and alter the meaning of what is written, so care must be taken to check the meaning and/or the spelling of a word when using these terms.

Some common homonyms used in dentistry are:

die	tooth or bridge pattern used in prosthodontic dentistry
dye	coloring material; may be used to indicate plaque
auxiliary	helping subsidiary, such as a dental assistant
axillary	underarm site; may be used to obtain body temperature
esthetics	pertaining to beauty
aesthesia	loss of pain sensation
facial	(a) pertaining to the face; (b) front surface of incisor tooth
fascial	pertaining to the fibrous membrane on muscles
palpation	use of hand or finger pressure to locate/examine
palpitation	condition of racing or increased heartbeat
suture	area or line where two bones unite, such as coronal suture
suture	stitch or staple repairing or closing wound (see Figure 1-1)

Sometimes dental terminology denotes the name of the person who developed the procedure, discovered the anatomical area, designed the instrument, named the disease, and the like. Examples are *Nasmyth membrane*, *Sharpey's fibers*, or *Bass technique*. These terms are called **eponyms** (**EP**-oh nims).

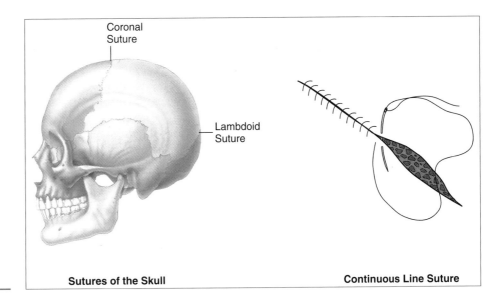

Coronal
Suture

Lambdoid
Suture

Sutures of the Skull **Continuous Line Suture**

FIGURE 1-1
The word suture
may have two or
more meanings.

PRONOUNCE THE DENTAL WORD

After locating the word, it has to be pronounced. In this book, each dental term is broken into "sounds like" syllables or elements that appear in parentheses. **BOLD** upper case letters are used to indicate the syllables that are to receive the most emphasis when pronouncing the word. If the word has a secondary syllable or element of stress, it is printed in **bold** lower case letters. All other elements are printed in the phonetic "sounds like" manner.

To pronounce a word, say it just as it is spelled out within the parentheses. For example, in periodontitis (**pear**-ee-oh-don-**TIE**-tis), the syllable **TIE** receives the most emphasis, and secondary, or lesser, stress is also placed on the first syllable, **pear**. In gingivitis (**jin**-jih-**VIE**-tis), the main emphasis is placed on **VIE**, with secondary stress on the first syllable, **jin**.

Pronunciation rules are standard. Some vocal accents, however, show regional/geographic differences or differences related to the school where they learned the words.

ANALYZE THE STRUCTURE OF THE DENTAL WORD

Dental terminology involves the study of words and terms related specifically to the dental sciences. Every science has its own unique terminology. Rules and conventions are standardized for the formation, pronunciation, pluralization, and meaning of terms.

In medical terminology, many words refer to the proximity or nearness to anatomical structures. A good share of dental terms, too, originate from bones or structures, but more often, from dental procedures or practical approaches.

Dental terms usually are formed by a combination of small words or syllables linked in a "building block" or word chain. Knowing the basic small divisions and the combining methods can help you understand word meanings. When broken into smaller parts, most longer terms reveal a prefix that modifies the term, a single- or double-root structure that provides the foundation to the term, and a suffix that qualifies the word's meaning.

When analyzing the structure of a word, some considerations to observe are the following.

▶ A *prefix* qualifies the word by indicating things such as the quantity, color, size, condition, or location. A word may or may not have a prefix.
▶ A *root* provides the basic foundation for the word. A dental term may have more than one root. When two roots are combined, a *combining vowel* (usually o) is used to connect them.
▶ A *suffix* sometimes is added to a root(s) to qualify or describe the meaning. The combining vowel (o) is placed ahead of the root, and the suffix is not used when the suffix itself begins with a vowel.
▶ A word may be easier to analyze by beginning with the suffix and working toward the beginning of the word.

Prefix

A prefix (**PRE**-fix) is the first building block of a word division that begins a term. A prefix alters the word's meaning by indicating number, color, size, location, or condition. Some common prefixes used in dental terminology are listed in Tables 1-1 through 1-5. Table 1-1 gives examples of prefixes denoting quantity or number. A more complete listing of prefixes may be found in the appendix.

TABLE 1-1   Examples of Prefixes Denoting Quantity or Number

PREFIX	MEANING	EXAMPLE	SOUNDS LIKE
/a-/an-	without	*a*nemia	(ah-**NEE**-me-ah)
bi-	two/double	*bi*furcation	(**bye**-fur-**KAY**-shun)
hemi-	half	*hemi*section	(**HEM**-ee-**sec**-shun)
mon/o-	one	*mono*mer	(**MON**-oh-mer)
poly-	many	*poly*merization	(pahl-ih-**mer**-ih-**ZAY**-shun)
prim/i-	first	*prim*ary	(**PRY**-mary)
quad/quat-	four	*quad*rant	(**KWAH**-drant)
semi-	half	*semi*luminal	(sem-eh-**LOOM**-in-all)
tri-	three	*tri*geminal	(try-**JEM**-in-al)
uni-	one	*uni*lateral	(you-nih-**LAT**-er-ol)

EXERCISE 1-1
Underline the prefix used in the following words, and specify what number or amount each represents:

1. **bicuspid**   _____cusps
2. **anesthesia**   _____feeling
3. **trifurcation** _____divisions
4. **unilateral**   _____sided
5. **polypnea**   _____breathing
6. **hemisphere** _____sphere
7. **monocyte**   _____cell
8. **primate**   _____beginning
9. **semicoma**   _____coma
10. **quaternary** _____elements

Occasionally, a root has more than one prefix with the same meaning. One meaning may stem from Latin and another may be a Greek version. For example, *alba*, from the Greek word *albus*, refers to the color white, such as in *albumen* and *albino*. *Leuko* is a prefix meaning white and is used in *leukoplakia* (a white, precancerous patch found inside the cheek). Although *leuko* may be more popular, both prefixes are correct. Table 1-2 gives examples of prefixes denoting color.

TABLE 1-2   Examples of Prefixes Denoting Color

PREFIX	COLOR	EXAMPLE	SOUNDS LIKE
albus	white	*albumen*	(al-**BU-men**)
chlor/o	green	*chloroform*	(**KLOR-oh-form**)
cyan/o	blue	*cyanosis*	(**sigh**-ah-**NO**-sis)
erythr/o	red	*erythrocyte*	(eh-**RITH**-row-site)
leuk/o	white	*leukoplakia*	(**loo**-koh-**PLAY**-key-ah)
melan/o	black	*melanoma*	(**mel**-ah-**NO**-ma)
xanth/o	yellow	*xanthoma*	(zan-**THO**-ma)

EXERCISE 1-2
Match each prefix in Column A with the color it represents in Column B.

Column A
1. xanth/o_____
2. cyan/o_____
3. erythr/o_____
4. leuk/o_____
5. melan/o_____
6. alba_____

Column B
a. red
b. yellow
c. blue
d. black
e. white
f. violet

Some prefixes are used to qualify the size or degree of development of the root term. Table 1-3 gives examples.

TABLE 1-3   Examples of Prefixes Denoting Size or Degree

PREFIX	MEANING	EXAMPLE	SOUNDS LIKE
hyper-	over/excess	*hyper*trophy	(high-per-**TROH**-fee)
hypo-	under/below	*hypo*plasia	(high-poe-**PLAY**-zee-ah)
macro-	large	*macro*dontia	(**mack**-row-**DON**-she-ah)
micro-	small/minute	*micro*be	(**MY**-crobe)
pan-	all around	*pan*oramic	(**pan**-oh-**RAM**-ic)
ultra-	extreme/beyond	*ultra*sonic	(**ul**-trah-**SON**-ic)

EXERCISE 1-3

Give the meaning of the prefix underlined in the following words:

1. <u>macro</u>glossia   =   _____tongue
2. <u>hyper</u>trophy   =   _____development
3. <u>hypo</u>thermia   =   _____temperature
4. <u>micro</u>organism =   _____germ
5. <u>pan</u>oramic   =   _____view
6. <u>ultra</u>violet   =   _____violet color range

   Some prefixes are used to specify the location or the position of the root term and the involvement, such as treatment occurring inside (*endo*) the tooth or treatment around (*peri*) the gingiva. Table 1-4 contains some examples of prefixes referring to location or direction.

TABLE 1-4   Examples of Prefixes Denoting Location or Direction

PREFIX	MEANING	EXAMPLE	SOUNDS LIKE
ab-	away from	*ab*sent	(**AB**-sent)
ad-	toward/near	*ad*jacent	(ad-**JAY**-cent)
ana-	apart	*ana*lysis	(an-**AL**-ah-sis)
ante-	in front	*ante*rior	(an-**TEE**-ree-or)
de-	down from	*de*hydration	(**dee**-high-**DRAY**-shun)
dia-	complete	*dia*lysis	(die-**AL**-ih-sis)
ecto-	outside	*ecto*pic	(eck-**TOP**-ic)
endo-	within	*endo*dontic	(**en**-doe-**DON**-tic)
epi-	upon/over	*epi*dermis	(ep-ih-**DER**-miss)
ex/o-	out from	*ex*cretion	(ex-**KREE**-shun)

continues

PREFIX	MEANING	EXAMPLE	SOUNDS LIKE
im-	into/position	*im*plant	(**IM**-plant)
in-	into/in	*in*cision	(in-**SIH**-zhun)
infra-	under/below	*infra*orbital	(**in**-frah-**OR**-bih-tal)
inter-	in midst of	*inter*dental	(in-ter-**DEN**-tal)
mes/o-	mid, among	*mesio*clusion	(**me**-zee-oh-**CLUE**-shun)
para-	near/besides	*par*entral	(par-**EN**-ter-al)
peri/o-	around	*perio*dontal	(pear-ee-oh-**DON**-tal)
post-	after/later	*post*erior	(pahs-**TEE**-ree-or)
pre/ante-	before	*pre*molar	(pree-**MOLE**-ar)
retro-	behind/back	*retro*molar	(rhe-tro-**MOLE**-ar)
sub-	lesser than	*sub*dermal	(sub-**DER**-mal)
supra-	above/over	*supra*orbital	(**sue**-pra-**OR**-bih-tal)
syn-	together	*syn*ergism	(**SIN**-er-jizm)
trans-	through	*trans*plant	(**TRANS**-plant)

EXERCISE 1-4

Using the prefix list given, choose the prefix that best describes the meaning of the term:
ab ad ecto endo ex in infra peri post retro supra trans

1. toward = _____
2. outside = _____
3. within = _____
4. under = _____

5. out from = _____
6. around = _____
7. after = _____
8. through = _____

9. above = _____
10. away from = _____
11. into = _____
12. behind = _____

Some prefixes are used to denote the condition of the root element. These prefixes may indicate that the condition is new (*neo*) or that the root term is not in effect as in the word, *infertile* (not fertile). Some examples denoting condition are presented in Table 1-5.

TABLE 1-5   Examples of Prefixes Denoting Condition

PREFIX	MEANING	EXAMPLE	SOUNDS LIKE
a-, an-	without	*an*odontia	(an-oh-**DON**-she-ah)
anti-	opposite	*anti*septic	(an-tih-**SEP**-tick)
brady-	slow	*brady*cardia	(bray-dee-**CAR**-dee-ah)
con-	with	*con*nective	(con-**ECK**-tif)
contra-	against	*contra*ngle	(**con**-tra-**ANG**-gl)

continues

TABLE 1-5   (continued)

PREFIX	MEANING	EXAMPLE	SOUNDS LIKE
dis-	remove	*dis*infect	(**dis**-in-**FECT**)
in-	not	*in*soluble	(in-**SOL**-you-bull)
mal-	bad	*mal*occlusion	(**mal**-oh-**CLUE**-shun)
neo-	new	*neo*plasm	(**NEE**-oh-plazm)
tachy-	fast	*tachy*cardia	(**tack**-ee-**CAR**-dee-ah)
un-	non/not	*un*erupted	(un-eh-**RUP**-ted)

EXERCISE 1-5

Match the prefix in Column A to the term it best describes in Column B:

Column A
 1. neo_____
 2. anti_____
 3. con_____
 4. contra_____
 5. dis_____
 6. a or an_____
 7. mal_____
 8. brady_____
 9. un or in_____
10. tacky_____

Column B
a. without
b. bad
c. fast
d. against
e. slow
f. new
g. opposite to
h. not/non
i. with
j. removal

Root Word

The main section or division of a term that provides the foundation or basic meaning is called the root word. A word may have one or more root sections. When a root section is combined or connected with other word elements, it may take on a combining vowel and become a **combining form**. The most common **combining vowel** is *o*. For example, the word *temporal* refers to the temporal bone in the skull and the word *mandible* is the lower jaw bone. Independently, these are two separate words, but they can be combined to form the word *temporomandibular*, as in temporomandibular joint (TMJ). Note that the combining vowel *o* is inserted in place of the *al* in *temporal*.

As another example, two roots are combined to designate specific areas of teeth. In referring to the back chewing surface of a tooth, the root term for back or distant is *distal* and the term *occlusal* designates the chewing or occluding area. When combining these two roots with the combining vowel *o*, we have distocclusal, the back chewing surface.

Other examples of terms with two roots are thermometer, cementoenamel junction, and radiograph. Table 1-6 gives examples of common root words and combining forms used in dental terminology. More examples of root words may be found in the appendix.

TABLE 1-6   Common Dental Root/Combining Forms

ROOT WORD	SOUNDS LIKE	COMBO FORM	PERTAINS TO
alveolar	(al-**VEE**-oh-lar)	alveo	alveolus
apical	(**AY**-pih-kal)	apic/o	apex of a root
axis	(**ACK**-sis)	ax/o	midline
buccal	(**BUCK**-al)	bucc/o	cheek
cheilo	(**KEY**-loh)	cheil/o	lip
coronal	(ko-**ROW**-nal)	coron/o	crown
dens	(**DENZ**)	dent/o	tooth
distal	(**DIS**-tal)	dist/o	farthest from center
enamel	(ee-**NAM**-el)	ename/o or amel/o	tooth, enamel tissue
fluoride	(**FLOOR**-eyed)	fluor/o	the chemical
frenum	(**FREE**-num)	frene	frenum
gingiva	(**JIN**-jih-vah)	gingiv/o	gum tissue
glossa	(**GLOSS**-ah)	gloss/o or gloss/a	tongue
incisor	(inn-**SIGH**-zor)	incis/o	incisor tooth
labial	(**LAY**-bee-al)	labi/o	lip area
lingua	(**LING**-wa)	lingu/o	tongue
mandible	(**MAN**-dih-bull)	mandibu/a	lower jaw
maxilla	(**MACKS**-ill-ah)	maxilla/o	upper jaw
mesial	(**MEE**-zee-al)	mesi/o	middle, mid-plane
mucosa	(myou-**KO**-sa)	muc/o	tissue lining an orifice
occlude	(oh-**KLUDE**)	occlus/o	occluding, jaw close
orthos	(**OR**-thohs)	orth/o	straight, proper order
stoma	(**STOH**-mah)	stoma	mouth/opening
temporal	(**TEM**-por-al)	tempor/o	temporal bone

EXERCISE 1-6

Place a root element for the given words in the blanks provided.

1. lower jaw   _____
2. tongue   _____
3. jaw closing   _____
4. tooth   _____
5. gum tissue   _____
6. lip   _____
7. middle   _____

8. frenum   _____
9. far from center _____
10. mouth   _____

Suffix

An element added to the end of a root word or combining form to describe or qualify the word meaning is a **suffix** (**SUF**-icks). A suffix cannot stand alone and usually is united with a root element by inserting a combining vowel (*o*) unless the suffix begins with a vowel. In that case, the combining form or vowel is dropped. For example, the surgical removal of gum tissue is the meaning of *gingivectomy* from the root word *gingivo* (gum) and suffix *ectomy* (surgical excision). Dropping the ending vowel in *gingivo* and adding *ectomy* to make *gingivectomy* unites these two word elements.

Word endings can act as an adjective or indicate time and size, condition, agents, or specialists. Some examples of common suffixes used in dental terminology are given in Tables 1-7 to 1-10. A more complete listing of common suffixes is contained in the appendix.

Suffixes used as adjectives are word endings that describe or show a relationship. Suffixes have the ability to transform a noun or verb into an adjective or verbs into nouns by the addition of a word ending. The suffixes in Table 1-7 transform the root word to indicate relationship or description to the root foundation.

TABLE 1-7   Examples of Suffixes in Adjective Use

SUFFIX	SHOWS RELATION TO THE ROOT	SOUNDS LIKE
-ac	cardi*ac* (heart)	(**CAR**-dee-ack)
-al	gingiv*al* (gum tissue)	(**JIN**-**jih**-**vahl**)
-ar	alveol*ar* (alveolus)	(al-**VEE**-oh-lar)
-ary	maxill*ary* (maxilla)	(**MACK**-sih-**lair**-ee)
-eal	pharyng*eal* (pharynx)	(fair-**IN**-gee-al)
-form	fusi*form* (spindle shape)	(**FUE**-sif-orm)
-gram	radio*gram* (x-ray),	(**RAY**-dee-oh-gram)
-graphy	sialo*graphy* (saliva measurement)	(sigh-ah-**LOG**-rah-fee)
-ic or tic	cariogen*ic* (start of decay)	(**care**-ee-oh-**JEN**-ick)
-ior	poster*ior* (in the rear)	(pahs-**TEE**-ree-or)
-oid	coron*oid* (crown)	(**KOR**-oh-noyd)
-ous	ven*ous* (vein)	(**VEE**-nus)

EXERCISE 1-7
Underline the suffix indicating relationship in each given word and write it in the blank next to the word.

1. dental _____
2. anterior _____
3. sonogram _____
4. ovoid _____
5. axillary _____
6. caustic _____

7. cardiac _____
8. mucous _____
9. dentoform _____
10. malar _____
11. radiograph _____
12. pharyngeal _____

A suffix added to a root may indicate the condition of the root foundation. It may denote disease (*pathy*) or inflammation (*itis*) occurs or just merely indicate that the condition exists (*tion*). Table 1-8 gives examples.

TABLE 1-8   Examples of Suffixes Indicating Condition

SUFFIX	CONDITION OF ROOT FOUNDATION	SOUNDS LIKE
-ant	etch*ant* (etching)	(**EH**-chent)
-cle	vesi*cle* (small blister)	(**VES**-ih-cull)
-cule	mole*cule* (small bit of matter)	(**MAHL**-eh-cule)
-ia	anesthes*ia* (without feeling)	(**an**-es-**THEE**-zee-ah)
-ible, ile	revers*ible* (change to or from)	(reh-**VERSE**-ih-bull)
-id	cusp*id* (cusp shape)	(**CUSS**-pid)
-ion,	occlus*ion* (bite)	(oh-**CLUE**-shun)
-itis	arthr*itis* (joint inflammation)	(ar-**THRY**-tis)
-ity	acid*ity* (acid)	(ah-**SID**-ih-tee)
-ium	bacter*ium* (germ)	(back-**TEER**-ee-um)
-olus	alve*olus* (air sac)	(al-**VEE**-oh-lus)
-oma	lip*oma* (fat tumor)	(lie-**POE**-mah)
-pathy	myo*pathy* (muscle disease)	(my-**OP**-ah-thee)
-sion	inci*sion* (surgical cut)	(in-**SIH**-zhun)
-tic	necro*tic* (dead tissue)	(neh-**KRAH**-tic)
-tion	mastica*tion* (chewing)	(mass-tih-**KAY**-shun)

EXERCISE 1-8
Insert the correct suffix to complete the root element.

1. Condition of being acid is acid_____.
2. Surgical cut is inci_____.
3. Term for a germ is bacter_____.

4. Fatty tumor is lip_____.
5. Act of chewing is mastica_____.
6. Dead tissue is necro_____.
7. Muscle damage disease is called myo_____.
8. A small bit of matter is a mole_____.

Some suffixes are added to the root element to indicate an agent or a person concerned with or trained in that specialty. The suffixes in Table 1-9 are some of the more familiar ones, and many more are used to indicate specialization.

TABLE 1-9   Suffixes Denoting Agent or Person Concerned

SUFFIX	AGENT OR PERSON
-ent	pati*ent*, recipi*ent*, resid*ent*
-eon	surg*eon*
-er	subscrib*er*, examin*er*, practition*er*
-ician	phys*ician*
-ist	dent*ist*, orthodont*ist*
-or	doct*or*, don*or*

EXERCISE 1-9

List five agents and/or persons concerned with a specialty area and underline the suffix denoting their position.

1._____   4._____
2._____   5._____
3._____

Some suffixes are added to root elements to show processes, uses, or healing. When analyzing a long dental word, starting backwards, the suffix may indicate something happening to the root element, such as *ectomy* (surgical removal) or *trophy* (development). Other suffixes are added to indicate pain (*algia*) or bleeding (*rrhage*) and so on. Table 1-10 gives some examples.

TABLE 1-10   Suffixes Expressing Medical Terms, Processes, Uses

SUFFIX	MEANING	SAMPLE WORDS
-algia	pain	odont*algia*, neur*algia*, my*algia*
-ate, -ize	use/action	vaccin*ate*, lux*ate*, palp*ate*, visual*ize*
-cyte	cell	leuco*cyte*, osteo*cyte*
-ectomy	surgical removal	apico*ectomy*, append*ectomy*

continues

SUFFIX	MEANING	SAMPLE WORDS
-ology	study of	hist*ology*, bi*ology*
-opsy	view	bi*opsy*, aut*opsy*
-phobia	dread, fear	claustro*phobia*
-plasty	surgical repair	gingivo*plasty*
-rrhea	discharge	hemmo*rrhea*, sialo*rrhea*
-scope	instrument	micro*scope* (micro), laryngo*scope* (larynx)
-tomy	incision	myo*tomy* (muscle)
-trophy	development	osteo*trophy* (bone development)

EXERCISE 1-10

Examine the boldfaced words in each sentence and circle the suffix denoting a medical procedure, use, or condition of the root element.

1. A **gingivoplasty** may be the correct treatment for an infected third molar area.
2. The dentist examined Mr. Smith's teeth for **odontalgia** after his accident.
3. The assistant prepared the biopsy slide for the **microscope**.
4. Mary Hughes's health records showed a history of **myopathy**.
5. Tissue **hemorrhage** may be an indicator of a serious blood disease.
6. The dentist will **cauterize** the patient's gingiva during the procedure.
7. The patient was referred to an oral surgeon for the **apicoectomy**.
8. To avoid bone and tooth damage, the dentist will **luxate** the tooth before removal.
9. Some patients claim to suffer **claustrophobia** when visiting the dental office.
10. The dentist retained a sample of the removed tissue to send for a **biopsy**.

▌ DEFINE THE MEANING OF THE DENTAL WORD

After providing the word and its pronunciation, this text gives the meaning of the word, including the definition and any relevant feature that occurs within or about the word. For example:

▶ Syncope (**SIN**-koh-pee): a temporary loss of consciousness resulting from an inadequate supply of blood to the brain; also know as swooning or fainting.
▶ Xerostomia (zee-roh-**STOH**-me-ah; xeros = *dry*, stoma = *mouth*): dryness of the mouth caused by the lack of normal saliva secretion.

In the first example, synonyms (e.g., fainting) are provided for *syncope*. The second example contains information about the derivation of the word *xerostomia; xeros* is Greek for dry, and *stoma* is the word for mouth.

PLURALIZE THE DENTAL WORD

Because much of the dental terminology originates from Latin and Greek, the rules for changing terms from singular to plural are predetermined by the conventions of those languages. Occasionally we find English plural terms and, whenever possible, encourage the use of these endings. The standard method to understand plural forms of words is to learn the basic rules for changing word endings, bearing in mind a few terms will not conform to the rules given in Table 1-11. Whenever you are not sure of a spelling, look it up in a dictionary or reference book.

TABLE 1-11 Guidelines for Plural Forms

WORD ENDINGS	CHANGE TO	SINGULAR	PLURAL
a	*ae* (add *e* to end)	gingiva	gingivae
ex, ix	*ices* (drop *x*, add *ices*)	apex	apices
itis	*ides* (drop *s*, add *des*)	pulpitis	pulpitides
sis	*sis* (change *sis* to *ses*)	cementosis	cementoses
nx	*nges* (change *nx* to *nges*)	larynx	larynges
on	*a* (change *on* to *a*)	ganglion	ganglia
oma	*omas* (add *s* to the end)	dentinoma	dentinomas
um	*a* (change *um* to *a*)	frenum	frena
us	*i* (change *us* to *i*)	sulcus	sulci
y	*ies* (drop *y*, add *ies*)	biopsy	biopsies

EXERCISE 1-11

Provide the plural form for each singular word listed below.

Singular   **Plural**
  1. index   _____
  2. ganglion   _____
  3. bacterium   _____
  4. fungus   _____
  5. calculus   _____
  6. iris   _____
  7. biopsy   _____
  8. prosthesis   _____
  9. vertebra   _____
 10. carcinoma   _____

USE THE DENTAL WORD

After reading and pronouncing each word, the student should determine the structure of the term. An examination of the meaning of the given word will help to determine if the student's structure analysis was correct and will reinforce word meanings. To strengthen knowledge of the dental term, the student should practice incorporating the dental term into a sentence or statement. Completing the review exercises that appear at the end of each chapter will help in obtaining this objective.

REVIEW EXERCISES

MATCHING
Match the following word elements with their meanings:

1. _____glossa
2. _____supra-
3. _____peri-
4. _____-trophy
5. _____mesial
6. _____ab-
7. _____stoma
8. _____-oma
9. _____retro-
10. _____dys-
11. _____mal
12. _____itis
13. _____gingiva
14. _____dens
15. _____-otomy

a. tumor
b. from, away from
c. tongue
d. mouth
e. above
f. bad, difficult
g. gum tissue
h. middle, mid-plane
i. around or about
j. inflammation
k. development, growth
l. evil, sickness, disorder, poor
m. cutting into, incision into
n. backward
o. tooth

DEFINITIONS
Using the selection given for each sentence, choose the best term to complete the definition.

1. The root/combining word for cheek is _____.
   a. glossa
   c. frenum
   a. labial
   d. buccal

2. Which suffix means pain or ache_____?
   a. -algia
   c. -ous
   b. -oma
   d. -soma

3. Which prefix means toward or increase? _____
   a. an-
   c. ad-
   b. ab-
   d. in-

4. The abbreviated form for high volume evacuation is: _____
   a. HIV
   c. HEE
   b. HVE
   d. HCC

5. Which prefix means before (in time or place)? _____
   a. ante-
   c. retro-
   b. anti-
   d. chrono-

6. The root or combining word for lower jaw is: _____.
   a. maxilla
   c. mesial
   b. mandible
   d. megial

7. Which suffix means tissue death, decay?_____
   a. -plasty
   c. -necrosis
   b. -pathogy
   d. -ectomy

8. The combining form for straight or for proper order is _____.
   a. occlus/o
   c. oppos/o
   b. orth/o
   d. anti/e

9. Which suffix means graph or picture (especially in radiology)? _____
   a. -gram
   c. -grate
   b. -photo
   d. -trophy

10. Which prefixes determine the number to be two? _____
    a. bi- and di-
    c. tri- and bi-
    b. bi- and dye-
    d. bi- and sou-

11. Which combining form means apex of the root? _____
    a. apix/o   b. apic/o
    c. axi/o   d. axium

12. A pattern used in prosthodontic dentistry is _____.
    a. die   b. dye
    c. dys-   d. dial

13. The combining form meaning lip is _____.
    a. dist/o   b. cheil/o
    c. bucc/o   d. bucca

14. Which prefix means less than, below, or under? _____
    a. hypo-   b. hyper-
    c. trans-   d. hydro-

15. Which suffix designates a specialist in a given study? _____
    a. -ology   b. -ologist
    c. -ier   d. -teur

BUILDING SKILLS

Locate and define the prefix, root/combining form, and suffix (if present) in the following words.

1. **anodontia** (an-oh-**DON**-she-ah)— condition of being without teeth.
   prefix _____
   root or combining form _____
   suffix _____

2. **frenectomy** (freh-**NECK**-toh-mee)— surgical cutting of any frenum or a division of a frenum.
   prefix _____
   root or combining form _____
   suffix _____

3. **interproximal** (in-ter-**PROCKS**-ih-mal)— between two adjoining surfaces.
   prefix _____
   root or combining form _____
   suffix _____

4. **gingivectomy** (jin-jih-**VEK**-toe-me)— excision and removal of gum tissue.
   prefix _____

root or combining form _____
suffix _____

5. **periodontitis** (pear-ee-oh-don-**TIE**-tis)— inflammation/degeneration of dental periosteum.
   prefix _____
   root or combining form _____
   suffix _____

6. **malocclusion** (**mal**-oh-**CLUE**-zhun)— imperfect occlusion of the teeth, improper closure.
   prefix _____
   root or combining form _____
   suffix _____

7. **submandibular** (sub-man-**DIB**-you-lar)— beneath the lower jaw or mandible.
   prefix _____
   root or combining form _____
   suffix _____

8. **cheilosis** (kee-**LOW**-sis)—morbid condition of lips, such as occurs with vitamin B deficiency.
   prefix _____
   root or combining form _____
   suffix _____

9. **exodontia** (**ecks**-oh-**DAHN**-she-ah)— extraction or removal of a tooth.
   prefix _____
   root or combining form _____
   suffix _____

10. **orthodontist** (**or**-thoh-**DON**-tist)—a specialist dealing with tooth arrangement.
    prefix _____
    root or combining form _____
    suffix _____

PLURALS

Use the blank space to write the plural form of each given word.

1. maxilla _____

2. matrix _____

3. alveolus _____

4. cellulitis _____

5. pharynx   _____

6. axion   _____

7. necrosis   _____

8. osteoma   _____

9. bacillus   _____

10. fulcrum   _____

11. exotosis   _____

12. index   _____

13. meatus   _____

14. calculus   _____

15. appendix   _____

WORD USE

Read the following sentences and define the bold-faced word.

1. After reading the posted compliance notice on the wall, Ms. Gilligan requested an explanation for the **acronym** OSHA.

   _____

2. The hygienist explained to the new patient that a **gingivectomy** is a common treatment for her dental disease.

   _____

3. The dentist wrote a prescription for therapeutic vitamin B complex for the patient suffering from **cheilosis**.

   _____

4. A calcium deposit in the **sublingual** salivary duct caused a large and uncomfortable swelling in the mouth.

   _____

5. The emergency patient who called this morning complaining of **odontalgia** has arrived for his appointment.

   _____

AUDIO LIST

This list contains selected new, important, or difficult terms from this chapter. You may use the list to review these terms and to practice pronouncing them correctly. When you work with the audio for this chapter, listen to the word, repeat it, and then place a checkmark in the box. Proceed to the next boxed word and repeat the process.

- ❏ acronym (**ACK**-roh-nim)
- ❏ -algia (**AL**-jee-ah)
- ❏ ante- (**AN**-tea)
- ❏ anti- (**AN**-tie)
- ❏ dys- (**DIS**)
- ❏ -ectomy (**ECK**-toh-me)
- ❏ endo- (**EN**-doe)
- ❏ homonym (**HAHM**-oh-nim)
- ❏ hyper- (**HIGH**-per)
- ❏ hypo- (**HIGH**-poh)
- ❏ infra- (**INN**-frah)
- ❏ intra- (**INN**-trah)
- ❏ -itis (**EYE**-tiss)
- ❏ -oid (**OYD**)
- ❏ -ologist (**AH**-loh-jist)
- ❏ -ology (**AH**-loh-jee)
- ❏ -otomy (**AH**-toh-mee)
- ❏ peri- (**PEAR**-ee)
- ❏ -plasty (**PLAS**-tee)
- ❏ prefix (**PREE**-fix)
- ❏ poly- (**PAHL**-ee)
- ❏ retro- (**REH**-troh)
- ❏ suffix (**SUFF**-icks)
- ❏ supra (**SOO**-prah)
- ❏ -trophy (**TROH**-fee)

CHAPTER 2

Anatomy and Oral Structures

Upon completion of this chapter, the reader should be able to identify and understand terms related to the:

1. **Anatomy of the skull.** Name and identify the major bones of the face and skull.
2. **Anatomical features of the skull.** Locate the sinus cavities, sutures, processes, and foramina of the skull.
3. **Landmarks and features of the mandible.** Locate the major structural points of the mandible and explain their functions or purposes.
4. **Muscles of mastication.** Identify the names and locations of the major muscles of mastication and explain the function of each.
5. **Trigeminal nerve location and functions.** Describe the principal branches of the trigeminal nerve and explain the functions of each division.
6. **Blood supply of the cranium.** Locate and identify the major blood vessels to and from the cranium.
7. **Locations and purposes of the salivary glands.** Describe the placement and functions of the major salivary glands.
8. **Functions and agents of the lymphatic system.** Explain the function of the lymphatic system and the major lymphatic agents present in the body.
9. **Important structures in the oral cavity.** Locate and explain features in the oral cavity, such as the labia, frena, tongue, and palate structures and miscellaneous tissues.

ANATOMY OF THE SKULL

Medical terminology deals with the entire body and all its systems, whereas the language of dentistry is related mostly to the head region. The skull area is composed of two main bone divisions: the cranium and the facial section.

Cranium

The cranium (**KRAY**-nee-um) is the portion of the skull that encloses the brain. Eight bones make up this section of the skull (Figure 2-1).

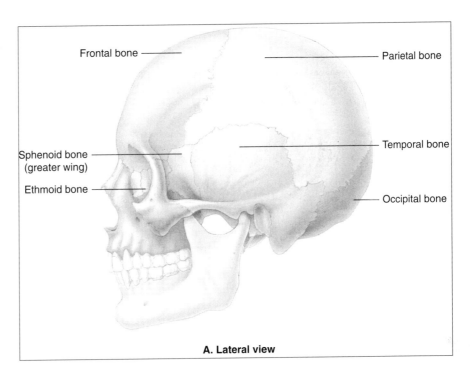

Frontal bone — Parietal bone

Sphenoid bone
(greater wing) — Temporal bone

Ethmoid bone — Occipital bone

A. Lateral view

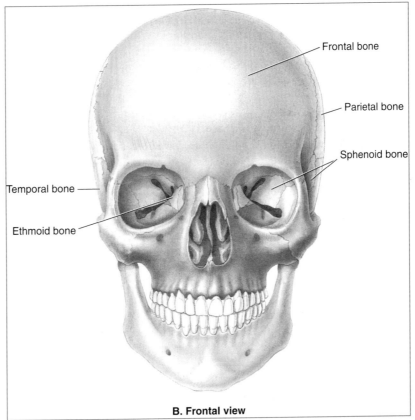

Frontal bone

Parietal bone

Sphenoid bone

Temporal bone

Ethmoid bone

FIGURE 2-1
Cranial bones

B. Frontal view

temporal (**TEM**-pore-al): two fan-shaped bones, one on each side of the skull, in the temporal area above each ear.

parietal (pah-**RYE**-eh-tal): two bones, one on each side, that make up the roof and side walls covering the brain.

frontal (**FRON**-tal): a single bone in the frontal or anterior region that makes up the forehead.

occipital (ock-**SIP**-ih-tal): one large, thick bone at the lower back of the head that forms the base of the skull and contains a large opening for the spinal cord passage to the brain.

ethmoid (eth-**MOYD**): a spongy bone located between the eye orbits that helps form the roof and part of the anterior nasal fossa of the skull.

sphenoid (**SFEE**-noyd): a large bone at the base of the skull, situated between the occipital and ethmoid bones in front of and between the parietal and temporal bones on each side.

Facial Bones

Fourteen bones make up the facial division of the cranium (see Figure 2-2). All are paired with one on each side, except there is only one vomer in the nose and one

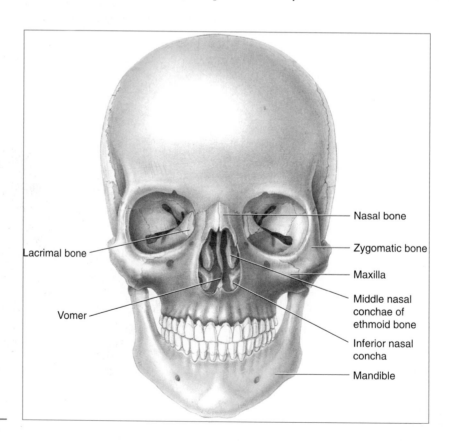

FIGURE 2-2
Facial bones

mandible extending from right to left. The facial bones are:

zygomatic (**zye**-goh-**MAT**-ick): two facial bones, one under each eye, that form and give shape to the cheekbone. The zygomatic bones are also called the malar (**MAY**-lar) bones.

maxilla (max-ILL-ah): two facial bones, one under each eye, that unite in the center to form the upper jaw and support the maxillary teeth.

palatine (**PAL**-ah-tine): two bones, one each on the left and the right, that form the hard palate of the mouth and the nasal floor.

nasal (**NAY**-zal): two bones, one left and one right, that form the arch or bridge of the nose.

lacrimal (**LACK**-rih-mal): two bones, one each, at the inner side or nose site of the orbital cavity.

inferior nasal conchae (**KONG**-kah in singular use; **KONG**-kee in plural use): two thin, scroll-like bones that form the lower part of the interior of the nasal cavity.

mandible (**MAN**-dih-bul): the strong, horseshoe-shaped bone that forms the lower jaw.

vomer (**VOH**-mer): a single bone that forms the lower posterior part of the nasal septum.

Miscellaneous Bones of the Skull

Although the **auditory** ossicles (**AHS**-ih-kuls), small bones in the ear, are not considered bones of the face or cranium, they are present in the head or skull (Figure 2-3). The three auditory ossicles are:

malleus (**MAL**-ee-us): largest of the three ossicles in the middle ear; commonly called the ear mallet.

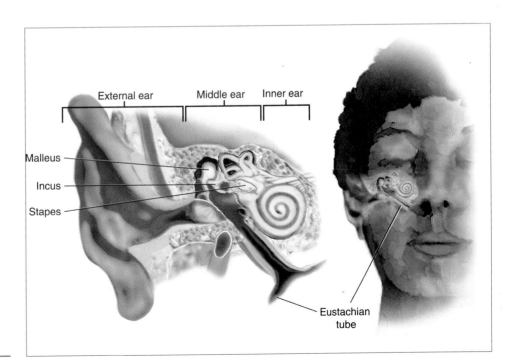

FIGURE 2-3
Bones of the ear

incus (**IN**-kus): one of three ossicles in the middle ear; commonly called the anvil.

stapes (**STAY**-peez): one of the three ossicles in the middle ear; commonly called the stirrup.

Another bone of interest and closely related to the dental field but not located in the skull is the hyoid (**HIGH**-oyd), a horseshoe-shaped bone lying at the base of the tongue. It does not articulate with any other bone.

ANATOMICAL FEATURES OF THE SKULL

Many anatomical features are present in the cranial and facial bones. These include the sinuses, bone sutures, processes of the skull bones, and major foramina. Each feature has a specific location and purpose.

Sinus

A sinus (**SIGH**-nus) is an air pocket or cavity in a bone that lightens the bone, warms the air intake, and helps form sounds. These sinus cavities receive their names from the bone in which they are situated. The four pairs of **paranasal sinuses** are (Figure 2-4):

ethmoid: located in the ethmoid bone at the side of each eye.

sphenoid: located in the sphenoid bone situated behind the eyes.

frontal: located in the frontal bone or the forehead above each eye.

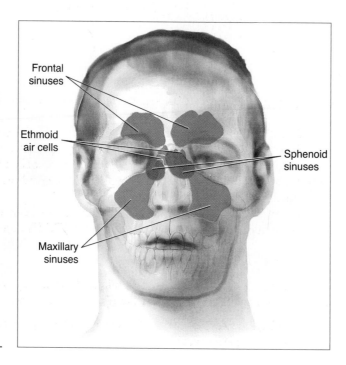

FIGURE 2-4
Sinuses

maxillary: located in the maxilla; the maxillary sinus is the largest and is called the **atrium** (**A**-tree-um) **of Highmore;** this cavity is easily seen and is used as a landmark for identifying radiographs in the mounting of films.

Sutures of the Skull

A **suture** (**SOO**-chur) is a line where two or more bones unite in an immovable joint. Several main sutures are located in the cranium (Figure 2-5).

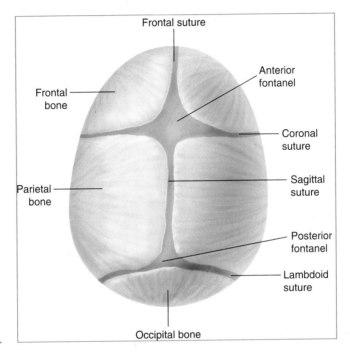

FIGURE 2-5
Sutures

sagittal (**SAJ**-ih-tal): the union line between the two parietal bones on the top of the skull.
coronal (**KOR**-oh-nal): junction of the frontal and the parietal bones; this area is soft at birth and shortly afterward, and has been called the baby's "soft spot" or fontanel (fon-tah-**NELL** = *little fountain*), sometimes spelled *fontanelle*.
lambdoid (**LAM**-doyd): located between the parietal bone and the upper border of the occipital bone.
temporoparietal (**tem**-poe-roe-pah-**RYE**-eh-tal): located between the temporal and parietal bones; also known as the squamous (**SKWAY**-mus) suture.

Sutures of the Mouth

Oral cavity sutures are unions of bones occurring in the mouth, places where the left and right bone pairs meet. The four main sutures of the mouth are.

posterior (pos-**TEE**-ree-or) nasal spine: located in the upper arch between the nasal bone and superior maxilla.

median palatine suture: the union between the palatine bones.

incisive (in-**SIGH**-siv) suture: located in the anterior area of the pre-maxilla and palatine processes.

nasion (**NAY**-zhun): a point where the nasofrontal suture is cut across by the middle plane of the skull.

Processes of the Cranium

A process (**PROS**-es) is a projection or outgrowth of bone or tissue. This bone excess is not to be confused with the fusion line where two bones develop into one, such as the mandible. The symphysis (**SIM**-fih-sis) in the center of the mandible, forms the chin, and is called the **mental** or chin protuberance (pro-**TOO**-ber-ans = *projection*). The mandible has eight main processes or bony growths related to dentistry.

alveolar (al-**VEE**-oh-lar): bone growth or border of the maxilla and the mandible; makes up and forms the tooth sockets.

condyloid (**KON**-dih-loyd): posterior growth on the ramus (**RAY**-mus) of the mandible; articulates with the temporal bone in the temporomandibular (**tem**-poe-roe-man-**DIB**-you-lar) joint (TMJ).

coronoid (**KOR**-oh-noyd): anterior growth on the ramus of the mandible that serves as the attachment position for the temporalis muscle.

frontal (**FRON**-tal): projection of maxilla meeting with the frontal bone to form the eye orbit.

infraorbital (**in**-frah-**OR**-bih-tal): growth process from the zygomatic bone that articulates with the maxilla to form the lower side of the eye orbit.

mastoid (**MASS**-toyd): growth on the temporal bone behind the ear that is used for muscle attachment.

pterygoid (**TER**-ih-goyd = *wing-shaped*): growth of the sphenoid bone extending downward from the bone; the most inferior end of the process is known as the pterygoid hamulus (**HAM**-you-lus), a hook-like end that serves as a site for muscle attachment.

styloid (**STY**-loyd): small, pointed growth from the lower border of the temporal bone; serves as a bone position for attachment of some tongue muscles.

Foramina of the Cranium

A foramen (for-**RAY**-men) is an opening or hole in the bone for nerve and vessel passage. A foramen is not to be confused with the external auditory meatus (mee-**AY**-tus), a large opening in the temporal bone used for the passage of auditory nerves and vessels. The nine main foramina (foh-**RAY**-min-ah = *plural of foramen*) of the head related to dentistry are.

magnum (**MAG**-num): opening in the occipital bone for spinal cord passage.

mandibular (man-**DIB**-you-lar): located on the lingual side of the ramus of the mandible; permits nerve and vessels passage.

mental (MEN-tal = *Latin for chin*): opening situated on left and right anterior areas of the mandible; used for passage of nerve and vessels (see Figure 2-6).

lingual (**LIN**-gwal): small opening in the center of the mental spine for nerve passage to the incisor area.

incisive (**in-SIGH**-siv): an opening in the maxilla behind the central incisors on the midline.

supraorbital (**soo**-prah-**OR**-bih-tal): an opening in the frontal bone above the eye orbit.

infraorbital: an opening in the maxilla under the eye orbit.

palatine: anterior and posterior openings in the hard palate.

zygomaticofacial (**zye**-goh-**MAT**-ee-coe-**fay**-shal): an opening in the zygomatic bone.

All bones are covered by a fibrous membrane called the periosteum (pear-ee-**AHS**-tee-um). This membrane forms a lining on all surfaces, except the areas of articulation. When this layer has a mucous surface, it is called mucoperiosteum (**MYOU**-koh-**pear**-ee-**AHS**-tee-um). The oral cavity has three types of oral mucosa (**MU**-ko-sa):

lining mucosa: mucous membrane that lines the inner surfaces of the lips (**labial mucosa**) and the cheeks (**buccal mucosa**).

masticatory (**mass-TIH-kah-toe-ree**) mucosa: elastic type of mucous membrane that undergoes stress and pull; located around the alveolar area of the teeth and lines the hard palate.

specialized mucosa: smoother mucous tissue found on the dorsal side of the tongue.

▌LANDMARKS AND FEATURES OF THE MANDIBLE

The mandible is the only movable bone in the skull. It is the strongest bone in the face and supports many features (see Figure 2-6). The mandible has seven major anatomical parts:

ramus (**RAY**-mus): ascending part of the mandible that arises from the curved, lower arch.

angle of the mandible: area along the lower edge of the mandible where the upward curve of the mandible forms.

sigmoid notch: S-shaped curvature between the condyle and coronoid processes.

mylohyoid (my-loh-**HIGH**-oyd) ridge: bony ridge on the lingual surface of the mandible.

oblique (oh-**BLEEK**) line: slanted, bony growth ridge on the facial side of the mandible.

retromolar (**ret**-trow-**MOLE**-ar) area: the space located to the rear of the mandibular molars.

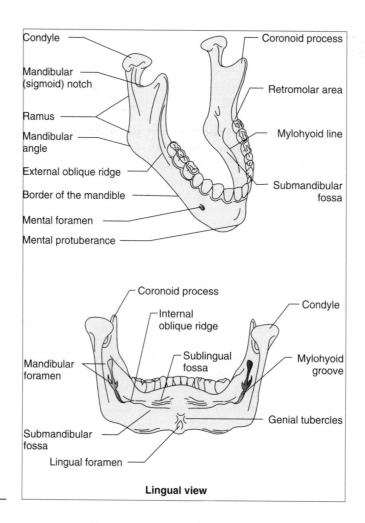

FIGURE 2-6
Lateral view of mandible with major landmarks noted.

Labels (top figure):
Condyle
Mandibular (sigmoid) notch
Ramus
Mandibular angle
External oblique ridge
Border of the mandible
Mental foramen
Mental protuberance
Coronoid process
Retromolar area
Mylohyoid line
Submandibular fossa

Labels (bottom figure):
Coronoid process
Internal oblique ridge
Sublingual fossa
Mandibular foramen
Submandibular fossa
Lingual foramen
Condyle
Mylohyoid groove
Genial tubercles

Lingual view

mandibular notch: an indentation on the lower border of the mandible, near the angle where the ramus starts into its upright position.

The mandible **articulates** (are-**TICK**-you-lates), or comes together, as a joint with the temporal bone of the cranium. This temporomandibular joint is commonly abbreviated as TMJ. The **condyle** (**KON**-dial) of the mandible rests in a depression in the temporal bone called the **glenoid** (**GLEE–noyd) or mandibular fossa** (**FAH**-sah). The **articular eminence** (ar-**TICK**-you-lar **EM**-in-ence) forms the anterior boundary of the fossa and helps maintain the mandible in position. Between the contact area of these two bones is the articular disc, a **meniscus** (men-**IS**-kus) and **synovial** (sin-**OH**-vee-al) **fluid** that cushions and lubricates the joint as it works in a hinge action movement.

MUSCLES OF MASTICATION

Mastication (mass-tih-**KAY**-shun = *chewing*) is controlled by paired (left–right) muscles, named for their placement area. Each performs a specific function. The four major muscles of mastication (Figure 2-7) are:

temporal: a fan-shaped muscle on each side of the skull; elevates and lowers the jaw and can draw the mandible backward.
masseter (mass-**EE**-ter): the muscle that closes the mouth; the principal mastication muscle.
internal pterygoid (**TER** -ih-goyd = *wing-shaped*): muscle that raises the mandible to close the jaw.
external pterygoid: muscle that opens the jaw and thrusts the mandible forward; assists with lateral movement.

Several other muscles of the head are important to dentistry. These essential muscles relate to or control some of the anatomy concerned with dental care (Figure 2-8).

orbicularis oris (or-bick-you-**LAIR**-iss **OR**-iss). Also known as the "kissing muscle," a circular muscle surrounding the mouth that compacts, compresses, and protrudes the lips.
buccinator (**BUCK**-sin-ay-tor): principal cheek muscle; compresses the cheek, expels air through the lips, and aids in food mastication.
mentalis (men-**TAL**-is): muscle of the chin (mental) that moves the chin tissue and raises or lowers the lower lip.

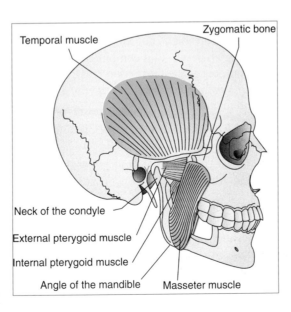

FIGURE 2-7
Muscles of mastication

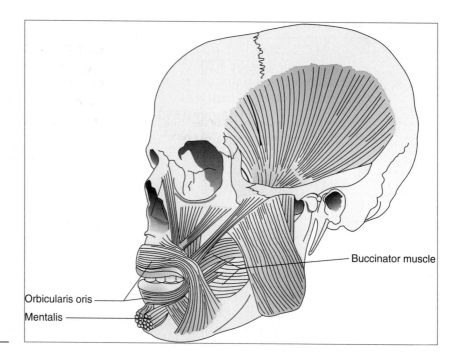

FIGURE 2-8
Muscles of facial
expression

Buccinator muscle

Orbicularis oris

Mentalis

TRIGEMINAL NERVE LOCATION AND FUNCTIONS

Muscle movement and the registration of sensations is accomplished by nerves, the communication lines to the brain. The head contains twelve pairs of cranial nerves. Each pair is numbered, and one of each pair is on the left and one on the right. Table 2-1 lists the cranial nerves, type (sensory, motor, or mixed) meaning, function, and example malfunction(s).

The most important nerve connected with dentistry is the fifth cranial nerve, the **trigeminal** (try-**JEM**-in-al) nerve. This combined motor and sensory nerve emerges from the brain and branches at the **Gasserian** (gas-**AIR**-ee-un), or semilunar, **ganglion** (**GANG**-lee-un = *mass of nerves*). The trigeminal nerve divisions are the ophthalmic, maxillary, and mandibular.

ophthalmic (off-**THAL**-mick): a sensory nerve division with three branches.

> **lacrimal:** provides sensation for the lacrimal gland and eye conjunctiva.
> **frontal:** provides sensation for the forehead, scalp, upper eyelid, and nasal root.
> **nasociliary** (**nay**-zoh-**SIL**-ee-air-ee): provides sensation for nose, eye, and eyebrow.

maxillary: a sensory division of the trigeminal nerve, with several branches.

> **anterior palatine:** provides sensation for the hard palate, **periosteum** (pear-ee-**AH**-stee-um), and mucous membrane for molars and premolar teeth.
> **middle palatine:** provides sensation for the soft palate, the **uvula** (**YOU**-view-lah), and upper or soft part of the palate.

TABLE 2-1   The Cranial Nerves and Their Functions

NERVE	TYPE	MEANING	FUNCTION	EXAMPLE MALFUNCTION(S)
I Olfactory (ol-**FACK**-toh-ree)	S	olfact = *smell*	smell	**Anosmia** (an-OZ-mee-ah) = loss of sense of smell
II Optic	S	optic = *eye*	vision	**anopia (an-OH-pee-ah)** = blindness
III Oculomotor (ock-you-low-MOE-tor	M	oculo = *eye* motor = *movement*	upper eyelid and eyeball movement	**strabismus** (stra-BIZ-mus) = eyes not fixing at the same point **ptosis** (TOE-sis) = eyelid droop **diplopia (dip-LOW**-pee-ah) = double vision
IV Trochlear (**TRAH**-klee-ur)	M	trochle = *small pulley*	eye movement and sensation	vertical droop of eye
V Trigeminal (try-**JEM**-in-al)	M	tri = *three* geminal = *branches*	dental and face nerve	teeth and facial sensation, tongue movement
VI Abducens (**AB**-due-senz)	M	ab = *away* ducens = *to lead*	lateral eye sense and movement	eyeball cannot move laterally; stays medial
VII Facial (**FAY**-shal)	M	facial = *pertaining to the face*	taste sense and facial expression	**Bell's palsy** = face contraction, taste loss, decreased saliva
VIII Vestibulocochlear (vest-**tib**-you-low-**COCK**-lee-ar); also termed Acoustic Nerve	M	vestibulo = *small opening or cavity,* cochlear = *snail-like*	equilibrium, hearing, sensation	acoustic loss, **vertigo (VER-tih-go)** = dizziness **tinnitus (tin-EYE-tuss)** = ear ringing **ataxia** (ah-**TACK**-see-ah) = muscle incoordination
IX Glossopharyngeal (**gloss**-oh-fair-an-**JEE**-al)	M	glosso = *tongue* pharyngeal = *throat area*	taste sensation, swallowing, regulation of O_2 and CO_2 breaths	Loss of taste sensatiom, swallowing difficulty reduced saliva flow of parotid gland
X Vagus (**VAY**-gus)	M	vaga = *vagrant, wander*	taste sensation of epiglottis, pharynx, blood pressure, smooth muscle of gastrointestinal system, heart rate, digestion	paralysis of vocal cords; heart rate increase sensation interference with swallowing, gastrointestinal organs
XI Accessory (ack-**SESS**-orree)	M	access = *assist, help out*	body sensation, muscles of shoulders	difficulty raising shoulders and move head
XII Hypoglossal (**high**-poe-**GLOSS**-al)	M	hypo = *under* glosso = *tongue*	body sensation, tongue movement in speech and swallowing	difficulty chewing, speaking, and swallowing

Note: S = sensory
    M = motor

posterior palatine: provides sensation for the tonsils and the soft palate.

nasopalatine (nay-zo-PAL-ih-tine): provides sensation for the nose and the palate.

infraorbital (in-fra-OR-bih-tal): subdivides into three parts: anterior, middle, and posterior.

> ▸ **anterior:** provides sensation to maxillary centrals, laterals, and canines.
> ▸ **middle:** provides sensation to the maxillary premolars and the mesiobuccal root of the maxillary first molar.
> ▸ **posterior:** provides sensation to the maxillary second and third molar, and to the remaining roots of the maxillary first molar.

zygomatic (zye-goh-MAT-ick): provides sensation to the lacrimal and upper cheek area.

sphenopalatine (sfee-no-PAL-ih-tine): sensory nerve ending for the maxillary anterior mucosal and palatine tissues.

mandibular: mixed nerve division that registers sensation and causes movement (see Figure 2-9). It has six branches:

inferior alveolar: provides sensation to the mandibular teeth.

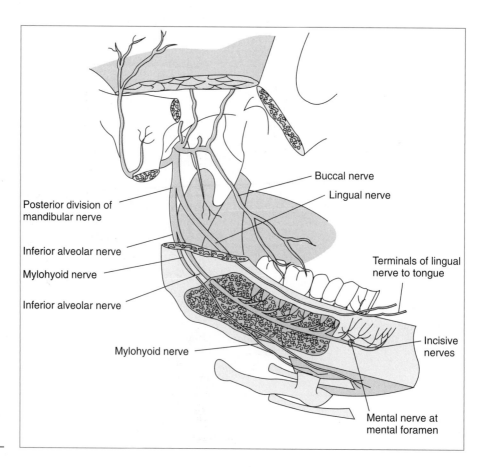

FIGURE 2-9
Mandibular branch of trigeminal nerve

mylohyoid: provides sensation to some muscles in the floor of the mouth.

mental: provides sensation to the skin of chin and the lower lip.

incisive: provides sensation to the anterior teeth and alveoli.

lingual: provides some sensation to the tongue and causes some movement.

buccal: provides sensation to the buccal gingiva and mucosa.

▐ BLOOD SUPPLY OF THE CRANIUM

Blood is supplied to the head by a vascular (**VAS**-cue-lar = *small vessels*) system of arteries and veins. An artery (**AR**-ter-ee) carries blood away from the heart, and a vein (**VAYN**) takes blood to the heart. Knowledge of the vascular system is important for control of bleeding and also for administration of local anesthesia. The major blood supply vessels to the head that are of interest in dentistry are the carotid artery, jugular vein, and capillaries.

carotid (care-**OT**-id) artery: rises from the aorta right and left and divides in the neck to form two arteries (Figure 2-10).

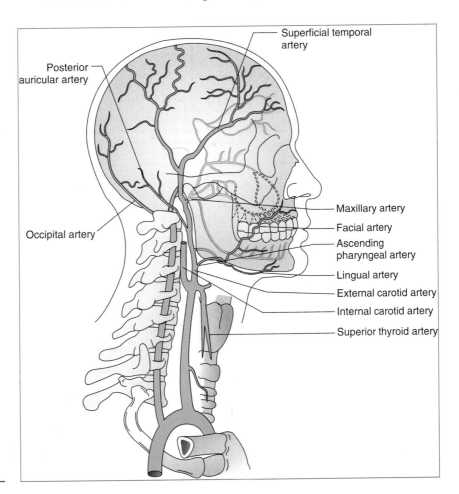

FIGURE 2-10
Carotid arteries

internal carotid: blood supply to the brain and eyes

external carotid: branches to the throat, face, tongue, and ears; these branches are:

> ▶ **infraorbital** (under eye orbit): provides blood to the maxillary anterior teeth.
> ▶ **inferior alveolar** (lower alveolar process): provides blood to the mandibular teeth.
> ▶ **facial** (pertaining to face): provides blood to the face, tonsils, palate, and submandibular gland.
> ▶ **lingual** (tongue): divides into branches to serve the tongue, tonsil, soft palate, and throat.
> ▶ **maxillary** (upper jaw): provides blood to the maxillary teeth.

jugular (**JUG**-you-lar) **vein:** transports blood from the head to the heart; drains to the internal jugular through three divisions (Figure 2-11).

facial division: carries blood from the face structures.
maxillary division: carries blood from the maxillary region.
pterygoid venus plexus (**PLECK**-sus = *network*): collects the blood supply from the head.

capillaries (**KAP**-ih-lair-eez): tiny blood vessels that help to transport blood from the veins to the arteries.

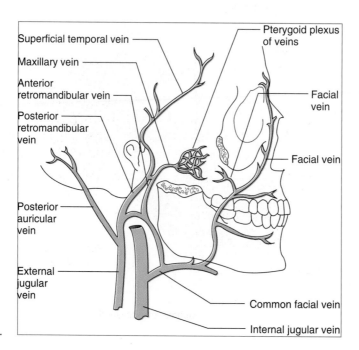

FIGURE 2-11
Jugular veins

LOCATIONS AND PURPOSES OF THE SALIVARY GLANDS

Salivary glands supply secretions to the oral cavity that protect the lining of the mouth, help moisten food, assist in speech, and make saliva to expectorate (ex-**PECK**-toe-rate = *spit*). The major salivary glands produce large amounts of secretions, and the minor salivary glands maintain moist oral tissue. Secretions may produce serum (**SEAR**-um = *watery fluid*) or mucin (**MYOU**-sin = *sticky, slimy secretion*) that forms mucus. Some glands produce both with enzymes (**EN**-zimes = *body-produced chemicals*) to digest food. In dentistry, three major salivary glands are of interest (Figure 2-12):

parotid (pah-**ROT**-id): the largest salivary gland, located near the ear; produces serus saliva, which empties into the mouth near the maxillary second molar through the Stenson's duct (**DUCKT** = *to lead*).

submandibular: a smaller gland located on the lower side of the face that secretes mucin and serus fluids with enzymes; empties through the Wharton's, or submandibular, duct openings under the tongue on each side of the lingual frenum.

sublingual: smallest major salivary gland, situated in the floor of the mouth; secretes mucin through multiple ducts; many other small glands are nearby, functioning to keep the mouth tissues moist.

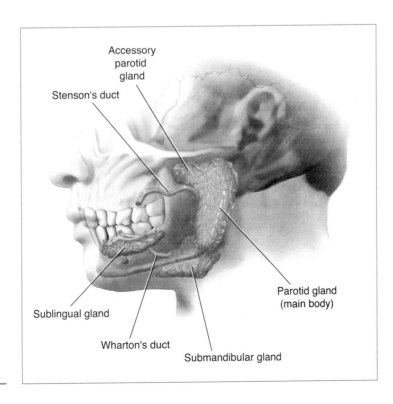

FIGURE 2-12
Salivary glands, lateral view

FUNCTIONS AND AGENTS OF THE LYMPHATIC SYSTEM

Present throughout the body, the lymphatic system helps protect the body from disease and assists with immunity. This lymphatic system is composed of a variety of structures:

lymph (LIMF): vessels that transport lymph fluid of plasma, water, and waste products.
lymph capillaries: tiny vessels or tubes that carry lymph fluid.
lymph node: a mass of lymph cells forming a unit of lymphatic tissue that are named after the formation site, for example:

axillary (**ACK**-sih-lair-ee = *pertaining to the armpit*): lymph nodes located under the armpit.
cervical (**SIR**-vih-kul = *pertaining to the neck*): lymph nodes located in the neck.
inguinal (**IN**-gwee-nal = *pertaining to the groin*): lymph nodes found in the abdomen.

tonsil (**TAHN**-sil): a lymphatic tissue mass found in the posterior of the throat between the anterior and posterior fauces and on the back of the tongue; tonsils act as filters, aid in the production of disease-fighting immune responses, and may help immunity.
adenoid (**ADD**-eh-noyd): lymphatic tissue found in the nasopharynx area; may provide protection similar to tonsils.

Agents of the Lymphatic System

The main action of the lymphatic system is to defend the body against disease and infection caused by antigens (**AN**-tih-jens), foreign, pathogenic substances introduced into or produced by the body. An antigen accomplishes this function through a variety of agents of the immune response.

antibody (**AN**-tie-bah-dee): protein material, manufactured by the body, that destroys antigens; antibodies are the basis for the immune response.
lymphocytes (**LIM**-foe-sites): lymph cells that assist in body defenses; the two types are:
B-lymphocytes: produce antibodies to destroy antigens.
T-lymphocytes: also called T-cells; produced in the thymus; assist with the immune system to destroy foreign cells and pathogens.

immunoglobulin (im-you-no-**GLOB**-you-lin): plasma-made proteins, produced in lymph tissue, that are capable of acting as antibodies in the immune response.
interferon (in-ter-**FEAR**-on): proteins produced by cells exposed to viruses; help to provide immunity to unaffected cells.
phagocytes (**FAG**-oh-sites): white blood cells that ingest and destroy antigens in a process called phagocytosis (**fag**-oh-sigh-**TOE**-sis). The two classes or forms are:

macrophages (**MACK**-roe-fayges): large phagocyte cells that ingest antigens and inflammatory bodies.
microphanges (**MY**-crow-fanges): neutrophilic cells that ingest smaller matter, such as bacteria.

IMPORTANT STRUCTURES IN THE ORAL CAVITY

The composition of the oral cavity involves many different tissues and forms. Each structure is designed for a specific purpose and function. The more important landmarks of note in the dental field are described next.

Labia

The lips, or labia (**LAY**-bee-ah = *lips*), have several sections or divisions:

superior oris (**OR**-iss): upper lip.
inferium oris: lower lip.
labial commissure (**KOM**-ih-shur): area at the corners of the mouth where the lips meet.
vermilion (ver-**MILL**-yon) border: area where the pink-red lip tissue meets the facial skin.
philtrum (**FIL**-trum): median groove in the center external surface of the upper lip.
caruncle (**CAR**-unk-ul); small, fleshy mucous tissue elevations under the tongue.

Frenum

The tongue and each lip and cheek attach to the oral membrane with a triangular piece of tissue called a frenum (**FREE**-num). The oral cavity has five major frena (**FREE**-nah = *plural of frenum*):

labial frenum (2): tissue that attaches the inside of the lip to the mucous membrane in the anterior of the oral cavity. They occur in both the maxillary and the mandibular arches. The maxillary labial frenum is a common site for a maxillary frenectomy.
lingual frenum (1): attaches the lower side of the tongue to the floor membrane. Openings to Wharton's duct are found on each side of this frenum. If the lingual frenum is too short, ankyloglossia (**ang**-key-loh-**GLOSS**-ee-ah), a "tongue-tied" condition, can result.
buccal frenum (2): attaches the inside of the cheek to the oral cavity in the maxillary first molar area. This frenum occurs on the left and the right sides.

Tongue Structures

The tongue is an important organ in the oral cavity that performs many necessary functions. The tongue, or glossa (**GLOSS**-ah = *Latin for tongue*), is a strong muscular organ that aids in chewing, talking, and deglutition (**dee**-glue-**TISH**-un = *swallowing*). A median sulcus (**SULL**-kus = *groove, depression*) divides the tongue's top surface into two parts. The tongue also has many papillae (pah-**PIH**-lie = *tissue growths*) or taste buds situated on the dorsal (**DOOR**-sal = *back*) surface of the tongue. The major papillae are illustrated in Figure 2-13.

circumvallate (sir-kum-**VAL**-ate): the largest, V-shaped papillae, situated on the dorsal aspect of the tongue; sense bitter tastes.
filiform (**FIL**-ih-form): the smallest, hair-like papillae covering the entire dorsal aspect of the tongue; do not sense taste.

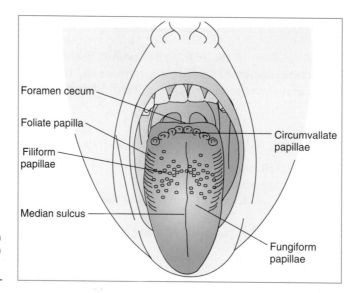

FIGURE 2-13
View of tongue with taste buds (papillae) noted.

fungiform (**FUN**-jih-form): small, dark-red papillae on the middle and anterior dorsal surface and along the sides of the tongue; sense sweet, sour, and salty tastes.

foliate (**FOE**-lee-ate): on the posterior lateral borders of the tongue, and can be seen if the tongue is grasped with gauze and extended; sense sour tastes.

Palate Structures

The palate (**PAL**-at), or roof of the mouth, is composed of assorted structures. It is divided into two main divisions—hard palate and soft palate.

hard palate: composed of the palatine processes of the maxillae bones; covered with mucous membrane and has rugae (**RUE**-guy), irregular folds or bumps on the surface.

> incisive papilla: tissue growth situated at the anterior portion of palate behind the maxillary centrals; the site for infiltration injection of local anesthesia.
> palatine raphe (**RAH**-fay = *ridge between the union of two halves*); white streak in the middle of the palate.

soft palate: flexible portion of the palate; area where the gag reflex is present.

Miscellaneous Oral Cavity Structures

uvula: tissue structure hanging from the palate in the posterior of the oral cavity.
vestibule (**VES**- tih-byul): open gum area between the teeth and the cheek.
fauces (**FOE**-sèz): constricted opening or passage leading from the mouth to the oral pharynx, bound by the soft palate, the base of tongue, and the palatine arches. The fauces have two pillars.

glossopalatine (gloss-oh -**PAL**-ah-tine = *glossa* and *palate* area) arch: anterior pillars.

pharyngopalatine (fare-in-goh-**PAL**-ah-tine = *pharynx* and *palate* area): posterior pillars.

The palatine tonsils lay between these pillars.

REVIEW EXERCISES

MATCHING

Match the following word elements with their meaning:

1. _____cranium
2. _____jugular
3. _____philtrum
4. _____superius oris
5. _____magnum
6. _____parotid
7. _____buccinator
8. _____glossa
9. _____node
10. _____mastication
11. _____mental
12. _____suture
13. _____uvula
14. _____frontal
15. _____incus

a. foramen in occipital bone for spinal cord passage
b. tissue structure hanging from posterior of palate
c. another word for tongue
d. portion of skull that encloses the brain
e. mass of lymph cells forming body named for area site
f. takes blood from head to heart
g. upper lip
h. act of chewing
i. groove on external middle surface of upper lip
j. principal cheek muscle
k. forehead bone
l. bone of middle ear
m. another word for chin
n. immoveable junction of two bones
o. largest salivary gland

DEFINITION

Using the selection given for each sentence, choose the best term to complete the definition.

1. Which of the following papillae do not sense taste?
   a. circumvallate   b. filiform
   c. foliate   d. fungiform

2. A mass of lymph cells forming a unit of lymphatic tissue is called a lymph:
   a. antigen   b. parietal
   c. node   d. forama

3. A body-produced chemical helping to break down food for digestion is called an:
   a. infragen   b. enzyme
   c. expectorant   d. antigen

4. Which artery carries the blood supply to the head and brain?
   a. jugular   b. carotid
   c. capillary   d. radial artery

5. Branch of the ophthalmic nerves that provides sensation for the tear gland is the:
   a. lacrimal   b. nasociliary
   c. maxillary   d. plexus

6. The principal muscle of mastication that closes the mouth is the _____
   a. internal pterygoid   b. external pterygoid
   c. masseter   d. common pterygoid

7. Which of the following three is not an auditory ossicle?
   a. stapes   b. malleus
   c. tympanic   d. anvil

8. The protective mucous layer covering the bone surface is the:
   a. periosteum   b. mucoperiosteum
   c. calcisopenum   d. osteoplasta

9. The fusion line in the center/middle of the mandible is the:
   a. symphysis   b. condyle
   c. ramus   d. orbit

10. The suture between the two parietal bones is called the:
    a. sagittal   b. coronal
    c. temporoparietal d. symphysis

11. The atrium of Highmore is another name for the:
    a. opening in the occipital bone
    b. oral cavity free space between the cheek/lips
    c. maxillary sinus cavity
    d. opening in the frontal bone

12. Which of the following is not considered a facial bone?
    a. temporal   b. maxilla
    c. zygomatic   d. vomer

13. The bone that lies in suspension between the larynx and the mandible is the:
    a. lambdoid   b. hyoid
    c. sigmoid   d. frontal

14. The large bone growth behind the ears on the temporal bone is the:
    a. coronoid   b. sublingual
    c. mastoid   d. occipital

15. An opening or passage through a bone that is used for nerve or vessel passage is called a/an:
    a. foramen   b. transvessel
    c. alveolar crest   d. sinus

16. An inferior end of a process that has a hooked end is called a:
    a. plexus   b. hamulus
    c. protuberance   d. forama

17. The S-shaped curvature between the condyle and the coronoid process is the:
    a. ramus   b. angle of mandible
    c. sigmoid notch   d. coronoid

18. A protein produced by cells exposed to viruses is a/an:
    a. interferon   b. antigen
    c. immunoglobulin   d. phagocyte

19. The area located to the rear of the mandibular molars is the:
    a. retromolar area
    b. suborbital area
    c. supramandibular area
    d. hyoid area

20. The median sulcus divides the tongue into how many sections?
    a. none   b. one
    c. two   d. three

BUILDING SKILLS

Locate and define the prefix, root/combining form, and suffix (if present) in the following words:

1. **infraorbital**
   prefix   _____
   root/combining form   _____
   suffix   _____

2. **periosteum**
   prefix   _____
   root/combining form   _____
   suffix   _____

3. **mastication**
   prefix   _____
   root/combining form   _____
   suffix   _____

4. **sublingual**
   prefix   _____
   root/combining form   _____
   suffix   _____

5. **expectorate**
   prefix   _____
   root/combining form   _____
   suffix   _____

FILL-INS

Write the correct word in the blank space to complete each statement.

1. The skull is composed of two main bone divisions, the _____ and the facial bones.

2. A/an _____ is a protein material manufactured by the body to destroy an antigen.

3. The _____ gland is the smallest of the major salivary glands.

4. The _____ foramen is located in the maxilla behind the central incisors.

5. The _____ is the tissue membrane covering the bones of a mucous surface.

6. The ascending part of the mandible is called the _____.

7. The junction of the frontal and parietal bones at birth are soft and sometimes called the baby's "soft spot" or the _____.

8. Another name for the circular muscle surrounding the mouth is _____.

9. The trigeminal nerve emerges from the brain and branches at the semilunar mass of nerves called the _____.

10. The division of the trigeminal nerve that registers sensation to the lower jaw is the _____ division.

11. The internal carotid artery supplies blood to the eyes and the _____.

12. The parotid salivary gland empties into the mouth through the _____ duct.

13. The lymphatic system helps protect the body from disease and assists with _____.

14. A/an _____ is a lymph cell that ingests and destroys antigens.

15. _____ lymph cells ingest bacteria.

16. Taste buds are also called _____.

17. The _____ papillae are small, dark red papillae on the middle and anterior dorsal surface and along the sides of the tongue.

18. The _____ is the muscular tissue structure that hangs down from the palate in the rear of the oral cavity.

19. The mucus membrane in the roof of the mouth that forms irregular folds and bumps on the surface is called _____.

20. The palatine tonsils lay between the _____ pillars.

WORD USE

Read the following sentences and define the bold-faced word.

1. Mr. John Clancey has been referred to our office for a second opinion regarding the possible diagnosis of **temporomandibular** joint disorder.

   _____

2. A partial eruption of the left mandibular third molar was charted and an inflammation of the **retromolar** area was noted.

   _____

3. X-ray examination revealed a fracture of the left **coronoid** process and the presence of an unerupted maxillary tooth.

   _____

4. The patient was given a prescription for treatment of enlarged tonsils and an acute infection in the **pharyngopalatine** area.

   _____

5. Mrs. Barbara Timmins called to confirm the time and date scheduled for her son's oral surgery treatment of **ankylogossia.**

   _____

AUDIO LIST 💿

This list contains selected new, important, or difficult terms from this chapter. You may use the list to review these terms and to practice pronouncing them correctly. When you work with the audio for this chapter, listen to the word, repeat it, and then place a checkmark in the box. Proceed to the next boxed word and repeat the process.

- ❑ abducens (**AB**-due-senz)
- ❑ adenoid (**ADD**-eh-noyd)
- ❑ alveolar (al-**VEE**-oh-lar)
- ❑ alveolus (al-**VEE**-oh-lus)
- ❑ ankyloglossia (**ang**-key-loh-**GLOSS**-ee-ah)
- ❑ anopia (an-**OH**-pee-ah)
- ❑ anosmia (an-**OZ**-mee-ah)
- ❑ antibody (**AN**-tie-bah-ee)
- ❑ antigens (**AN**-tih-jens)
- ❑ articular eminence (ar-**TICK**-you-lar **EM**-ih-nense)
- ❑ Bell's palsy (**PAUL**-zee)
- ❑ buccinator (**BUCK**-sin-ay-tor)
- ❑ capillaries (**KAP**-ih-lair-eez)
- ❑ carotid (care-**OT**-id)
- ❑ cervical (**SIR**-vih-kul)
- ❑ circumvallate (sir-kum-**VAL**-ate)
- ❑ commisure (**KOM**-ih-shur)
- ❑ conchae (**KONG**-kee) (pl. of concha)
- ❑ condyle (**KON**-dial)
- ❑ condyloid (**KON**-dih-loyd)
- ❑ coronal (kor-**OH**-nal)
- ❑ coronoid (**KOR**-oh-noyd)
- ❑ cranium (**KRAY**-nee-um)
- ❑ diplopia (die-**PLOH**-pee-ah)
- ❑ ethmoid (eth-**MOYD**)
- ❑ expectorate (ex-**PECK**-toe-rate)
- ❑ fauces (**FOH**-sez)
- ❑ filiform (**FIL**-ih-form)
- ❑ foliate (**FOH**-lee-ate)
- ❑ foramen (foh-**RAY**-men)
- ❑ frenum (**FREE**-num)
- ❑ frontal (**FRON**-tal)
- ❑ ganglion (**GANG**-lee-un)
- ❑ glenoid fossa (**GLEE**-noyd **FAH**-sah)
- ❑ glossa (**GLOSS**-ah)
- ❑ glossopharyngeal (gloss-oh-fair-an-**JEE**-al)

- ❑ immunoglobulin (im-you-no-**GLOB**-you-lin)
- ❑ incisive (in-**SIGH**-siv)
- ❑ incus (**IN**-kus)
- ❑ infraorbital (in-frah-**OR**-bih-tal)
- ❑ interferon (in-ter-**FEAR**-on)
- ❑ jugular (**JUG**-you-lar)
- ❑ lacrimal (**LACK**-rih-mal)
- ❑ lambdoid (**LAM**-doyd)
- ❑ lymph (**LIMF**)
- ❑ lymphocytes (**LIM**-foe-sites)
- ❑ malleus (**MAL**-ee-us)
- ❑ mandible (**MAN**-dih-bull)
- ❑ masseter (mass-**EE**-ter)
- ❑ mastoid (**MASS**-toyd)
- ❑ maxillary (**MACK**-sih-lairee)
- ❑ meatus (mee-**AY**-tus)
- ❑ meniscus (men-**IS**-kus)
- ❑ mentalis (men-**TAL**-is)
- ❑ mucin (**MYOU**-sin)
- ❑ mucoperiosteum (**myou**-koh-pear-ee-**AHS**-tee-um)
- ❑ mylohyoid (my-loh-**HIGH**-oyd)
- ❑ nasal (**NAY**-zel)
- ❑ nasion (**NAY**-zhun)
- ❑ nasociliary (**nay**-zoh-**SIL**-ee-air-ee)
- ❑ occipital (ock-**SIP**-ih-tal)
- ❑ oculomotor (ock-you-low-**MOE**-or)
- ❑ olfactory (ol-**FACK**-toh-ree)
- ❑ ophthalmic (off-**THAL**-mick)
- ❑ orbicularis oris (or-**bick**-you-**LAIR**-iss **OR**-iss)
- ❑ palatine (**PAL**-ah-tine)
- ❑ papillae (pah-**PIH**-lie) (plural of papilla)
- ❑ parietal (pah-**RYE**-eh-tal)
- ❑ parotid (pah-**ROT**-id)
- ❑ periosteum (pear-ee-**AH**-stee-um)
- ❑ phagocytes (**FAG**-oh-sites)
- ❑ philtrum (**FIL**-trum)

- ❏ posterior (pahos-**TEE**-ree-or)
- ❏ protuberance (proh-**TOO**-ber-ans)
- ❏ pterygoid (**TER**-eh-goyd)
- ❏ ptosis (**TOE**-sis)
- ❏ ramus (**RAY**-mus)
- ❏ raphe (**RAH**-fay)
- ❏ retromolar (ret-trow-**MOLE**-ar)
- ❏ rugae (**RUE**-guy)
- ❏ sagittal (**SAJ**-ih-tal)
- ❏ sigmoid (**SIG**-moyd)
- ❏ sphenoid (**SFEE**-noyd)
- ❏ sphenopalatine (sfee-no-**PAL**-ah-tine)
- ❏ squamous (**SKWAY**-mus)
- ❏ stapes (**STAY**-peez)
- ❏ strabismus (strah-**BIZ**-muss)
- ❏ styloid (**STY**-loyd)
- ❏ sulcus (**SULL**-kus)
- ❏ symphysis (**SIM**-fih-sis)
- ❏ synovial (sin-**OH**-vee-al)
- ❏ temporal (**TEM**-pore-al)
- ❏ temporomandibular (**tem**-poe-roe-man-**DIB**-you-lar)
- ❏ temporoparietal (**tem**-poe-roe-pah-**RYE**-eh-tal)
- ❏ tinnitus (tin-**EYE**-tuss)
- ❏ tonsil (**TAHL**-sill)
- ❏ trigeminal (try-**JEM**-in-al)
- ❏ trochlear (**TRAH**-klee-ur)
- ❏ uvula (**YOU**-view-lah)
- ❏ vagus (**VAY**-gus)
- ❏ vermillion border (ver-**MILL**-yon **BORE**-der)
- ❏ vertigo (**VER**-tih-go)
- ❏ vestibule (**VES**-tih-byul)
- ❏ vestibulocochlear (ves-**tib**-you-low-**COCK**-lee-ar)
- ❏ vomer (**VOH**-mer)
- ❏ zygomatic (zye-goh-**MAT**-ick)
- ❏ zygomaticofacial (zye-goh-**MAT**-ee-coe-fay-shal)

CHAPTER 3

Tooth Origin and Formation

OBJECTIVES   Upon completion of this chapter, the reader should be able to identify and understand terms related to the:

1. **Classification of the human dentition.** Discuss the various dentitions and terms related to them.

2. **Histological stages of tooth development.** Identify each developmental stage of tooth formation from initiation to attrition.

3. **Tissue structure of the teeth.** Identify and determine the makeup of each of the tooth tissues and conditions related to their development.

4. **Tissue composition of the periodontium.** Name and discuss the various tissues and membranes that make up the periodontium.

5. **Odontology.** Discuss the attributes and characteristic terms that are common to the teeth in the human dentition.

6. **Tooth surfaces.** Name and identify the tooth surfaces and characteristic landmarks.

CLASSIFICATION OF THE HUMAN DENTITION

Each human receives two sets of teeth. The first set, or deciduous (deh-**SID**-you-us = *falling off*) teeth, is followed by the permanent dentition (den-**TISH**-un = *tooth arrangement*). The twenty deciduous teeth that erupt first are commonly called "baby teeth" or primary teeth. The thirty-two permanent teeth that erupt and replace the deciduous teeth are commonly called secondary teeth. The permanent teeth are also termed succedaneous (suck-seh-**DAY**-nee-us) because these teeth, with the exception of the molars, replace the deciduous teeth when the latter exfoliate (ecks-**FOH**-lee-ate = *scale off*).

Mixed dentition occurs from ages six to sixteen, when the dentition contains both deciduous and secondary teeth. Figure 3-1 illustrates mixed dentition. Although

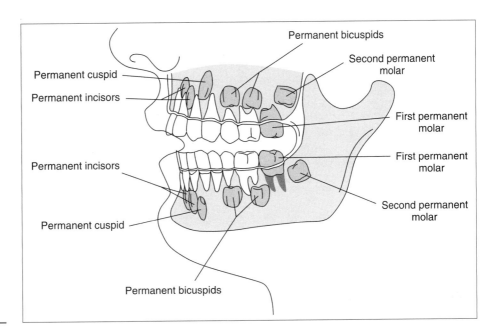

FIGURE 3-1
Mixed dentition

human teeth are considered heterodont (**HET**-er-oh-dahnt = *teeth of various shapes*), all teeth go through the same stages of development.

HISTOLOGICAL STAGES OF TOOTH DEVELOPMENT

The term odontogenesis (oh-**dahn**-toh-**JEN**-eh-sis, odont = *tooth*, genesis = *production*) refers to the formation and the origin of the tooth. During its evolution and growth, each tooth begins and passes through the developmental stages shown in Figure 3-2.

First Stage of Development

The first, or bud, stage of development is termed the initiation (ih-**nish**-ee-**AY**-shun = *beginning*). At the fifth or sixth week in utero (in **YOU**-ter-oh = *in uterus*), the dental lamina (**LAM**-ih-nah = *membrane band containing organs of future teeth*) develops in the primitive oral cavity epithelium (**ep**-ith-**EE**-lee-um = *mucous tissue covering and connective tissue layer*). At various points of fetal and age development, these organs present buds or seeds of future teeth.

Second Stage of Development

The second stage of development, called proliferation (pro-**lif**-er-**AY**-shun = *reproduction of new parts*), includes the bud and early cap stages. Proliferation begins during the fourth or fifth month in utero, when small buds appear at different time periods until all deciduous teeth are apparent. Permanent teeth follow the same pattern but begin development in utero and after birth.

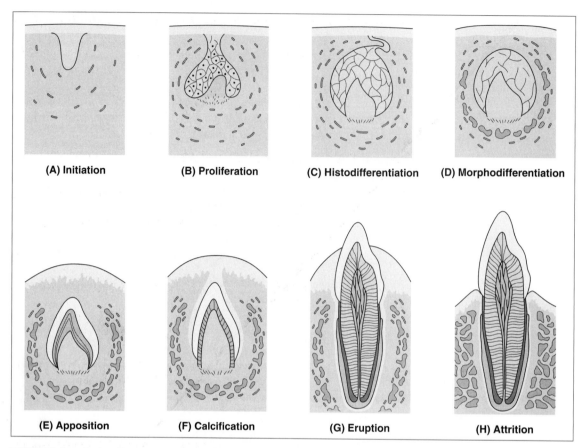

(A) Initiation **(B) Proliferation** **(C) Histodifferentiation** **(D) Morphodifferentiation**

(E) Apposition **(F) Calcification** **(G) Eruption** **(H) Attrition**

FIGURE 3-2   The histological stages of tooth development.

The tooth bud consists of three parts.

dental organ (*enamel organ*): derived from the ectoderm (**ECK**-toh-derm = *outer layer of development*), gives the tooth bud its covering;

dental papilla (pah-**PILL**-ah = *tissue development giving rise to dentin, pulp*): makes up the inner structures of the tooth, such as the dentin and the pulp, and is derived from the mesoderm (**MESS**-oh-derm = *middle layer*), in particular from the mesenchyme (**MEZ**-en-kime = *connective tissue cells*);

dental sac (**SACK** = *pocket covering*): derived from the mesoderm, makes up the surrounding covering for the dental organ and papilla; gives rise to the cementum, or root-covering tissue, the periodontal ligaments that hold the tooth in the alveolar socket, and the alveolar bond; also called the *dental follicle*.

Third Stage of Development

The differentiation (**dif**-er-en-she-**AY**-shun = *acquiring different functions from the original*) stage (C and D in Figure 3-2) causes changes in the tooth bud shape and makeup. It occurs in two ways.

1. histodifferentiation (his-toh-dif-er-en-she-**AY**-shun = *branch into different tissues*), and
2. morphodifferentiation (more-foh-diff-er-en-she-**AY**-shun = *change into other shape*).

Tooth Development.   After the makeup and shape change from the tooth cap to the early bell stage, the various tissues of the tooth begin to develop and function. This process occurs because of the appearance of specialized germ cells:

odontoblasts (oh-**DAHN**-toh-blasts = *dentin forming cells*): encourage cell growth to form the dentin, the bulk of the tooth.
ameloblasts (ah-**MEAL**-oh-blasts = *enamel forming cells*): encourage cell growth to form the enamel covering tissue of the tooth.
cementoblasts (see-**MEN**-toh-blasts = *cementum forming cells*): encourage cell growth to form the root-covering cementum tissue.
fibroblasts (**FIE**-broh-blasts = *fiber forming germ cells*): encourage cell growth to form the periodontal ligaments.
osteoblasts (**AHS**-tee-oh-blasts = *bone forming germ cells*): encourage cell growth to form alveolar bone and the alveolar plate.

Fourth Stage of Development

In the fourth stage, apposition (ap-oh-**ZIH**-shun = *addition of parts*), mineral salts and organic matter are set down in place for tissues and tooth formation.

Fifth Stage of Development

The fifth phase of development, calcification (**kal**-sih-fih-**KAY**-shun = *deposit of lime salts*) is characterized by the hardening and setting of tooth tissues. It continues after eruption (the sixth stage) until total development is accomplished, which takes approximately two years.

Sixth Stage of Development

Eruption (ee-**RUP**-shun = *breaking out*), the sixth phase of tooth development, is commonly called "cutting of the teeth." It occurs when the tooth moves toward the oral cavity and enters through the tissues.

Final Stage of Development

Attrition (ah-**TRISH**-un = *chafing or abrasion*) is the last stage of development. This wearing away occurs where teeth interact through mastication and speech.

Specialized Cells

The stages of tooth development occur at different times according to the tooth involved and its normal developmental schedule, from the first growth stage at the fourth or fifth week in utero to the final calcification of the permanent third molars.

In addition to the constructive developing actions, some degenerative periods are necessary to remove the deciduous teeth, making room for the permanent dentitions. Several specialized cells cause root **resorption** (ree-**SORP**-shun = *removal of hard tooth surface*) and degeneration of deciduous teeth.

odontoclasts (oh-**DAHN**-toh-klasts): cells that bring about absorption of primary tooth roots.

cementoclasts (see-**MEN**-toh-klasts): cells that destroy tooth cementum.

osteoclasts (**AHS**-tee-oh-klasts): cells that destroy or cause absorption of bone tissue.

Tooth Abnormalities

Changes or disturbances during any of the development stages can cause a variety of tooth irregularities or abnormalities, called **anomalies** (ah-**NOM**-ah-leez = *not normal*).

amelogenesis (**ah-meal-oh-JEN-ih-sis** = *process of forming tooth enamel*) imperfecta: a genetic disorder resulting in the formation of defective enamel.

anodontia (an-oh-**DON**-she-ah = *absence of teeth*): partial or total lack of teeth.

dens in dente (**DENZ** in **DEN**-tay = *tooth in tooth*): a tooth enfolding on itself to form a small cavity that holds a hard structure or mass; found most commonly on the lingual surface of the maxillary laterals.

dentinogenesis imperfecta (**den**-tin-oh-**JEN**-eh-sis = *occurring in dentin formation*; im-per-**FECK**-tuh =*inadequacy*): a genetic disorder characterized by weakened or gray-colored teeth or shell teeth resulting from poor formation.

enamel hypoplasia (high-poh-**PLAY**-zee-ah = *underdevelopment of tissue*): lack of enamel covering.

fluorosis (floor-**OH**-sis = *reaction to overfluoridation*): described as "mottled enamel."

fusion (**FEW**-zhun = *joining together*): union of tooth buds resulting in large crown or root.

germination (**jerm**-ih-**NAY**-shun = *development of germ cell*): single tooth germ separating to form two crowns on a single root.

Hutchinsonian incisors: saw-like incisal edges of maxillary incisors, caused by maternal syphilis during tooth formation.

hypocalcification (**high**-poh-kal-sih-fih-**KAY**-shun = *underbonding* or *incomplete calcification*): lack of hardening of tooth tissue, resulting in weak, susceptible teeth.

macrodontia (**mack**-roh-**DAHN**-she-ah): abnormally large teeth.

microdontia (**my**-kroh-**DAHN**-she-ah): unusually small teeth.

peg-shaped teeth: a condition of small, rounded teeth that usually occurs in the maxillary lateral incisors.

supernumerary (**sue**-per-**NEW**-mer-air-ee = *extra*): more than the normal amount of teeth.

TISSUE STRUCTURE OF THE TEETH

Although there are four different types of teeth—incisors, canines/cuspids, premolars, and molars—all teeth possess the same tissues formations, anatomical basics, and structural landmarks.

Enamel

Enamel (eh-**NAM**-el) is a hard tooth covering that is 96 percent inorganic. Tooth enamel exhibits a variety of unique structures and characteristics.

cuticle (**KYOU**-tih-kul): also called Nasmyth's (**NAHS**–myth) **membrane,** a tissue layer covering tooth surfaces; wears away soon after eruption.

stripes of Retzius (**RET**-zee-us = *Swedish anatomist*): lines in enamel; also called bands or striae of Retzius.

lamellae (lah-**MEL**-ah = *thin plate or scale*): developmental cracks or imperfections in enamel tissue extending toward or into the dentin.

tuft (*abnormal clump of rods*): irregular grouping of undercalcified enamel.

spindles (**SPIN**-duls = *spindle-like processes*): end areas of union for odontoblasts and enamel rod endings.

rods: slightly curved, prism-like structures that extend from dentinoenamel junction to the outer surface; tightly packed with an organic matrix material to give a smooth, hard surface (see Figure 3-3).

gnarled enamel (**NARL**-ed = *twisted*): enamel rod twisting and curving within the tooth tissue.

Dentin

Dentin (**DEN**-tin), the main tissue of tooth surrounding the pulp, is less inorganic (70 percent) than enamel. It is slightly yellow-brown in color and gives bulk to the tooth. Dentin is present in both the crown and the root and may exhibit two unique characteristics.

tubules (**TOO**-bules = *small tubes*): also known as **Tomes' dentinal tubules,** small, S-shaped tubes or channels extending from the dentinoenamel wall to the pulp chamber. The tubules (see Figure 3-3) transmit pain stimuli and nutrition throughout the tissues

fibers (**FIGH**-bers = *threadlike films/elements*): also known as **Tomes' dentinal fibril,** fibers lying within the dentin tubule that help the dentin to nourish and register sensation.

Dentin gives shape to the tooth. It is softer than enamel but harder than the pulp tissue. The three different types of dentin tissue are:

primary dentin: dentin in newly formed tooth, the original dentin.

regular secondary dentin: occurs during regular development and maturing of tooth.

irregular secondary dentin: occurs as protection from irritation, decay, trauma, attrition, and the like. This irregular secondary dentin is also called "reparative dentin," or tertiary (**TERR**-shee-air-ee = *third*) dentin, the third type of dentin.

Pulp

Pulp (= *soft, vascular tooth tissue*) is found in the center of the tooth. It is encased in the **pulp chamber** in the crown, and in the **pulp canal,** located in the root section of the

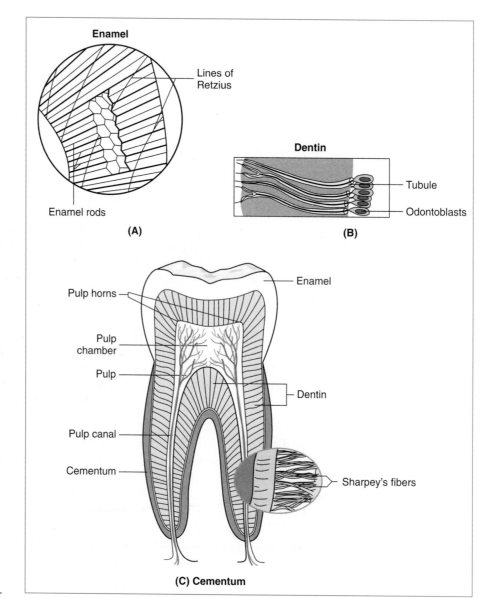

FIGURE 3-3
Posterior tooth with enlargement views of (a) enamel, (b) dentin, and (c) cementum with periodontal attachment and pulp horns, pulp chamber, and pulp canal.

tooth. **Pulp** horns are pointed edges or boundaries of the pulp chamber extending toward the chewing surfaces (see Figure 3-3). The most organic tooth tissue, pulp performs four main functions:

1. nourishment,
2. defense,
3. registration of sensation/pain, and
4. dentin protection.

The tooth pulp is composed of multiple cells called **fibroblasts** that are capable of developing connective tissue.

Four common diseases of the pulp are:

pulpitis (pul-**PIE**-tis = *pulp inflammation*): also called toothache; occurs for many reasons.
pulp stone: also known as denticle (**DEN**-tih-kul), a small growth on a tooth.
pulp cyst **(SIST):** a closed, fluid-filled sac within the pulp tissue.
granuloma (gran-you-**LOH**-mah) = *granular tumor or growth*): a growth or tumor usually found in the root area.

Cementum

Cementum (see-**MEN**-tum = *tissue covering of tooth root*) is approximately 55 percent inorganic, rough in texture, and meets the enamel tissue at the **cementoenamel** (cement-enamel union) **junction** that is located at the neck of the tooth. The function of cementum is to protect the root and provide rough surface anchorage for attachment of **Sharpey's fibers,** that are connective tissue fibers of the periodontal ligament. There are two kinds of cementum.

1. **primary cementum**: original cementum that does not contain bone-type cells and is uniform in surface texture; also called **acellular** (ay-**SELL**-you-lar = *without cells*) **cementum.**
2. **secondary cementum**: contains bone-type cells and usually forms on the lower root surface as a result of stimulation, attrition, and wear; also called **cellular cementum.**

In addition to matrix material and cementoblasts, other features may be present in cementum.

lacuna (lah-**KYOU**-nah = *small open space*): tiny cavities that may contain cementocytes (see-**MEN**-toh-sites = *irregular cementum forming cells*).
canaliculi (kan-ah-**LICK**-you-lie): small channels or canals.
hypercementosis (**high**-per-**see**-men-**TOH**-sis = *overgrowth of cementum tissue*): an anomaly resulting in thickening of cementum; usually occurs as a result of constant stress or occlusal trauma.

▌ TISSUE COMPOSITION OF THE PERIODONTIUM

The anchorage, support, and protection of the teeth is provided by various tissues collectively called the **periodontium** (**pear**-ee-oh-**DANT**-ee-um = *tissues surrounding teeth*). The periodontium is composed mainly of four separate tissues:

periodontal (pear-ee-oh-**DAHN**-tahl = *around tooth*): membrane, fibers that anchor the tooth in the alveolar socket.
alveolar (al-**VEE**-oh-lar): bone, bony sockets, or crypts for teeth placement in the maxillae and the mandibular bones; alveolar bone also gives support to the teeth.

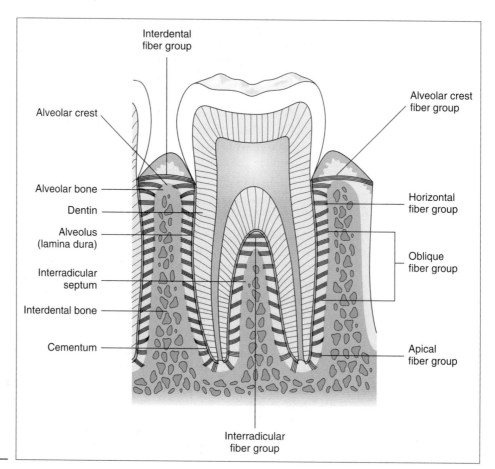

FIGURE 3-4
Principal fibers of
the periodontium.

gingiva (**JIN**-jih-vah = *mouth tissue*): mucous tissue surrounding the teeth; also gives
protection to the teeth and underlying tissues.

Although we have discussed **cementum** as a tissue covering for the tooth root
structure, this tissue also is considered an essential element of the periodontium.

Periodontal Membranes

Periodontal membranes, also called periodontal ligaments, are made up of connective tissues arranged in bundles and dense fibrous tissue groupings. There are five
principal types of periodontal membranes or ligaments (Figure 3-4). The functions
of each are as follows.

alveolar crest fibers: found at the cementoenamel junction, they help to retain the
tooth in its socket and to provide protection for the deeper fibers.
horizontal fibers: connect the alveolar bone to the upper part of the root and assist
with control of lateral movement.

oblique fibers: attach the alveolar socket to the majority of the root cementum and assist in resistance of the axial forces.

apical fiber bundles: running from the apex of the tooth to the alveolar bone, they help prevent tipping and dislocation, as well as protect the nerve and blood supply to the tooth.

interradicular fiber bundles: present in multirooted teeth, extending apically from the tooth furcation; help the tooth resist tipping, turning, and dislocation.

Alveolar Bone   The alveolar bone, also called the alveolar process, is composed of an alveolar socket and a dense covering of compact bone with an inner and outer growth called **cortical plate**. Lining the alveolar socket is a thin **cribriform** (**KRIB**-rih-form = *sieve-like*) **plate** covering called the **lamina dura** (**LAM**-ih-nah **DUR**-ah = *hard lining*). This outline is easily viewed on radiographs.

Gingiva   Also known as gum tissue, the gingiva protects the tooth root and underlying tissues. It is composed of various epithelial layers, some of which are attached and some of which are free gingiva. These tissue layers are described as:

attached: the portion that is firm, dense, stippled, and bound to the underlying periosteum, tooth, and bone.

keratinized (**KARE**-ah-tin-ized = *hard* or *horny*): hard tissue, also called *masticatory mucosa*, the area where the gingiva and mucous membrane unite; indicated by color changes from pink gingiva to red mucosa, called the **mucogingival** (myou-koh-**JIN**-jih-vahl) border.

marginal: the portion that is unattached to underlying tissues and helps to form the sides of the gingival crevice; also called the free margin gingiva, forming the gingival **sulcus**, approximately 1 to 3mm in depth.

papillary: the part of the marginal gingiva that occupies the interproximal spaces; normally triangular and filling the tooth embrasure area; also called interdental **papilla**.

Cementum.   The function of the cementum in the periodontium is to provide anchorage for the tooth in the alveolar socket. This is accomplished by the covering of **Sharpey's fibers** that extend between the rough cementum surface and the alveolar wall.

ODONTOLOGY

Although teeth differ in size and shape, they have many attributes and characteristics in common. They are composed of the same four tissues arising from the same germ cells, and share many common features in form and structure. The study of teeth and their form is called **odontology** (oh-dahn-**TAHL**-oh-jee).

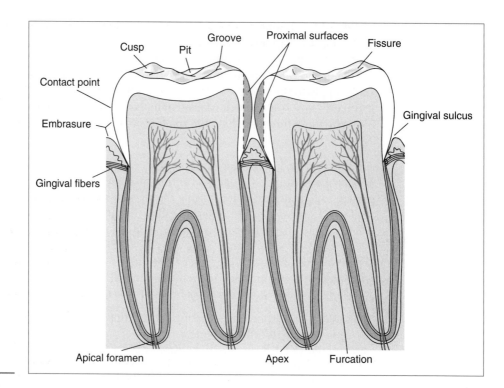

FIGURE 3-5
Examples of common tooth terms.

Characteristics

Teeth share the characteristics and terminology shown in Figure 3-5.

maxillary: upper tooth area.
mandibular: lower tooth area.
arch (*curved or bow-like outline*): half of the mouth, either maxillary or mandibular.
quadrant (**KWAH**-drant = *one fourth*): half of an arch, right or left, and containing eight teeth.
anterior (an-**TEE**-ree-or = *before or in front of*): front area of the mouth, from canine (cuspid) to canine (cuspid).
posterior (pos-**TEE**-ree-or = *toward the rear*): area back from the corners of the mouth, not including the canine (cuspid) or incisor teeth.

Types of Teeth

The four types of teeth are incisors, canines, premolars, and molars.

1. **Incisors** (in-**SIGH**-zors = *cutters*) are single-rooted anterior teeth with a sharp cutting edge. Maxillary incisors are larger than mandibular incisors. The central incisor gives character to the face and smile. The lateral incisors resemble the central ones but are smaller and the incisal edge turns more distally. The laterals may show irregularities such as a peg-shape and frequently are missing as a result of genetic

origin. The mandibular laterals are wider than their centrals, and the maxillary centrals are wider than their laterals.

2. The **canines** (**KAY**-nines = *eyetooth*) are single-rooted anterior teeth at the corners of the mouth, also called **cuspids** (**KUSS**-pids). The canine is the longest tooth in the mouth and divides the anterior from the posterior. The mandibular canine resembles the maxillary canine but is not as pointed and is thicker in the distal portion.

3. **Premolars** (pree-**MOE**-lar = *before a molar*) are the fourth and fifth teeth posterior from the center of the mouth. The maxillary teeth are sometimes called *bicuspids* because the cusps are large and well defined. The mandibular teeth are called premolars because they resemble a molar in form. Either name is correct. The maxillary first bicuspid exhibits two root canals even if the root's bifurcation is not apparent to the eye and it is normally smaller than its second bicuspid. The mandibular premolars are rounder and imitate the molar teeth to follow.

4. **Molars** (**MOE**-lars = *grinding teeth*) are the most posterior teeth, excluding the premolars. The maxillary molar teeth have three roots, termed **trifurcation** (**try**-fer-**KAY**-shun = *branching into three parts*). The mandibular molars have two roots, termed **bifurcation** (**bye**-fer-**KAY**-shun = *branching into two parts*). The maxillary first molar, the largest of the three, can exhibit an extra cusp on the meso-lingual cusp area that is called the **cusp of Carabelli**. The second molar resembles the first but is smaller. The mandibular second molar is smaller than the first molar but resembles it in shape. The maxillary and mandibular third molars are often mis-shaped or distorted because of their placement. These molars are termed "wisdom teeth" because their eruption dates are late, from 18 to 25 years of age (presumably when wisdom is supposed to come!)

Tooth Anatomy

The anatomy of the teeth involves a variety of parts:

crown: the top part of the tooth, containing the pulp chamber, dentin, and enamel covering. The crown is classified in one of two ways.

> **anatomical crown:** covered with enamel and may not be totally visible, but will be present the entire life of the tooth.
> **clinical crown:** surface visible in oral cavity; may not be totally visible for various reasons—impaction, hyperplasia, malposition, immaturity, and the like.

root: bottom part of tooth; may have single root, be bifurcated into two roots, or as in the maxillary molar teeth, trifurcated into three roots.

cervical line: the place where the enamel of the crown meets the cementum of the root; area is called the cementoenamel junction or **cervix** (**SIR**-vicks = *neck*) of the tooth.

apex (**AY**-pecks = *root end*): tip of a tooth; one apex is at each end of each root tip.

contact area: surface point or area where two teeth meet side by side (widest part of tooth); if no contact, the open area is referred to as a **diastema** (dye-ah-**STEE**-mah).

embrasure: V-shaped area between contact point of two teeth and gingival crest.

proximal surface: side wall of tooth that meets or touches side wall of another tooth.

axial surfaces: long-length surface of tooth.

line angle: meeting of three surfaces on a tooth, such as mesial, incisal, and labial.

midline: imaginary vertical line bisecting the head at the middle of the face; determines right and left sides.

antagonist (an-**TAG**-oh-nist = *opposing tooth*): tooth that counteracts, occludes, or contacts another tooth in the opposing arch.

TOOTH SURFACES

A tooth has six major surfaces, of which the apical surface end is actually only a tip. The following terms indicate the various surfaces of teeth.

facial (**FAY**-shal): surface of the tooth toward the cheek and lips; further defined as the buccal (cheek) or labial (lip) surface.

buccal (**BUCK**-al = *cheek*): posterior teeth surface toward the cheeks.

labial (**LAY**-bee-al = *lips*): anterior teeth surface toward the lips.

lingual (**LIN**-gwal = *tongue*): surface of teeth toward the tongue.

mesial (**ME**-zee-al = *to the middle*): side surface of tooth closest to midline (middle) of the face.

distal (**DIS**-tal = *to the distant, away*): side surface of the tooth farthest from the midline of the face.

chewing: surface that meets with the opposing teeth to complete the tooth's functions.

incisal (in-**SIGH**-zel = *to cut*): cutting edge of anterior teeth (centrals, laterals, and cuspids).

occlusal (oh-**KLOO**-zal = *to grind, meet*): grinding or chewing surface of premolars and molars (posterior area).

apical (**AY**-pih-kahl): relative to root-tip end of tooth (apex or root); **apical foramen** is a tiny opening in the apex or root that is used for the passage of nerves and vessels.

Tooth Landmarks

The teeth have some common landmarks, or anatomical markings. Because these are not present on all teeth, their placement assists us in identifying each tooth.

cingulum (**SIN**-gyou-lum): smooth, convex, or rounded bump on the lingual surface near the cervical line on anterior teeth; less noticeable on the mandibular anteriors than on the maxillary anteriors.

ridge: a linear elevation that receives its name from its location, such as *lingual ridge* and *marginal ridge*; ridges commonly found on teeth are:

> **marginal ridges:** rounded enamel elevations on occlusal surface of posteriors, linguals of anteriors, and mesial and distal surfaces of all teeth.

> **transverse ridge:** occurs on occlusal surface of posterior teeth at a point where two triangular ridges meet.

> **triangular ridge:** named after the cusps involved in the triangular ridge, from cusp tips to central groove on occlusal surface of posterior teeth.

> **oblique ridge:** a slanting ridge found on maxillary molars, and present more on the first molar than second molar.

fissure (**FISH**-er): a groove or natural depression, slit, or break; also may be an incomplete lobe union in enamel surface of a tooth.

fossa (**FAH**-sah): a shallow, rounded, irregular depression or concavity on lingual surface of anteriors and on occlusal surfaces of posterior teeth.

pit: pinpoint depression at junction of developed grooves or at the end of a groove.

sulcus (**SULL**-kus): long depression between ridges and cusps; valley on tooth surface.

groove: a rut, furrow, or channel; the two types of grooves are:

> **developmental:** grove between junction of crown or root parts; occurs during tooth development.

> **surface:** supplemental grooves occurring on occlusal surface of posterior teeth.

cusp: a point of the crown of a tooth, elevation, or mound on biting surface of crown; the **cusp of Carabelli** (kare-ah-**BELL**-ee) is an extra cusp on the lingual surface of the maxillary first molar, situated on the mesiolingual cusp, a distinguishing landmark of this tooth; this one also is called a **tubercle** (**TOO**-ber-kul), a small knob-like prominence.

lobe (**LOWB**): a well-defined part of an organ that develops into tooth formation; a developing cusp that eventually unites with other lobes to form a complete tooth.

furrow (**FER**-oh): a shallow, concave groove located on either the crown or the root; also called a "developmental depression."

eminence (**EM**-in-ence): a high place, projection, or prominence.

furcation (fur-**KAY**-shun = *fork or branch off*): the place where tooth roots branch apart.

mamelon (**MAM**-eh-lon): bumps forming a scallop border of the incisal edge of newly erupted anteriors; because of attrition, mamelons wear away shortly after eruption and become remnants of lobe forms.

REVIEW EXERCISES

MATCHING
Match the following word elements with their meanings:

1. _____cementum
2. _____odontology
3. _____exfoliate
4. _____heterodont

5. _____ameloblasts

6. _____fibroblasts
7. _____fusion

8. _____quadrant

9. _____molar

10. _____diastema
11. _____occlusal

12. _____lingual

13. _____succedaneous

14. _____deciduous

15. _____pulp

a. teeth of various shapes
b. pulp tissue cells
c. grinding tooth
d. chewing surface of posterior teeth
e. study of teeth and their form
f. permanent teeth
g. one fourth of oral cavity, one half of arch
h. surface of tooth touching tongue
i. tissue covering of root
j. primary teeth
k. soft, vascular tissue, center of tooth
l. joining together, union
m. open space between adjacent teeth, open contacts
n. enamel forming cell
o. scale off, shed

DEFINITIONS
Using the selection given for each sentence, choose the best term to complete the definition.

1. Which bicuspid/premolar exhibits two root canals even if the root bifurcation is not apparent to the eye?
   a. maxillary first bicuspid/premolar
   b. mandibular first premolar/bicuspid
   c. mandibular second premolar
   d. maxillary second bicuspid/premolar

2. The second stage of tooth development, in which the small tooth buds start to appear, is called:
   a. initiation   b. proliferation
   c. apposition   d. attrition

3. The building cell that forms the bulk tissue of the tooth is a/an:
   a. ameloblast   b. fibroclast
   c. odontoblast   d. cementoclast

4. A person exhibiting extremely large-sized teeth is said to have which condition?:
   a. microdontia   b. macrodontia
   c. anodontia   d. omnidontia

5. A small opening or cavity that may contain cememtocytes is called a/an:
   a. lacuna   b. forama
   c. lamella   d. tubule

6. Sharpey's fibers are _____
   a. connective tissues that make up and compose the pulp tissue.
   b. nerve fibers that register sensation.
   c. part of the periodontal ligament system.

7. Protection of the tooth and underlying tissues is the function of the:
   a. cementum   b. gingiva
   c. alveolar process   d. sulcus

8. Anchoring and support of the teeth is provided by the:
   a. periodontium   b. periodontosis
   c. cribriform plate   d. tubules

9. An overgrowth of cementum tissue on the root area is called:
   a. rootoexcession   b. hypercementosis
   c. hypocementosis   d. anacementa

10. Small channels or canals present in the cementum are called:
    a. vascular rows   b. cementovenus
    c. canaliculi   d. bands of Retzius

11. Dental papilla is derived from which developing tissue layer?
    a. mesoderm   b. estoderm

c. endoderm   d. bioderm

12. An overgrowth of cementum tissue is also known as:
    a. hypocementosis   b. hypercementosis
    c. primary cementum d. acellular cementum

13. The removal of the hard tooth surface and degeneration of the tooth is called____.
    a. germination   b. exfoliation
    c. resorption   d. calcification

14. The cusp of Carabelli may be found on which tooth?
    a. maxillary central incisor
    b. mandibular second molar
    c. mandibular lateral
    d. maxillary first molar

15. During tooth formation, the middle layer of tissue is called:
    a. mesoderm   b. ectoderm
    c. entoderm   d. bioderm

16. The surface of the tooth closest to the mid-line is called:
    a. distal   b. mesial
    c. occlusal   d. saggital

17. A groove, natural depression, or slit in the enamel of the tooth is called a:
    a. ridge   b. fissure
    c. mamelon   d. sulcus

18. A high place or projection of a tissue is called a/an:
    a. eminence   b. apex
    c. sulcus   d. occlusion

19. The single-rooted tooth found at the corner of the mouth is called a/an:
    a. bicuspid   b. incisor
    c. canine   d. lateral

20. Nasmyth's membrane is another word for the tooth:
    a. surface   b. periodontal tissues
    c. cuticle   d. enamel

BUILDING SKILLS

Locate and define the prefix, root/combining form, and suffix (if present) in the following words:

1. **hypercementosis**
   prefix   _____
   root/combining form   _____
   suffix   _____

2. **anodontia**
   prefix   _____
   root/combining form   _____
   suffix   _____

3. **microdontia**
   prefix   _____
   root/combining form   _____
   suffix   _____

4. **periodontitis**
   prefix   _____
   root/combining form   _____
   suffix   _____

5. **mucogingival**
   prefix   _____
   root/combining form   _____
   suffix   _____
   suffix   _____

FILL-INS

Write the correct word in the blank space to complete each statement.

1. Because the human dentition contains teeth of various sizes and shapes, the dentition is considered to be _____.

2. The fifth stage of tooth development is called _____.

3. The term for the condition of having more than the normal amount of teeth is _____.

4. A hard tooth-like mass that develops in a small cavity inside the tooth is called _____.

5. During the first stage of tooth development the _____ develops in the primitive oral cavity.

6. Another word for primary teeth is

   _____.

7. A tiny depression at the junction of a developed groove or at the end of the grooves is called a _____.

8. The reaction of overfluoridation to enamel is called _____.

9. Poor formation of teeth resulting in weak, gray, shell teeth is called:

   _____.

10. The main tissue of the tooth that surrounds the pulp is _____.

11. The small opening in the apex of the root that permits the passage of the nerve and vessels is called the _____.

12. Another word for pulp stones or small tooth growths is _____.

13. The lining of the alveolar socket is completed by the cribriform plate called the

   _____.

14. The site for the union of the mucous membrane and the gingival tissues is called the

   _____.

15. The presence of both deciduous and permanent teeth in the mouth is termed a/an _____dentition.

16. The _____molars will exhibit three roots.

17. A line angle is the union or junction of _____tooth surfaces.

18. The facial surface of the tooth that touches the lip is also called the _____ surface.

19. A convex, rounded bump on the lingual surface of anterior teeth is called a/an

   _____.

20. A tooth that comes in contact with or meets in occlusion with the opposing tooth is called a/an _____.

WORD USE

Read the following sentences and define the bold-faced word.

1. The oral surgeon will remove the **supernumerary** teeth before the placement of the orthodontic bands.

   _____

2. The presence of **mamelons** in the anterior region of a teenager can be an obvious symptom of malocclusion.

   _____

3. The endodontist has recommended root canal treatment for the **pulpitis** in the maxillary right central incisor.

   _____

4. Improper toothbrushing techniques can irritate and inflame the **gingival** tissue area.

   _____

5. The assistant prepared the anesthetic syringe to be used for the anesthesia of the left mandibular **quadrant**.

   _____

AUDIO LIST

This list contains selected new, important, or difficult terms from this chapter. You may use the list to review these terms and to practice pronouncing them correctly. When you work with the audio for this chapter, listen to the word, repeat it, and then place a checkmark in the box. Proceed to the next boxed word and repeat the process.

- ❏ acellular (ay-**SELL**-you-lar)
- ❏ alveolar (al-**VEE**-oh-lar)
- ❏ ameloblast (ah-**MEAL**-oh-blast)
- ❏ anodontia (an-oh-**DON**-she-ah)
- ❏ antagonist (an-**TAG**-oh-nist)
- ❏ apical (**AY**-pih-kahl)
- ❏ apposition (ap-oh-**ZIH**-shun)
- ❏ attrition (ah-**TRISH**-un)
- ❏ bifurcation (**bye**-fer-**KAY**-shun)
- ❏ buccal (**BUCK**-al)
- ❏ calcification (kal-sih-fih-**KAY**-shun)
- ❏ canaliculi (kan-ah-**LICK**-you-lie)
- ❏ cementoblasts (see-**MEN**-toh-blasts)
- ❏ cementoclasts (see-**MEN**-toh-klasts)
- ❏ cementum (see-**MEN**-tum)
- ❏ cervix (**SIR**-vicks)
- ❏ cingulum (**SIN**-gyou-lum)
- ❏ cuticle (**KYOU**-tih-kul)
- ❏ deciduous (deh-**SID**-you-us)
- ❏ dens in dente (**DENZ** in **DEN**-tay)
- ❏ denticles (**DEN**-tih-kuls)
- ❏ dentin (**DEN**-tin)
- ❏ dentinogenesis imperfecta (den-tin-oh-**JEN**-eh-sis im-per-**FECK**-tuh)
- ❏ dentition (den-**TISH**-un)
- ❏ diastema (dye-ah-**STEE**-mah)
- ❏ differentiation (dif-er-en-she-**AY**-shun)
- ❏ distal (**DIS**-tal)
- ❏ ectoderm (**ECK**-toh-derm)
- ❏ eminence (**EM**-in-ence)
- ❏ enamel (eh-**NAM**-el)
- ❏ epithelium (ep-ith-**EE**-lee-um)
- ❏ eruption (ee-**RUP**-shun)
- ❏ exfoliate (ecks-**FOH**-lee-ate)
- ❏ fibroblasts (**FIE**-broh-blasts)
- ❏ fissure (**FISH**-er)
- ❏ fluorosis (floor-**OH**-sis)
- ❏ fossa (**FAH**-sah)
- ❏ furcation (fur-**KAY**-shun)
- ❏ furrow (**FER**-oh)
- ❏ germination (jerm-ih-**NAY**-shun)
- ❏ gingiva (**JIN**-jih-vah)
- ❏ gomphosis (gahm-**FOH**-sis)
- ❏ granuloma (gran-you-**LOH**-mah)
- ❏ heterodont (**HET**-er-oh-dahnt)
- ❏ histodifferentiation (his-toh-dif-er-en-she-**AY**-shun)
- ❏ hypercementosis (high-per-see-men-**TOH**-sis)
- ❏ hypocalcification (high-poh-kal-sih-fih-**KAY**-shun)
- ❏ hypoplasia (high-poh-**PLAY**-zee-ah)
- ❏ incisal (in-**SIGH**-zel)
- ❏ keratinized (**KARE**-ah-tin-ized)
- ❏ labial (**LAY**-bee-al)
- ❏ lacuna (lah-**KYOU**-nah)
- ❏ lamellae (lah-**MEL**-ah)
- ❏ lamina dura (**LAM**-ih-nah **DUR**-ah)
- ❏ lingual (**LIN**-gwal)
- ❏ lobe (**LOWB**)
- ❏ macrodontia (mack-roh-**DAHN**-she-ah)
- ❏ mamelon (**MAM**-eh-lon)
- ❏ mesenchyme (**MEZ**-en-kime)
- ❏ mesial (**ME**-zee-al)
- ❏ mesoderm (**MESS**-oh-derm)
- ❏ microdontia (my-kroh-**DAHN**-she-ah)
- ❏ morphodifferentiation (more-foh-diff-er-en-she-**AY**-shun)
- ❏ mucogingival (myou-koh-**JIN**-jih-vahl)
- ❏ occlusal (oh-**KLOO**-zahl)
- ❏ odontoblasts (oh-**DAHN**-toh-blasts)
- ❏ odontoclasts (oh-**DAHN**-toh-klasts)
- ❏ odontogenesis (oh-**dahn**-toh-**JEN**-eh-sis)
- ❏ odontology (oh-dahn-**TAHL**-oh-jee)
- ❏ osteoblasts (**AHS**-tee-oh-blasts)
- ❏ osteoclasts (**AHS**-tee-oh-klasts)
- ❏ papilla (pah-**PILL**-ah)
- ❏ periodontal (pear-ee-oh-**DAHN**-tahl)
- ❏ periodontium (**pear**-ee-oh-**DANT**-ee-um)
- ❏ proliferation (pro-**lif**-er-**AY**-shun)
- ❏ pulpitis (pul-**PIE**-tis)
- ❏ quadrant (**KWAH**-drant)
- ❏ resorption (ree-**SORP**-shun)
- ❏ succedaneous (**suck**-seh-**DAY**-nee-us)
- ❏ sulcus (**SULL**-kus)
- ❏ supernumerary (sue-per-**NEW**-mer-air-ee)
- ❏ tertiary (**TERR**-shee-air-ee)
- ❏ trifurcation (try-fer-**KAY**-shun)
- ❏ tubercle (**TOO**-ber-kul)
- ❏ tubule (**TOO**-bule)

CHAPTER 4

Practice and Facility Setups

OBJECTIVES   Upon completion of this chapter, the reader should be able to identify and understand terms related to:

1. **Dental professionals.** Name and discuss the various roles of the professionals who render dental care.

2. **Places of employment.** Describe the various places and organizational structures in the field of dentistry where qualified and interested parties work.

3. **Dental hand instruments.** List and explain the use of the major hand instruments used in dental procedures.

4. **Rotary dental instruments.** List and explain the use of the major rotary instruments used in dental procedures.

5. **Dental facility operative equipment.** Describe the common operative equipment used in the dental operatory and office environments.

DENTAL PROFESSIONALS

Each profession speaks a language of its own, using terms or words connected with its common procedures, personnel, techniques, and instrumentation. People who are involved with, use the language, and participate in each of these occupations are said to be professionals of that occupation. Others who are not related to or familiar with this profession are called *lay people*. Each of the many types of personnel associated with the dental profession performs a special function or meets a particular need. Some are directly involved with the practice, and others provide support.

Dentist

The dentist, who is a Doctor of Dental Surgery (DDS) or a Doctor of Medical Dentistry (DMD), diagnoses, performs, and monitors the dental care of patients. Various specialists perform the following specific duties or skills within the dental profession.

prosthodontist (**prahs**-thoh-**DAHN**-tist): replaces missing teeth with artificial appliances such as a full mouth denture or partial bridgework.

periodontist (pear-ee-oh-**DAHN**-tist): treats diseases of periodontal (gingiva and supporting) tissues.

orthodontist (**or**-thoh-**DON**-tist): corrects malocclusion and improper jaw alignment.

pediatric (pee-dee-**AT**-rick) dentist: performs dental procedures for children; also called pedodontist (**PEE**-doh-**don**-tist).

endodontist (en-doh-**DAHN**-tist): treats the diseased pulp and periradicular structures.

oral and maxillofacial (**mack**-sill-oh-**FAY**-shul) surgeon: performs surgical treatment of the teeth, jaws, and related areas.

public health dentist: works on causes and prevention of common dental diseases and promotes dental health to the community or general population.

oral pathologist: studies the nature, diagnosis, and control of oral diseases.

oral and maxillofacial radiologist: is concerned with the production and interpretation of radiant energy images or data regarding the oral and maxillofacial regions.

forensic (for-**EN**-sick) dentist: discovers and uses pathological evidence for legal proceedings; forensic dentistry is not yet established as a recognized specialty but is organized and related to a particular type of dental care.

The official organization of dentists and dental specialists, the **American Dental Association (ADA)**, has branches on the state (constituent) and local (component) levels. As illustrated in Figure 4-1, the official seal of the ADA is a triangle containing the Greek letter D (triangle) for dentistry and a serpent on the staff indicating a healing art. The branch on one side contains twenty leaves for the deciduous teeth, and

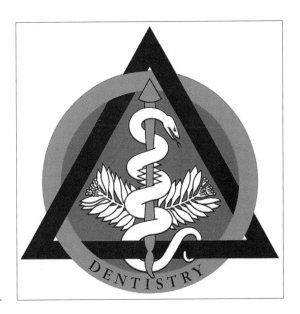

FIGURE 4-1
Logo for American Dental Association. (Courtesy of American Dental Association)

the branch with thirty-two leaves on the other side represents the permanent teeth. All symbols are encircled with the ring of health.

Registered Dental Hygienist

The **registered dental hygienist (RDH)** completes postsecondary education in dental hygiene instruction. An RDH is board-tested in theory and proficiency and state registered. The hygienist is concerned with the prevention of dental disease, specializing in the cleaning, polishing, and radiographing of teeth, periodontal treatment, and patient education. The hygienist may also perform some operative or supportive procedures if educated, tested, and certified as a state approved **expanded function dental auxiliary (EFDA)**.

In addition to these practice areas, a dental hygienist who completes the advanced ADHA educational curriculum that prepares the hygienist to provide diagnostic, preventive, restorative, and therapeutic services directly to the public may earn **ADHP (advanced dental hygiene practitioner)** certification. The official organization of hygienists is the **American Dental Hygienist's Association (ADHA)**, with branches at the state (constituent) and local (component) level.

Dental Assistant

The **dental assistant** aids the dentist in diagnosis, treatment, and dental care. The dental assistant may be an **RDA** (state-registered dental assistant) or a **CDA** (nationally certified dental assistant), or a state-registered dental assistant with expanded functions **(RDAEF)**. Each state regulates the permissible duties, functions, training, and designated titles for expanded duty personnel. Specialized certifications are offered by the **Dental Assisting National Board (DANB)**. These certifications include:

CDA = Certified Dental Assistant
RHS = Radiation Health and Safety
COA = Certified Orthodontic Assistant
CDPMA = Certified Dental Practice Management Assistant

The official dental assistant organization is the **American Dental Assistants Association (ADAA)**, with constituent, component, and local-level branches.

Dental Laboratory Technician

The **dental laboratory technician** performs dental lab procedures under written orders from a licensed dentist. The technician may receive OJT (on the job training) or education in a laboratory or school setting. The technician may be a **certified dental technician (CDT)**. The official organization of these professionals is the **National Association of Dental Laboratories (NADL)**, which also has state and local branches.

Denturist

The denturist (**DEN**-ture-ist) independently specializes in the construction of dentures and may practice only in those states that recognize, license, and permit this profession.

Other Dental Professionals

Other related dental professionals include dental supply/detail persons, dental equipment technicians, and dental manufacturers and suppliers. Some dental professionals dedicate their careers to research, education, and the development of oral medicine.

PLACES OF EMPLOYMENT

Qualified and interested parties work in various places and organizational structures in the field of dentistry.

solo: dental practice owned and operated by a single dentist or a practice that is owned by a dentist who contracts with another dentist (an associate) to work in the establishment with the owner.

partnership: dental practice owned and operated equally by two or more dentists.

group: dental practice employing a multitude of dentists; may be incorporated and owned by the working dentists or owned and operated by an outside corporation or dental health plan.

clinics and hospitals: a clinic setting or hospital care center that offers dentistry services. Many hospitals grant privileges to dentists to bring difficult or compromised patients for dental care using hospital services; oral surgeons may be staff members and work in the hospital and in their private offices.

specialty practice: various specialists working in private offices or facilities concerned with their training. Public health specialists may work in out-patient clinics, field establishments, schools, and offices. Forensic specialists may work in labs, the field, and courts.

miscellaneous practice sites: includes research, insurance companies, education, publication, specialty houses, charity clinics, and other areas.

DENTAL HAND INSTRUMENTS

Each profession employs its own type and kind of instrumentation. Just as a baseball team requires balls, bats, masks, gloves, and bases, dentistry requires specialized equipment for operation. Some tools are in common use in all aspects of dentistry, and others are constructed for various specialized procedures. Following are the standard instruments, grouped by their related family of use.

Hand Grasp Instruments

Hand instruments may have one working end (single-ended) or a working end at each of the opposite sides (double-ended). Working ends on the same instrument may vary in size, function, or location of operative sites. Many instruments are named for an inventor or school where they were designed. Instruments are grouped into families according to function and are constructed of various materials from stainless steel to hard resin. All instruments have the three components shown in Figure 4-2.

shaft or handle: used to grasp the instrument; supplied in various weights, diameters, and surfaces that may be smooth or serrated.

shank: connects the handle to the working end; sometimes called the *instrument neck*.

working end: also called *blade* or *nib*; rounded end is the *toe*, pointed end is the *tip*.

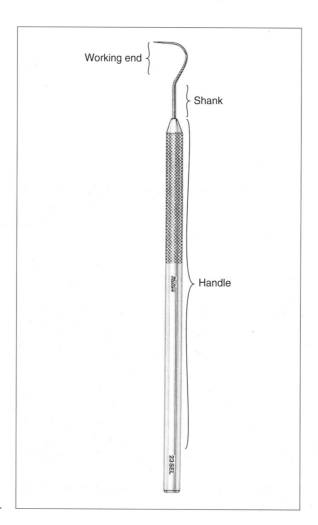

FIGURE 4-2
Parts of hand instruments. (Courtesy of Miltex Instrument Company, Inc. Lake Success, NY)

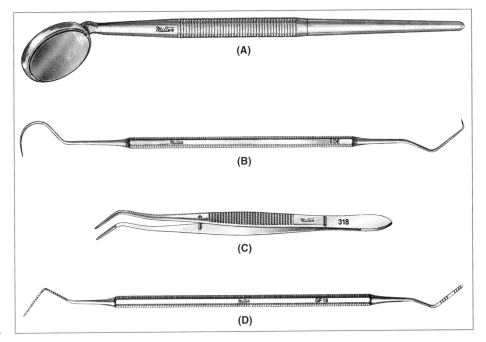

FIGURE 4-3
Basic dental setup.
(A) Mouth Mirror
(B) Explorer
(C) Cotton or
College Pliers
(D) Periodontal
Probe (in many
facilities). (Courtesy
of Miltex Instrument
Company, Inc.,
Lake Success, NY)

Basic Dental Setup

The basic dental setup is an instrument collection composed of a mouth mirror, explorer, periodontal probe, cotton forceps or pick-up, and a piece of 2×2 gauze. This setup, or **armamentarium** (ar-mah-men-**TARE**-ee-um), is used for most procedures. Illustrations of these instruments are shown in Figure 4-3.

mouth mirror: used for reflection, retraction, and visual observation; supplied in various sizes and may have plain faces or faces that magnify the view; some are solid, one piece; others have cone screw-in handles.

explorer: a sharp, flexible, pointed instrument used to detect caries and calculus, to explore restorations, surfaces and furcations, to make location marks, and to pick up cotton points or materials; supplied as single- or double-ended with an explorer edge on one side and another type of edge on the opposite side.

cotton forceps: tweezer-like pinchers used to transport materials to or from the mouth; also called *dressing pliers*; available with or without a serrated tip.

periodontal probe: a longer pointed instrument with measured marks on the tip; used to assess depth of tissue pockets; available with a round or flat blade and may be color-coded to help determine measurements.

expro (EX-pro): double-ended instrument with a diagnosing probe tip at one end and an explorer tip at the other end.

pen-probe: a double-ended instrument with a probe-marking tip on one end and a pen on the opposite end.

Periodontal Grouping

The periodontal group is a family of instruments used to treat and care for the gingival and periodontal tissues. They will be discussed more in Chapter 16, Periodontology.

scaler: thin-bladed hand instrument with pointed tip and two cutting edges; used to scale (scrape off) hard deposits from teeth.

sickle scaler: sharp blade in the shape of a sickle; used to remove calculus from tooth surfaces.

curette (kyou-**RETT**): round-tipped thin blade with a longer neck and two cutting edges; used to remove subgingival deposits, and termed *universal curette*. (Other curettes have one cutting edge and are designed for specific use, see Chapter 16, Periodontics.)

implant scaler/curette: non-metalic, resin-tipped instrument, designed to remove deposits around titanium implant abutments.

periodontal knife: hand instrument with flat-bladed incision tip of various shapes and angles; used to remove or recontour soft tissue.

scalpel (**SKAL**-pell): handle for attachment of blades of assorted sizes and shapes; used to incise (cut into) or remove tissue; also used in specialized dental procedures.

Restorative Grouping

The restorative grouping is an assortment of hand instruments used to remove decay, make preparations, and restore tooth surfaces. Figures 4-4 and 4-5 illustrate the instruments and parts below.

excavator (**ECKS**-kah-vay-tore): hand instrument with long-necked, cup-like, sharp-edged blades; used to remove soft, decayed tissue from preparations; also may be called *spoon excavator* (Figure 4-4A).

FIGURE 4-4
Restorative instruments for cutting and prepping. (Courtesy of Miltex Instrument Company, Inc., Lake Success, NY)
(A) Excavators
    Blade Excavator
    Spoon Excavator
(B) Gingival Margin Trimmers
(C) Hoe
(D) Enamel Hatchets
(E) Chisels
(F) Cleoid-Discoid Carver
(A = Courtesy of Miltex Instrument Company, Inc., Lake Success, NY; B – F = Courtesy of Hu-Friedy Mfg Co., Inc.)

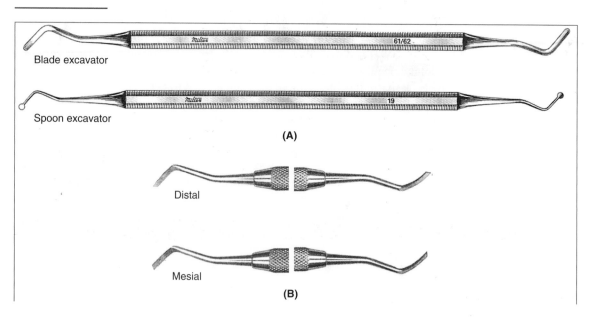

Blade excavator

Spoon excavator

(A)

Distal

Mesial

(B)

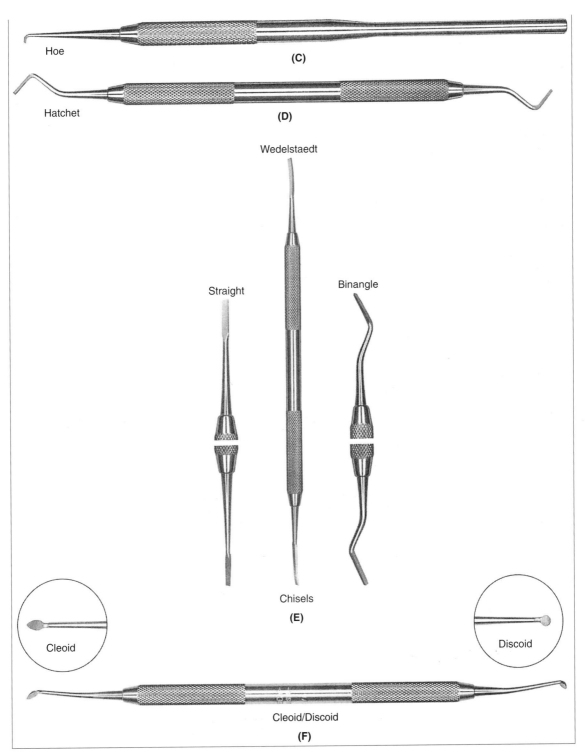

Hoe

(C)

Hatchet

(D)

Wedelstaedt

Straight

Binangle

Chisels

(E)

Cleoid

Discoid

Cleoid/Discoid

(F)

FIGURE 4-4 (continued)

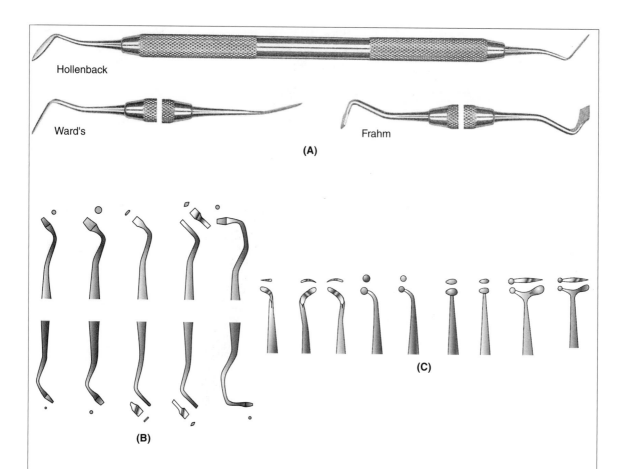

Hollenback

Ward's

Frahm

(A)

(B)

(C)

FIGURE 4-5
Restorative
instruments for
filling and refining.
(A) Carvers
(B) Condensers
(C) Burnishers
(D) Plastic and
Composite
Instruments
(E) Amalgam
Carriers (A–C =
Courtesy of Hu-
Friedy Mfg. Co.,
Inc., E = Courtesy of
Miltex Instrument
Company, Inc., Lake
Success, NY)

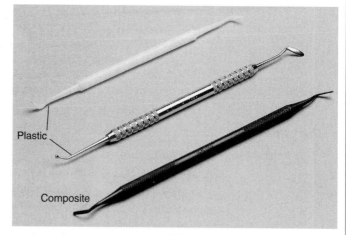

Plastic

Composite

(D)

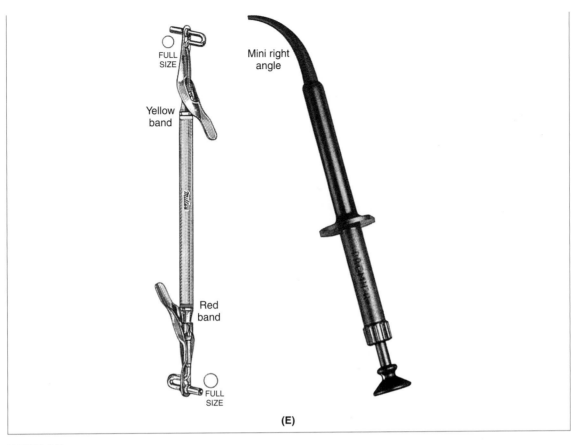

(E)

FIGURE 4-5
(continued)

gingival margin trimmer: hand instrument with long, slender, curved, flat blade; used to break away enamel margins during tooth preparations (Figure 4-4B).

hoe: smaller bladed instrument with a tip resembling a farm hoe; used to break or pull away enamel tissue during preparations (Figure 4-4C).

hatchet: hand instrument with a sharp-edged, hatchet-like tip; used to remove hard tissue (Figure 4-4D).

chisel: hand instrument with cutting edge that is used to cut away enamel tissue. Chisels have straight shafts, or a curved shaft, such as the Wedelstaedt chisel, as in Figure 4-4E, or may have an extra angled shaft, such as the biangle chisels in Figure 4-4E.

cleoid (**KLEE**-oyd)/ discoid (**DISK**-oyd) carver: double-ended, long-necked carving instrument with a pointed tip on one end (cleoid) and a disc-shaped blade on the other end (discoid); used to carve anatomy features in newly placed restorations, or can be used to remove decay and tooth tissue during cavity preparations (Figure 4-5A).

carver: thin-bladed hand instrument used to remove decay or carve newly placed restorative material; blade faces come in various shapes; a popular type is the Hollenback (Figure 4-5A).

plastic filling instrument (PFI): hand instrument with a flat blade; used to carry, transfer, and pack materials, or to carve restorative material (Figure 4-5D).

condenser: hand instrument with a thick, rounded or oval shaped, flat head that is sometimes serrated. It is used to pack or condense restorative material into the cavity preparation (Figure 4-5B).

burnisher: hand instrument with a smooth, rounded head that comes in various shapes; used to smooth out restorative material or other metal surfaces, such as a matrix strip.

beaver-tail burnisher: a burnisher with a beaver tail-shaped blade extending from the round nib or tip; used to smooth and carve restorative material while in the plastic, pliable shape, and to apply medication such as Dycal to a cavity preparation (Figure 4-5C).

amalgam carrier: hand instrument with holding cylinder for the transfer of amalgam material while in a plastic form; has a spring lever pusher to expel the material into the preparation. The instrument is supplied in assorted sizes with various cylinder materials on the end tips. Another type of amalgam carrier is the amalgam gun with a thumb spring push to expel the material (see Figure 4-5E). Both amalgam carriers may be loaded by pressing into the plastic load of restorative material in the amalgam well.

matrix (MAY-tricks) holder, matrix strip and **wedge:** holder device used to maintain artificial wall (matrix strip) around the tooth preparation. A wooden or resin triangular wedge is used to hold the strip in place and prevent the material from leaking.

file: hand instrument with a flat blade with serrated edging; used to smooth off and contour restorations or hard surfaces.

Evacuation

Evacuation of the mouth is accomplished by using tips that are inserted into suction tubing. These tips are placed in mouth and used to remove moisture, debris, and other matter. The two types of evacuator tips commonly used in saliva evacuation are:

high-volume evacuator (HVE): curved, metal or resin, beveled tip with a large hole; inserted into a high-evacuation tube system handle with off/on and intensity controls; used for gross removal of fluids and debris from the mouth.

saliva ejector tip: smaller suction tip that is inserted into the evacuation tubing from the dental unit; used for steady, constant fluid removal from the oral cavity.

Insertion of gauze pads or commercial absorbent pads near the saliva duct in the cheek can help to maintain fluid control. Some units have a **cuspidor (KUSS-pih**-dore = *basin*) nearby for patients to empty their mouth.

Assorted Instruments

Other instruments, such as scissors, spatulas, knives, and pliers, are used interchangeably in any family or instrument group. Each dental procedure calls for specific variations of the basic instruments mentioned previously, such as suture scissors, dressing pliers, gold knife, cement spatula, and so on.

Instruments may be color-coded by placing a colored band on the shaft to indicate the type of instrument, the operatory room of use, the type of setup, or any other way of grouping. These may be sterilized in colored trays arranged in a pre-setup to match this coding.

▌ROTARY DENTAL INSTRUMENTS

Rotary instruments are power-driven tools that operate in a circular motion at various speeds. The rate of speed, or rpm (rotations per minute) determines the classification of the instrument. The handpiece is a power device that holds and operates the inserted instrument. Depending upon its rpm, it is classified as slow speed, high speed, or ultra-high speed, Rotation is achieved by either a belt-driven, electric turbine or a compressed air system. Some handpieces also contain a fiberoptic light system to assist with observation in the oral cavity, and water spray to cool the operative field.

Individual handpieces that adapt to the power rotors are available in various shapes (see Figure 4-6).

straight handpiece (SHP): straight handpiece with no head; instruments are inserted directly into opening and held in place by engaging the manual or automatic tightening device in the unit's handpiece.

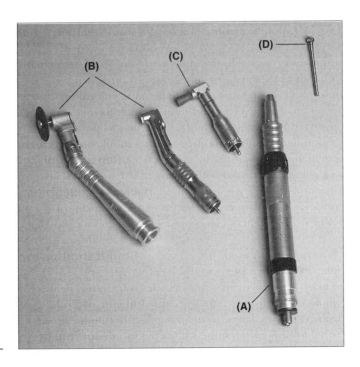

FIGURE 4-6
Low-speed handpiece with attachments.
(A) Handpiece
(B) Contra-Angle with and without Disk
(C) Right-Angle or Prophy Angle, with Rubber Cup
(D) Round Bur with Long Shank

contra-angle handpiece (CAHP): handpiece with an obtuse angled head (more than 90 degrees); is inserted into the power unit's straight handpiece and is used to gain access to posterior teeth and difficult areas.

right-angle handpiece (RAHP): handpiece with its head set at a 90-degree angle; is inserted and connects into the power unit's handpiece; employed in general use throughout the oral cavity.

prophy (PRO-fee) angle handpiece (PHP): small prophylaxis handpiece rotary angle with a 90-degree angle head; has a limited opening in the working end for polishing cups or brush placement. The PHP is inserted into slow-speed handpieces and is used to polish teeth. Many PHPs are disposable, and some may be battery-powered with swivel heads and optical light sources.

fiber optic handpiece: specific slow- or high-speed handpiece that supplies a light source to the operative site for improved vision.

rheostat (REE-oh-stat): a food petal or lever that is used to regulate the speed of the handpiece.

Although not considered standard operative power handpieces used in restorative and tissue-removing procedures, other dental instruments that are hand-held and attached to specialized dental units are termed handpieces. These instruments include:

air abrasion: air-powered handpiece delivering abrasive aluminum oxide powder or sodium bicarbonate under force to clean or prepare tooth surfaces or remove some carious tissue.

ultrasonic handpiece: high-speed vibration scaling tips used for scaling and curettage purposes, sometimes called *ultrasonic scaler*.

curing light handpiece: hand-held device that focuses a light beam to cure or "set" specified materials.

intraoral camera: handpiece with a small camera situated in the head; used to transmit various views of the oral setting.

electrosurgery handpiece: combination of assorted metal tips that fit into a probe handle; these tips pass electrical currents that incise and coagulate the blood in a surgical procedure.

laser handpiece: photon handpiece that emits a precise light-energy wavelength that is concentrated to perform specialized tasks; various wavelengths are utilized for a specific target or procedure, such as tooth whitening, caries removal, or surgical gingivectomy.

caries detection scanner: a non-invasive laser scan that detects early decay in occlusal areas.

implant drilling unit: lighted, digitally control drilling handpiece with sterile irrigation; used to smooth alveolar bone, drill operative sites, and install implants.

All dental handpieces are expensive items. They must be maintained, sterilized, and cared for in the manner specified by the manufacturer of the instrument.

Handpieces are used to hold the burs, mandrels, mounted stones, and discs that are used in restorations and chairside dental procedures. The dental bur is the most

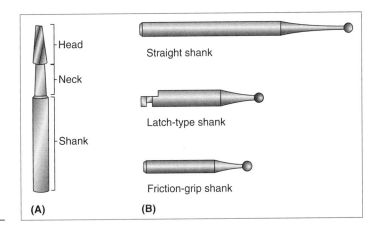

FIGURE 4-7
Parts of a bur.
(Courtesy of Miltex
Instrument
Company, Inc.,
Lake Success, NY)
(A) Parts of a bur
(B) Different bur
shanks

commonly used rotary item and is employed in cavity preparation and restorations. A bur has three parts (see Figure 4-7).

shank: the end of the bur that is inserted into the handpiece. The type of end is determined by the requirements of the power handpiece. The assortment of burs includes the friction grip (FG), right angle (RA), or handpiece (HP) that is placed directly into a straight handpiece. The length of the shank—long, short, or pedodontic—varies according to the type of bur or area involved.

neck: connecting area between the shank and the working end or head of the bur.

working end or head: end that cuts tissue or works on the tooth or material involved.

Each shape is designed for a specific purpose or position.

Bur Types

Rotary burs may be typed according to style or handpiece placement. Burs are supplied in graduated sizes and are numbered according to the shape of the head. Burs that have extra teeth in a crosscut pattern are called **dentated** (**DEN**-tay-ted = *dented, depressed*), and shortened burs are called **truncated** (**TRUN**-kay-ted = *cut part off, lop off*). Three types of burs are:

friction-grip bur: smooth-ended bur, held in the handpiece by the friction grip chuck.

latch-type bur: has grooved insertion bur end that hooks into the head of an RA handpiece.

straight handpiece: has a smooth, extended shaft that fits directly into the straight handpiece; available in mini, regular, or surgical lengths.

Bur Numbers

Bur numbers denote the shape of the rotary head. The desired cut of the tooth dictates which bur number is used in the procedure. The more popular shapes are the

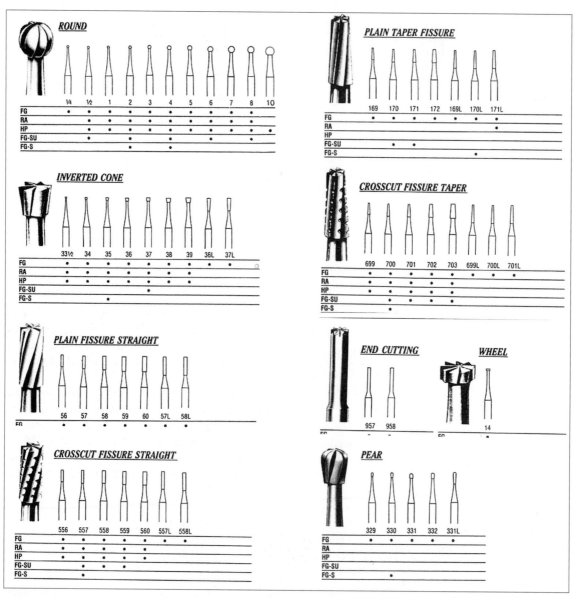

FIGURE 4-8
Bur shapes and number angles. (Courtesy of Miltex Instrument Company, Inc., Lake Success, NY)

round, inverted cone, and plain or tapered fissured burs. Each bur number is assigned a specific shape, but may be available in assorted ends to fit different handpieces. Specialized burs also include surgical burs with longer shafts, lab burs called vulcanite or acrylic, and finishing burs with a wide variety of cutting edges or blades in their working head. Figure 4-8 gives examples of burs.

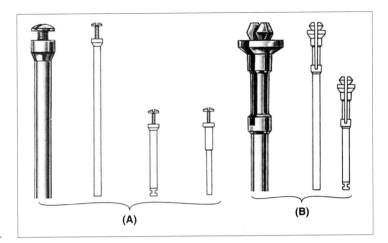

FIGURE 4-9
Mandrels with different heads and shanks. (Courtesy of Miltex Instrument Company, Inc., Lake Success, NY) (A) Screw-type Mandrels (B) Snap-on Mandrels

(A)   (B)

Miscellaneous Rotary Instruments

Several other instruments may be used in a rotary handpiece. These include:

mandrel (**MAN**-drell): a slim, metal holding device that fits into slow handpieces and is used to smooth and cut. They may have RA or HP end fittings and come in various lengths. Mandrels hold abrasive and rubber discs by a screw-on or snap-on method (see Figure 4-9). The Joe Dandy, a thick, carborundum disc, is a popular one.

stone, wheel, and discs: abrasive or chemically treated discs, wheels, cups, and points with various shapes that can be mounted permanently or glued on a shaft or placed on mandrels. They are supplied in assorted sizes and grit (abrasiveness) and are used for smoothing at chairside or in the lab (see Figure 4-10).

diamond rotary instruments: commonly called *burs* or *points*; used to cut, smooth, and reduce tissues; they follow the same numbering pattern and color coding as steel burs.

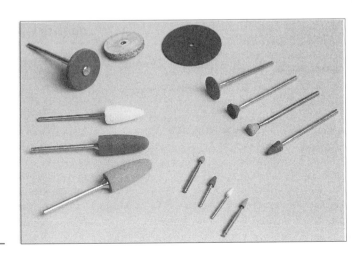

FIGURE 4-10
Various types of grits of stones, wheels, and points.

bur block: a tray device used to hold the small rotary instruments during use at the chair and while being sterilized; may be metallic or resin and have or not have a cover.

DENTAL FACILITY OPERATIVE EQUIPMENT

Each dental facility or clinic contains specialized dental equipment that is used to perform necessary treatments. Among the many items available, some for general dentistry and some for speciality use, all facilities need the basic items shown in Figure 4-11.

operatory (**AH**-purr-ah-tore-ee): small treatment room equipped with dental appliances. Some practices, such as orthodontic, and some clinics, have a large operatory area containing several chairs and necessary equipment separated with half-walls or room dividers.

dental chair: chair appliance, usually electrically powered, that raises, lowers, and tilts to provide easy access and proper vision; may be a lounge or upright chair style. Most chairs are operated by remote foot controls to eliminate hand use and contamination.

operatory light: viewing light for patient care; may be wall-mounted, on a floor stand, lowered from the ceiling, or attached to the chair unit. The light may be dimmed or the beam calibrated for specific vision needs. Some lights are activated by motion sensor devices, eliminating touching and contamination.

stools: movable seats for the dental personnel. Stools have height adjustment and back rests. Some stools have torso rests extending in front for forward-leaning support.

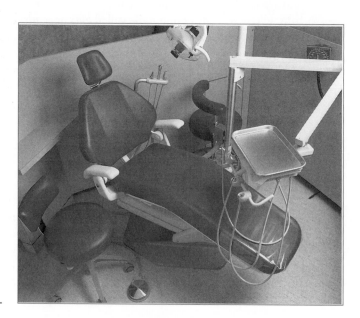

FIGURE 4-11
Basic dental unit.

dental unit: upright, stationary, or movable, table-style working appliance that provides handpiece power, aspiration, water, and air. Some units also provide electrosurgical power, a natural gas outlet, fiberoptic power, and custom appliances such as intraoral cameras, laser handpieces, perio-pocket depth sensors, air abrasion units, curing lights, air abrasion, pulp-depth indicators, and crown-shape fabricators.

cabinets: mobile, floor, or wall-mounted storage cabinets with drawer space for supplies and equipment.

radiographic units: various configurations; a dental practice may have a radiographic control unit in a central area with the x-ray head or power source in each operatory area; other facilities have head and control units in the operatory room or use a separate radiographic area; some have filmless, digitalized radiographic units using sensors and computer-assisted viewing and imaging.

diagnostic or auxiliary units: include perio-pocket detectors, newly developed electronic diagnostic devices used to assist with a patient survey; endodontic units that detect the depth of instrument probing to avoid accidental penetration of the apex. Laser dental surgery, electronic target anesthesia, computer interaction, ultrasonic cleaning methods, and other new units to aid the dental profession are being introduced each day.

REVIEW EXERCISES

MATCHING
Match the following word elements with their meanings:

1. _____orthodontist
2. _____PFI
3. _____shank
4. _____CDT
5. _____endodontist
6. _____DDS
7. _____hoe
8. _____FG
9. _____HVE
10. _____rpm
11. _____DANB
12. _____periodontist
13. _____probe
14. _____Joe Dandy
15. _____excavator

a. popular, useful disc; fits on a mandrel
b. Dental Assisting National Board
c. fine-pointed instrument with measuring marks
d. rotations per minute; speed of handpiece
e. specialist who corrects malocclusion
f. high-volume evacuation system
g. hand instrument used to remove, dig out decay
h. hand instrument used to break away or pull off enamel
i. specialist who treats diseased gingival tissues
j. Doctor of Dental Surgery
k. Certified Dental Technician
l. high-speed or friction-grip bur
m. connects instrument handle to working end
n. specialist who treats internal pulp tissues
o. hand instrument used to carry materials to the preparation

DEFINITIONS

Using the selection given for each sentence, choose the best term to complete the definition.

1. People who are trained in a specific field and are considered knowledgeable in that area are _____.
   a. lay people
   b. professionals
   c. expertizers
   d. apprentices

2. Which of the following are group members of the basic instrument setup? _____
   a. mirror, explorer, cotton pliers, probe
   b. mirror, excavator, matrix, probe
   c. periodontal probe, chart, mirror, hoe
   d. explorer, mirror, handpiece, matrix

3. Which part of an instrument is used to grasp or control the instrument? _____
   a. working end
   b. blade
   c. handle
   d. nib

4. Which of the following specialists replaces missing teeth with artificial appliances? _____
   a. prosthodontist
   b. periodontist
   c. pedodontist
   d. endodontist

5. Which of the following specialists works on common dental diseases in the community? _____
   a. public health dentist
   b. forensic dentist
   c. pediatric dentist
   d. surgeon

6. Which of the following may be certified as an ADHP? _____
   a. RDH
   b. CDA
   c. Certified Dental Technician
   d. RDA

7. A person who independently specializes in denture construction is a _____.
   a. dental detail person
   b. denturist
   c. dental practice consultant
   d. lab technican

8. A two-edged, rounded toe, cutting hand instrument used to remove subgingival calculus is a _____.
   a. scalpel
   b. universal curette
   c. gingival margin trimmer
   d. sickle scaler

9. A non-metallic, resin-tipped hand instrument used to clean / remove deposits around pegs and abutments is a/an _____.
   a. periodontal knife
   b. plastic filling instrument
   c. implant scaler /curette
   d. hatchet

10. A hand instrument used to smooth off and contour tooth tissue and materials is a ____.
    a. file
    b. scaler
    c. hatchet
    d. hoe

11. An intra-oral handpiece with the head set at a 90-degree angle is a _____.
    a. straight handpiece
    b. contra angle handpiece
    c. right-angle handpiece
    d. prophy angle

12. The end of the bur that is inserted into the handpiece is called the _____.
    a. shank
    b. neck
    c. head
    d. tip

13. Which of the following would not be inserted into the handpiece to become functional? _____
    a. mandrel
    b. matrix
    c. mounted stone
    d. bur

14. Which of the following may not be permanently bonded and placed in a mandrel? ____
    a. diamond bur
    b. abrasive wheel
    c. rubber disc
    d. steel bur

15. A hand instrument with a thick head, used to push or pack down material is a_____.
    a. condenser
    b. hatchet
    c. curette
    d. discloid-cleoid

16. A hand instrument used to smooth off or contour restorative material or metals is a _____.
    a. scaler
    b. condenser
    c. burnisher
    d. explorer

17. A retaining or holding device used to make an artificial wall in a restoration is a _____.
    a. retainer
    b. mandrel
    c. matrix
    d. dental dam

18. A hand instrument with a rounded ball end and a flat blade, used to smooth/carve is a_____.
    - a. carver
    - b. scalpel
    - c. beaver-tail burnisher
    - d. hatchet

19. The national organization for dental assistants is the _____.
    - a. ADHA
    - b. ADA
    - c. ADAA
    - d. AADA

20. A gingival margin trimmer is used to_____.
    - a. break away the enamel side of a tooth during preparation.
    - b. remove supra- and subgingival deposits from tooth margins.
    - c. maintain margin walls during the insertion and condensing of materials.

BUILDING SKILLS

Locate and define the prefix, root/combining form, and suffix (if present) in the following words:

1. **prosthodontist**
   prefix   _____
   root word/combining form   _____
   suffix   _____

2. **orthodontist**
   prefix   _____
   root word/combining form   _____
   suffix   _____

3. **endodontist**
   prefix   _____
   root word/combining form   _____
   suffix   _____

4. **periodontist**
   prefix   _____
   root word/combining form   _____
   suffix   _____

5. **pathologist**
   prefix   _____
   root word/combining form   _____
   suffix   _____

FILL-INS

Write the correct word in the blank space to complete each statement.

1. Persons who have not been trained or experienced in a particular trade or study are called _____.

2. Two initialed titles indicating that a person is trained as a dentist are: _____and _____.

3. When incision and immediate coagulation of the site is desired, the dentist will select the _____ handpiece.

4. A hand instrument that has a working head on each end is called a/an _____ instrument.

5. The three components of a hand instrument are _____, _____ _____ and _____.

6. A rounded blade end on a hand instrument is called a/an _____.

7. A pointed blade end on a hand instrument is called a/an_____.

8. The basic setup is composed of three instruments: _____, _____ and _____.

9. The purpose of the explorer instrument is to _____.

10. Three purposes for the use of a mouth mirror are _____, _____ and _____.

11. Cotton forceps or pickups are used to _____.

12. A hand instrument in the periodontal family with a blade in a semi-circle curve and used to remove supra gingival calculus is called a/n _____ scaler.

13. A hand instrument used to transfer amalgam while in a plastic stage is a/n _____.

14. Name at least two families of instruments: _____ and _____.

15. Three interworking items used to maintain artificial walls around a cavity prep are:

    _____,
    _____ and _____.

16. A CAHP handpiece has an obtused angle head. This handpiece is called a/an _____ handpiece.

17. Handpieces are made to hold _____,
    _____,
    and _____.

18. Three parts of a rotary instrument called a bur are:_____,
    _____, and _____.

19. Shortened burs are called _____.

20. Crosscut or extra teethed burs are called _____.

WORD USE

Read the following sentences and define the bold-faced word letters.

1. The dental assistant will use proper sterilization methods for all instruments, but give particular care to the expensive **handpiece**.

   _____

2. When faced with the gross removal of tooth structure, the dentist may choose a **dentated** type of rotary bur.

   _____

3. The chemical bleaching treatment of the pulp canal may be performed by the **endodontist**.

   _____

4. To include periodontal charting with the routine tooth-charting examination, many dental practices are placing the **periodontal probe** in the basic setup.

   _____

5. OSHA requirements for the handling and care of sharp items must be followed when dealing with the disposal of a **scalpel**.

   _____

AUDIO LIST

This list contains selected new, important, or difficult terms from this chapter. You may use the list to review these terms and to practice pronouncing them correctly. When you work with the audio for this chapter, listen to the word, repeat it, and then place a checkmark in the box. Proceed to the next boxed word and repeat the process.

- ❏ armamentarium (ar-mah-men-**TARE**-ee-um)
- ❏ cleoid (**KLEE**-oyd)
- ❏ curette (kyou-**RETT**)
- ❏ cuspidor (kuss-pih-**DORE**)
- ❏ denated (**DEN**-tay-ted)
- ❏ denturist (**DEN**-ture-ist)
- ❏ endodontist (en-doh-**DAHN**-tist)
- ❏ excavator (**ECKS**-kah-vay-tore)
- ❏ forensic (for-**EN**-sick)
- ❏ mandrel (**MAN**-drell)
- ❏ matrix (**MAY**-tricks)
- ❏ maxillofacial (**MACK**-sill-oh-fay-shul)
- ❏ operatory (**AH**-purr-ah-tore-ee)
- ❏ orthodontist (ore-thoh-**DON**-tist)
- ❏ pediatric (pee-dee-**AT**-rick)
- ❏ periodontist (pear-ee-oh-**DAHN**-tist)
- ❏ prosthodontist (prahs-thoh-**DAHN**-tist)
- ❏ rheostat (**REE**-oh-stat)
- ❏ scalpel (**SKAL**-pell)
- ❏ truncated (**TRUN**-kay-ted)

CHAPTER 5

Infection Control

OBJECTIVES   Upon completion of this chapter, the reader should be able to identify and understand terms related to:

1. **Disease conditions:** Discuss the meaning of disease with related signs and symptoms and the various classifications of disease conditions.
2. **Causes of disease and infection:** List and identify sources of disease and the pathogens that may be involved.
3. **Port of entry for disease:** Identify and explain the action of infectious agents and their method of causing disease.
4. **Immunity factors:** Explain immunity and the methods by which to acquire the various types of immunity.
5. **Disease prevention:** Discuss the importance of preventing disease, and list the common methods used to combat disease and infection.
6. **Agencies concerned with disease control:** List the principal agencies or government bodies concerned with the control of disease.

DISEASE CONDITIONS

Disease (*pathological condition of the body, abnormal condition*) manifests its presence through symptoms (**SIM**-tums = *perceptible change in the body or body function*), which may be objective or subjective. Objective symptoms, also called signs, are evidence observed by someone other than the patient—for example, edema (eh-**DEE**-mah = *swelling*). Subjective symptoms are evidence of a disease as reported by the patient— for example, odontalgia (oh-dahn-**TAHL**-jee-ah = *toothache*). An assortment of signs and symptoms grouped together that characterize a disease is called a syndrome (**SIN**-drome = *running together*).

The study of disease is called pathology (path-**AHL**-oh-jee). Pathologists search for disease etiology (ee-tee-**AHL**-oh-jee = *cause of the disease*). Symptoms and signs are used to form a **diagnosis** (**die**-agg-**NO**-sis = *denoting name of disease*), and a **prognosis** (prahg-**NO**-sis) is a prediction about the course of the disease.

Disease Terms

The condition of a disease or its intensity may be seen in various stages. Some terms used to describe the status of a current disease are:

acute (ah-**CUTE** = *sharp, severe*): describes immediate symptoms such as high fever and pain or distress.

chronic (**KRON**-ick = *not acute, drawn out*): describes a condition present over a long time, often without an endpoint, such as chronic fatigue and anemia.

remission (ree-**MISH**-un = *lessening or abating*): temporary or permanent cessation of a severe condition, such as sinusitis or some stage of cancer.

epidemic (**ep**-ih-**DEH**-mick = *among people or widespread*): a condition prevalent over a wide population, such as many cases of flu or typhoid in an area.

pandemic (pan-**DEM**-ick = *all people involved*): a disease that is more widespread than an epidemic, occurring over a large geographical area and populace, sometimes worldwide.

endemic (en-**DEM**-ick = *in people*): disease(s) occurring continuously in the same population or locality.

Classification of Diseases

Diseases may be classified further according to their actions. Some terms used to denote the origin or manifestations are:

exogenous (ecks-**AH**-jeh-nuss = *produced outside*): refers to causes outside the body, such as illnesses arising from trauma, radiation, hypothermia, and so on.

endogenous (en-**DAH**-jeh-nuss = *arising from within the cell or organism*): refers to causes arising from within the body, such as infections, tumors, and congenital and metabolic abnormalities.

congenital (kahn-**JEN**-ih-tuhl = *present from birth*): refers to conditions inherited from parents, such as cystic fibrosis.

degenerative (dee-**JEN**-er-ah-tiv = *breaking down*): refers to conditions resulting from natural aging of the body, such as arthritis.

opportunistic (ah-pore-too-**NISS**-tick = *taking advantage of*): refers to disease or infection occurring when body resistance is lowered, such as with fungal, bacterial, and viral infections.

nosocomial (**noh**-soh-**KOH**-mee-ahl = *disease in caregiving*): refers to diseases passed on from patient to patient in a health care setting, such as staphylococcal bacterial infections.

CAUSES OF DISEASE AND INFECTION

Diseases may be caused by a number of **pathogenic** (**path**-oh-**JEN**-ick = *disease-producing*) microorganisms, including bacteria, viruses, and other pathogens.

TABLE 5-1   Forms of Bacteria

OVAL/ROUNDED	ROD-SHAPED	SPIRAL
single form = *micrococci*	Called *bacilli.* If	rigid, spiral = *spirilla;*
paired form = *diplococci*	oval in shape = *coccobacilli*	
cluster form = *staphylococci*		flexible = *spirochetes;*
chain form = *streptococci*		
group of eight = *sarcinae*		curved rods = *vibrios*

Bacteria

Bacteria (back-**TEER**-ee-ah) (singular, **bacterium**) are one-celled, plant-like microorganisms lacking chlorophyll. These microorganisms have three principal forms: oval/rounded, rod-shaped, and spiral (see Table 5-1).

Other terms pertaining to specific characteristics of bacteria are:

aerobic (air-**OH**-bick): designates bacteria that require oxygen to live.
facultative aerobes: bacteria that can live in the presence of oxygen but do not require it.
obligate or **strict aerobes:** bacteria that cannot survive without oxygen, such as diphtheria.
anaerobic (an-ah-**ROH**-bick): bacteria that do not need oxygen for survival.
facultative anaerobes: bacteria that grow best without oxygen, but can survive in its presence; for example, bacterium fusiform (trench mouth).
obligate or **strict anaerobes:** bacteria that cannot live in the presence of oxygen.
flagella (flah-**JELL**-ah = *whips*): small, whip-like hairs that provide movement for some bacteria.

A **spore** is a thick walled reproductive cell. Some bacteria possess a capsule layer of slime, and a few rod-shaped bacteria develop an **endospore** for a resting stage when unfavorable conditions exist. This covering is difficult to destroy. Examples of bacteria that are capable of forming endospores include anthrax and tetanus.

Viruses.   Viruses (**VYE**-russes) are tiny parasitic organisms that cause diseases such as polio, hepatitis, smallpox, colds, HIV, herpes, and influenza, among many others. Viruses require living matter to reproduce and grow.

Other Pathogens.   Some other pathogens are listed below.

rickettsia (rih-**KET**-see-ah): microbes smaller than bacteria but larger than viruses, usually transmitted by **vectors** (**VEK**-tors = *carriers that transmit disease*), such as fleas, lice, and ticks. Rickettsia cause diseases such as Lyme and Rocky Mountain spotted fever.

fungi (**FUN**-guy = *a division of plants that include mold, yeasts, and slimes*) (singular, **fungus** = **FUNG**-us): Some fungi are beneficial, and others are pathogenic, the latter of which cause thrush, athlete's foot, and ringworm, for example. Fungi grow in two forms: **filamentous** (molds) and **unicellular** (yeasts).

protozoa (proh-toh-**ZOH**-ah = *small animal parasites or organisms*): must live upon another organism called the *host*. Protozoan organisms cause malaria, dysentery, and encephalitis, for example.

saprophytes (**SAP**-roh-fights): organisms living on decaying or dead organic matter, such as tetanus bacillus (lockjaw).

nematodes (**NEM**-ah-toads): small parasitic worms such as threadworms and roundworms.

commensal (koh-**MEN**-sahl = *living together*): microbes that live together on a host without harming it, such as mouth flora.

bloodborne pathogens: disease-producing microbes that are present in human blood.

PORT OF ENTRY FOR DISEASE

Disease or infection is contracted through various methods and ports of entry, as follows.

droplet infection: airborne infection in which pathogens discharged from the mouth or nose by coughing or sneezing are carried through the air and settle on objects.

indirect infection: infection resulting from improper handling of materials, contamination of articles or **fomes** (**FOH**-mez = *inanimate substances that absorb and transmit infection, such as doorknobs and bedding*). Poor sterilization methods permit passage of microbes from one person to another.

contact infection: infection that is passed directly through intimate relationships—contact with saliva, blood, or mucous membranes.

parenteral (pare-**EN**-ter-ahl = *injection*) entry: refers to piercing of the skin or mucous membrane; also called needle-stick.

carrier infection: exchange of disease by direct or indirect contact with an infected human or animal.

vector-borne infection: an infection that is transmitted by an organism such as a fly or mosquito.

food, soil, or water infection: infection passed along by microbes present in these media. In the dental office, water lines may harbor a **biofilm** containing bacterial cells that adhere to moist surfaces and form a protective slime that can carry pathogens or nematodes. Dust on surfaces also can transport pathogens.

For disease to occur and prosper, a **chain of infection** must be present. Any break or elimination of a link or factor in the chain will stop the disease or infection, as shown in Figure 5-1.

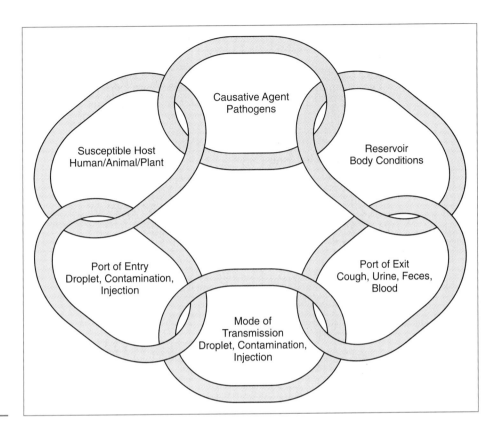

FIGURE 5-1
Chain of infection.

IMMUNITY FACTORS

Immunity (im-**YOU**-nih-tee = *resistance to organisms due to previous exposure*) may be affected by the **virulence** (**VEER**-you-lense = *power*) of a disease, the number or concentration of pathological organisms, and the patient's immune system.

Immunity can be classified according to either natural or artificial conditions, actively or passively.

natural immunity: inherited and permanent.

natural acquired immunity: obtained when a person is infected by a disease, produces antibodies, and then recovers from that disease.

artificial acquired immunity: obtained from inoculation or vaccination against a disease.

passive acquired immunity: results from receiving antibodies from another source, such as breast milk, or from injections of gamma globulin, antitoxins, or immune serum.

passive natural immunity: passes from mother to fetus congenitally or through antibodies in breast milk.

immunocompromised (**im**-you-no-**KAHM**-proh-mized): having a weakened immune system, resulting from drugs, irradiation, disease such as AIDS, or malnutrition.

Immunity may be acquired by inoculation or vaccination of an antigen that enables the body to produce an antibody to the disease. The vaccine used may contain killed pathogenic microbes or attenuated antigens. Terms related to acquired immunity are:

inoculation (inn-**ock**-you-**LAY**-shun): injection of microorganisms, serum, or toxin into the body.
vaccination (**vack**-sih-**NAY**-shun): inoculation with weakened or dead microbes.
antigen: substance that induces the body to form antibodies.
antibody: protein substance produced by the body in response to an antigen.
vaccine (**VAK**-seen): solution of killed or weakened infectious agents injected to produce immunity.
autogenous (**awe**-toh-**JEE**-nus) vaccine: vaccine produced from a culture of bacteria taken from the patient who will receive the vaccine.
attenuated (ah-**TEN**-you-**ate**-ed): diluted or reduced virulence of pathogenic microbes.

DISEASE PREVENTION

Prevention is the best protection method to combat disease and infection in the dental facility. Proper sanitation habits, effective sterilization, and careful handling are primary ways to obtain sanitary conditions. Relevant terminology includes the following.

asepsis (ay-**SEP**-sis): free from germs.
sanitation (san-ih-**TAY**-shun): application of methods to promote a favorable germ-free state.
disinfection (**dis**-inn-**FECK**-shun): application of chemicals to kill, reduce, or eliminate germs.
sterilization (stare-ill-ih-**ZAY**-shun): the process of destroying all microorganisms.

Procedures and Methods Used to Prevent Disease

Various methods and procedures are employed in the destruction of pathogens. Some of these are:

autoclave (**AWE**-toh-klave): apparatus for sterilization by steam pressure. Temperature (250 degrees), pressure (15 psi), and time (20 minutes) are regulated (see Figure 5-2).
"flash" autoclave: smaller autoclave with higher temperature setting (270 degrees) to lessen time (3–5 minutes) required to obtain sterilization.
dry heat sterilization: oven apparatus used for a hot air bake at high temperature (350 degrees) for a longer period of time (2 hours).

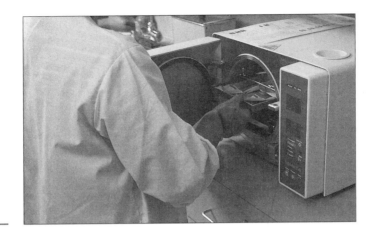

FIGURE 5-2
Dental assistant using autoclave.

chemical vapor: autoclave method using chemical vapor under pressure (20 psi) in place of water.

molten metal or **glass bead heat:** devices holding superheated (450 degrees) molten metal or small glass beads; used mainly in endodontic practice. (This method of sterilization is no longer recommended by the Centers for Disease Control and Prevention.)

germicidal gas: gas chamber apparatus for items that cannot withstand heat; requires long exposure and ventilation time before use; found mostly in hospitals.

chemical agents: liquids containing chemicals that kill microbes and spores and require longer immersion time. Some chemicals may be either disinfectants and/or sterilizers. Chemicals classified as sterilants require long (6–10 hours) immersion times to kill spores.

indicator strips or commercial spore vials: placed in or on wrapped items during the sterilization cycle to indicate the effectiveness of the sterilizing process. The two types of indication are:

process: Tapes or marked autoclave sleeves (see Figure 5-3) indicate that heat conditions have been obtained but do not guarantee that pressure and time have completed the sterilization. The markings on the autoclave bag or sleeve tape change color when exposed to the proper sterilizing conditions. The wrapping or sleeving of the articles provides protection from contamination in handling after sterilization.

biological: Vials with encased germs spore indicators assure that the sterilization process has been achieved.

Handpieces and other special handpiece items such as camera wands, probes, optic light ends, and so forth are expensive and should be lubricated and sterilized according to the manufacturer's directions. Figure 5-4 is an example of a handpiece maintenance system.

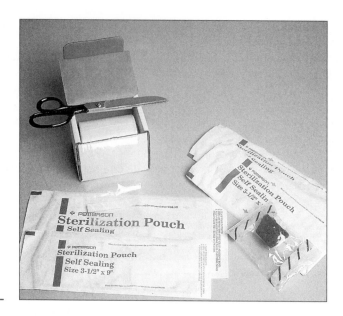

FIGURE 5-3
Autoclave bagging
materials.

Disinfection is the application of chemicals to kill, reduce, or eliminate germs. Terms related to this process are:

disinfectant (**dis**-inn-**FECK**-tant): chemical that kills many microbes, but not spore-forming bacteria. Although some chemicals may kill spores when used for a long period of time most are used for disinfecting.

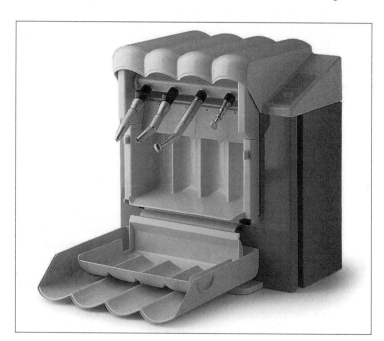

FIGURE 5-4
Handpiece
maintenance
system. (Courtesy
of Kavo Dental
Corporation)

antiseptic (an-tih-**SEP**-tick): usually a diluted disinfectant that inhibits growth of microbes.

bacteriostatic (back-tee-ree-oh-**STAT**-ick): inhibiting or retarding bacterial growth.

germicide (**JER**-miss-eyed): substance that destroys some germs.

holding solution: disinfectant solution with biodegradable (**bye**-oh-dee-**GRADE**-ah-bull = *chemical or metabolic material that breaks down protein material*) ingredient that is used to soak instruments until they are properly cleaned and sterilized.

ultrasonic cleaner: mechanical apparatus with a reservoir to contain a solution that cavitates (implodes = *bursts inwardly*) or bubbles off debris; this machine cleanses items prior to sterilization.

Miscellaneous Methods for Sanitation

Many items, procedures, and techniques, are employed to obtain a sanitized, clean area with protection for the patient and operator as well. To maintain sanitation and safety in a dental facility, the following are relevant.

PPE: *personal protective equipment* such as gloves, eyeglasses, clinical attire, and masks, to help protect the area and the wearer from disease microbes. Also included in PPE are hepatitis vaccinations (an OSHA requirement for health workers).

barrier techniques: drapes, covers, plastic instrument sleeves, and the like, to prevent contamination and help protect patients.

SOP: *standard operating procedures* for sanitation of operators and patients, including the training and use of proper handling and storing of dental equipment and supplies, hand washing and transfer methods, use of evacuation methods, rubber dams, and preoperative rinse of oral cavity with mouthwash.

standard precautions: treating each case as if the patient has a serious disease, including handling and sterilizing with each new use to prevent contamination; called maintaining a *sterile field*.

proper disposal techniques: disposing of all contaminated items in a marked biohazard bag; laundry and other materials used in patient care should be considered contaminated by splatter or aerosol matter.

sharps disposal unit: container used for collection and disposal of needles, broken glass, and sharp items.

biohazard container: labeled container for items contaminated with body fluids or life-threatening contaminates.

hazardous waste container: receptacle for used, unsanitary items.

MSDS papers: manufacturer's *material safety data sheet*; covers chemical content, labeling, storage, and safety advice; labels are marked with four colors to specify each danger potential.

saturate–wipe–saturate: disinfection cleaning of operative area. Many dental facilities fear that on a spray–wipe–spray method of disinfection, use of aerosol spreads and spatters germs from the contaminated sites. Instead, the personnel use disposable cloths saturated with a disinfecting solution to wipe up contaminated surfaces and then use another clean disposable, saturated cloth to leave behind a wet surface that is wiped dry after a 10-minute soak.

AGENCIES CONCERNED WITH DISEASE CONTROL

Boards of health at state and local levels apply restrictions and monitoring services to ensure proper health practices for service to the general public. Each state licenses and restricts the practice of dentistry within its borders. In addition, several government agencies and controlling bodies are involved with licensing, infection control, and hazard management in the dental facility. The following are federal agencies involved with disease control, and a national professional organization.

OSHA: Occupational Safety and Health Administration: issues and enforces restrictions and guidelines for infection control.

CDC: Centers for Disease Control and Prevention: sets regulations and issues suggestions for infection control.

EPA: Environmental Protection Agency: regulates and approves materials, equipment, medical devices, and chemicals used in dental practices.

FDA: Food and Drug Administration: regulates and approves marketing products and solutions used in infection control.

OSAP: Organization for Safety and Asepsis Procedures: national organization of health professionals; studies and makes suggestions for regulations and guidelines for infection control.

REVIEW EXERCISES

MATCHING
Match the following word elements with their meanings.

1. _____disease
2. _____fungus
3. _____droplet infection
4. _____pathology
5. _____antigens
6. _____immunity
7. _____germicide
8. _____asepsis
9. _____SOP
10. _____MSDS
11. _____acute
12. _____implode
13. _____PPE
14. _____symptom
15. _____sign

a. objective symptom
b. standard operating procedures
c. personal protective equipment
d. condition free from microbes
e. division of plants, includes molds, slimes
f. substance that induces the body to form antibodies
g. sharp, severe
h. study of disease
i. burst inwardly
j. pathological body state; abnormal condition
k. perceptible change in body or body function
l. manufacturer's safety data sheet
m. substance that destroys germs
n. resistance to microbes because of previous exposure
o. method of airborne carriage of germs

DEFINITIONS

Using the selection given for each sentence, choose the best term to complete the definition.

1. Which agency is concerned primarily with the safety and health of the environment?
   a. OSHA
   b. SPCA
   c. SDPA
   d. EPA

2. Symptoms of a disease that are reported by the patient are considered to be:
   a. subjective
   b. objective
   c. cumulative
   d. chronic

3. One-celled, plant-like microorganisms lacking chlorophyll are:
   a. viruses
   b. bacteria
   c. fungi
   d. cocci

4. A solution of weakened attenuated or weakened infectious agents used to produce immunity is a/an:
   a. vaccine
   b. disinfectant
   c. antibiotic
   d. toxin

5. Immunity that is obtained by an actual attack of the disease is called:
   a. passive
   b. active
   c. natural
   d. neutral

6. A protein substance that induces the body to form antibodies is called:
   a. biodegradable
   b. immunity
   c. antigen
   d. T-bar

7. Which of the following is not considered a harbor for microbes?
   a. sunlight
   b. water
   c. soil
   d. food

8. The process of destroying all micro-organisms is called:
   a. sterilization
   b. disinfection
   c. sanitation
   d. soaking

9. An oven apparatus used to bake or heat microorganisms to attain sterilization is a/an:
   a. autoclave
   b. dry heat sterilizer
   c. chemiclave
   d. ultrasonic cleaner

10. The use of drapes, wraps, and foil covering is considered to be what kind of technique?
    a. wrap
    b. ultrasonic
    c. barrier
    d. sepsis

11. A disease that occurs continuously in the same population or location is termed a/an:
    a. pandemic
    b. epidemic
    c. chronic
    d. endemic

12. A container marked Hazardous Waste Materials is used for:
    a. bloody gauze
    b. used facial tissues
    c. used saliva ejector tips
    d. used gum

13. Used needles and broken glass are disposed of in a:
    a. container marked biohazardous
    b. special sharps container
    c. bin for hazardous materials
    d. wastebasket or trash bag

14. Instruments are precleaned before sterilization in a/an:
    a. ultrasonic cleaner
    b. autoclave unit
    c. chemiclave machine
    d. hot oil bath

15. A pathological condition of the body is called:
    a. immunity
    b. treatment
    c. disease
    d. asepsis

16. A toothache would be considered a:
    a. sign
    b. symptom
    c. stimulate
    d. condition

17. A submicroscopic organism, requiring living matter is a:
    a. virus
    b. bacteria
    c. fungus
    d. cocci

18. Improper handling of equipment in the dental facility is an example of:
    a. airborne infection
    b. droplet infection
    c. indirect infection
    d. cross-infection

19. Protozoa are:
    a. members of the fungus family
    b. special types of bacteria
    c. members of the animal parasite family
    d. virus strains

20. The application of methods to promote a favorable germ-free state is called:
    a. sanitation
    b. sterilization
    c. germicidal condition
    d. sepsis

BUILDING SKILLS
Locate and define the prefix, root/combining form, and suffix (if present) in the following words.

1. **asepsis**
   prefix   _____
   root/combining form   _____
   suffix   _____

2. **sterilization**
   prefix   _____
   root/combining form   _____
   suffix   _____

3. **pathology**
   prefix   _____
   root/combining form   _____
   suffix   _____

4. **biodegradable**
   prefix   _____
   root/combining form   _____
   suffix   _____

5. **odontalgia**
   prefix   _____
   root/combining form   _____
   suffix   _____

FILL-INS
Write the correct word in the blank space to complete each statement.

1. Data sheets covering safety features of a product supplied by the manufacturer are called _____ sheets.

2. A container for items contaminated with body fluids or life-threatening contaminants is labeled _____.

3. A machine used to bubble or cavitate clean instruments before sterilization is called a/an _____.

4. A pathological condition of the body or a body function is called a/an _____.

5. Resistance to organisms because of previous exposure is called _____.

6. Direct passage of germs through an intimate relationship is called _____ infection.

7. Indicator strips are used to test the effect of the _____ process.

8. A/an _____ is an objective symptom, seen by someone other than the patient.

9. Microbes smaller than a bacterium and larger than a virus are termed _____.

10. Another word for airborne infection is _____ infection.

11. The study of disease is called _____.

12. A prediction of the course of a disease is a/an _____.

13. A carrier that transmits a disease is called a/an _____.

14. A/an _____ is a solution of kills or weakens infectious agents.

15. Short-term immunization by injection from antibodies is called _____ immunization.

16. Pathogenic microbes that have been weakened or reduced in virulence are said to be _____.

17. The term for a disease affecting a patient is called a/an _____.

18. The method of s microorganism's entrance into the body is termed the _____.

19. A/an _____ is a group of common symptoms / signs of a disease.

20. A/an _____
    is an injection of microorganisms, serum,
    or toxin into the body to produce immunity.

WORD USE

Read the following sentences and define the bold-faced word.

1. The dental receptionist questioned Mrs. Bailer regarding all the **symptoms** she had stated in the phone conversation.

   _____

   _____

2. Improper use and control of needles can cause a **parenteral** injury.

   _____

   _____

3. The dental assistant read that this specific disinfectant was not effective when dealing with **anaerobic** bacteria.

   _____

   _____

   _____

4. The dentist's report stated that the disease condition resulted from an **endogenous** source. _____

   _____

5. When placing an order for a new material, the office manager will request an **MSDS** sheet that applies to the item.

   _____

   _____

AUDIO LIST

This list contains selected new, important, or difficult terms from this chapter. You may use the list to review these terms and to practice pronouncing them correctly. When you work with the audio for this chapter, listen to the word, repeat it, and then place a checkmark in the box. Proceed to the next boxed word and repeat the process.

- ❑ **aerobic** (air-**OH**-bick)
- ❑ **anaerobic** (an-ah-**ROH**-bick)
- ❑ **antiseptic** (an-tih-**SEP**-tick)
- ❑ **asepsis** (ay-**SEP**-sis)
- ❑ **attenuated** (ah-**TEN**-you-ate-ed)
- ❑ **autoclave** (**AWE**-toh-klave)
- ❑ **autogenous** (awe-toh-**JEE**-nus)
- ❑ **bacteriostatic** (back-tee-ree-oh-**STAT**-ick)
- ❑ **biodegradable** (bye-oh-dee-**GRADE**-ah-bull)
- ❑ **commensal** (koh-**MEN**-sahl)
- ❑ **congenital** (kahn-**JEN**-ih-tuhl)
- ❑ **degenerative** (dee-**JEN**-er-ah-tiv)
- ❑ **diagnosis** (die-agg-**NO**-sis)
- ❑ **disinfectant** (dis-inn-**FECK**-tant)
- ❑ **disinfection** (dis-inn-**FECK**-shun)
- ❑ **endemic** (en-**DEM**-ick)
- ❑ **endogenous** (en-**DAH**-jeh-nuss)
- ❑ **etiology** (ee-tee-**AHL**-oh-jee)
- ❑ **exogenous** (ecks-**AH**-jeh-nuss)
- ❑ **flagella** (flah-**JELL**-ah)
- ❑ **fomes** (**FOH**-mez)
- ❑ **fungus** (**FUNG**-us)
- ❑ **immunocompromised** (im-you-no-**KAHM**-proh-mizd)
- ❑ **inoculation** (inn-ock-you-**LAY**-shun)
- ❑ **nematodes** (**NEM**-ah-toads)
- ❑ **nosocomial** (noh-soh-**KOH**-mee-ahl)
- ❑ **odontalgia** (oh-dahn-**TAHL**-jee-ah)
- ❑ **opportunistic** (ah-pore-too-**NISS**-tick)
- ❑ **pandemic** (pan-**DEM**-ick)

- ❏ parenteral (pare-**EN**-ter-ahl)
- ❏ pathogenic (path-oh-**JEN**-ick)
- ❏ pathology (path-**AHL**-oh-jee)
- ❏ prognosis (prahg-**NO**-sis)
- ❏ protozoa (proh-toh-**ZOH**-ah)
- ❏ rickettsia (rih-**KET**-see-ah)
- ❏ sanitation (**san-ih-TAY**-shun)

- ❏ saprophyte (**SAP**-roh-fight)
- ❏ sterilization (**stare**-ill-ih-**ZAY**-shun)
- ❏ symptom (**SIM**-tum)
- ❏ syndrome (**SIN**-drome)
- ❏ vaccination (vack-sih-**NAY**-shun)
- ❏ virulence (**VEER**-you-lense)
- ❏ virus (**VYE**-russ)

CHAPTER 6

Emergency Care

Emergency Care

OBJECTIVES Upon completion of this chapter, the reader should be able to identify and understand terms related to:

1. **Emergency prevention techniques.** Discuss the importance of prevention, the procedures for preparing for emergencies, and taking vital signs.

2. **Emergency prevention equipment and materials.** List and identify the major equipment and materials needed in emergency prevention and treatment.

3. **Airway obstruction and CPR protocol.** Discuss methods to clear the airway, and define the terms related to CPR.

4. **Classifications of shock.** List and discuss the various types of shock.

5. **Common medical emergencies.** List and describe the most common medical emergencies and conditions affecting dental care.

6. **Common dental emergencies.** Describe the most common emergencies occurring in the dental facility.

EMERGENCY PREVENTION TECHNIQUES

The best treatment for emergencies is to prevent them from happening. With careful training, observation, and preparation, many medical and dental emergencies can be averted. Two of the fundamental methods employed in facility readiness are:

1. patient health history: written and oral communication regarding the patient's present and past health status, including medication, treatment, allergies, and health concerns.

2. vital signs: body indications of the patient's present health status, including blood pressure, pulse, respiration, temperature, and the patient's concept of pain.

Blood Pressure

Blood pressure (BP) is an indication of the pulsating force of blood circulating through the blood vessels at rest **diastolic** (dye-ah-**STAHL**-ick) and while under the highest pressure of the circulating blood, the **systolic** (sis-**TAHL**-ick) pressure. BP is recorded in even numbers, with systolic pressure numbers placed before diastolic pressure numbers—for example, 120/80 (systolic/diastolic). Relevant terms are:

stethoscope (**STETH**-oh-scope): device employed to intensify body sounds. It has a set of earpieces inserted into rubber tubing that combines the two ear tubes into one and extends to a metal, bell-shaped or flat disk diaphgram. Stethoscopes used in training sometimes have two earpieces combined in one diaphragm for instruction purposes.

diaphragm (**DYE**-ah-fram = *thin covering*): a thin layer over the disk end of the stethoscope that enlarges or amplifies pulse and body sounds.

sphygmomanometer (**sfig**-moh-man-**AHM**-eh-ter): an instrument employed to determine the arterial blood pressure. Available in portable, wall-mounted, or mobile floor units; consists of a squeeze bulb on rubber tubing, an arm cuff, and a pressure or **aneroid** (**AN**-er-oyd = *air pressure*) dial or a marked, graduated, mercury column.

antecubital fossa (an-tee-**CUE**-bee-tal **FAH** sah): interior depression or bend of the elbow; the approximate area for placing the stethoscope diaphragm to determine blood pressure sound.

Pulse

Pulse is the beating force for blood circulating through arteries, classified according to rate, rhythm, and condition. Pulse counts may be taken at various body areas. Figure 6-1 shows the sites for taking pulse and blood pressure readings. Abnormal pulse rates can be:

▶ accelerated: faster pulse rate than normal or expected, also called "rapid."
▶ alternating: changing back and forth of weak and strong pulsations.

Other terms related to pulse are:

arrhythmia (ah-**RITH**-mee-ah): irregular heartbeat or pulsations.

bradycardia (**bray**-dee-**KAR**-dee-ah): pulse rate under 60 beats per minute (bpm).

tachycardia (**tack**-ee-**KAR**-dee-ah): an abnormal condition of pulse rates over 100 bpm (except in children).

deficit (**DEF**-ih-sit = *lacking*): lower pulse rate at the wrist than at the heart site; "heart flutter."

febrile (**FEEB**-ril): normal pulse rate becoming weak and feeble with prostration or illness.

frequency: pulse count; number of pulsations differ with age, sex, body position, and health of patient; it can be:

intermittent: occasional skipping of heartbeats.
irregular: variation of force or frequency in pulse rate.
regular: uniform pulse force, frequency, and duration.
thready: a fine, hard to locate, barely perceivable pulse.

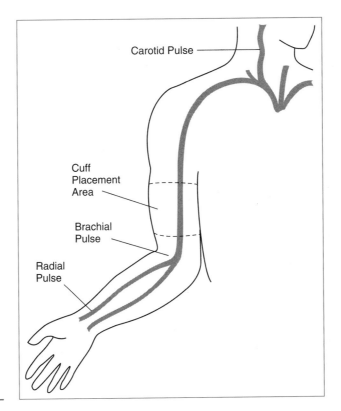

FIGURE 6-1

Pulse sites used in blood pressure readings and pulse counts.

Note: The pulse point at the wrist is the radial pulse; in the elbow, the brachial pulse; and in the neck, the carotid pulse.

In the figure: Carotid Pulse, Cuff Placement Area, Brachial Pulse, Radial Pulse

Respiration

Respiration is the inhaling or breathing in of oxygen and the exhaling or expelling of carbon dioxide. One respiration count requires an inspiration (in-spur-**AY**-shun = *breathing in*) and an expiration (ecks-purr-**AY**-shun = *breathing out*). Respirations are described according to rate, character, and rhythm as:

absent: suppressed respiratory sounds.
apnea (APP-nee-ah): cessation of breathing, usually temporary.
Cheyne-Stokes: respirations gradually increasing in volume until climax, then sub-
siding and ceasing for a short time before starting again; may be noted in dying.
deep: strong inhalation of air with exhalation.
dyspnea (**DISP**-nee-ah): out of breath; difficult or labored breathing.
frequent: rapid breathing that may be noted in children, those with disease, with
hysteria, or may be drug induced.
rales: noisy, bubbling sounds from lung mucus; heard on inhalation.
shallow: short inhalation with small rise in chest.
slow: fewer than 12 respirations per minute.
stertorous (**STARE**-toe-rus): rattling, bubbling, or snoring sounds that obscure
normal breaths.

TABLE 6-1   Normal Ranges in Vital Signs

AGES	BLOOD PRESSURE	PULSE	RESPIRATION	TEMPERATURE
Infants	70–100/50–70	80 to 160 bpm	30 to 70 bpm	99.2–99.8
2–5 years	82–110/50–75	80 to 120 bpm	22 to 35 bpm	98.5–99
6–12 years	84–120/54–80	75 to 110 bpm	18 to 25 bpm	98–98.5
13–18 years	90–140/62–88	60 to 90 bpm	16 to 20 bpm	97–99
Adults	90–140/60–90	60 to 100 bpm	15 to 20 bpm	97–99
Geriatric +70	90–140/60–90	60 to 100 bpm	15 to 20 bpm	96–99

Temperature

Temperature is the balance of heat loss and production in a body; may be taken at various sites, such as oral, rectal, **axillary** (**ACK**-sih-lair-ee = *armpit*), and **aural** (**ORE**-ahl = *pertaining to the ear*). Terms relating to temperature are:

fever: elevated body temperature, usually considered over 100–103 degrees F. (38.3C).
hyperthermia (high-per-**THER**-mee-ah): body temperature exceeding 104 degrees F (40 degrees C).
hypothermia (high-poh-**THER**-mee-ah): body temperature, below 95 degrees F (35 degrees C).
tympanic (tim-**PAN**-ick = *pertaining to eardrum*): measurement of body heat registered by an ear thermometer.

The normal ranges of four vital signs are listed in Table 6-1.

Patient's Concept of Pain

A sixth vital sign, the patient's concept of his/her pain, is added to the patient's assessment. Recording the patient's concept of pain endured can be used as a measurement in determining the patient's condition. The patient rates the level of pain on a scale of 1–10 in intensity. Any increase or decrease in this pain concept may indicate the course of the disease. This vital sign is subjective (because it is received from the patient) while the other five listed are objective (can be seen by others and recorded).

▌EMERGENCY PREVENTION EQUIPMENT AND MATERIALS

All facilities should maintain the basic equipment and materials necessary to deal with emergencies. Knowledge of the location and use of these emergency items is essential.

emergency call list: important phone numbers necessary in an emergency, located in a prominent position near every available phone.

oxygen source: container with oxygen gas, colored green; obtained in various sizes and may be centrally supplied to each work station.

oxygen regulator: device used to control the flow of oxygen.

oxygen flowmeter: gauge used to adjust the flow amount of oxygen.

oxygen mask: device placed over a patient's nose and mouth to administer gas; may be clear or tinted plastic or rubber material.

demand-valve resuscitator: device attached to an oxygen mask to apply pressure to the oxygen flow and thereby inflate the lungs.

AMBU-bag: hand-held squeeze device with a mask placed over the patient's nose and mouth; used to force atmospheric air into the patient's lungs; may be attached to the oxygen supply to force oxygen into lungs.

emergency tray: a tray assembled with materials and items necessary for emergencies; often supplied in kit form with medicines, administration items, and chemicals to be used for various emergency events. Emergency trays must be updated frequently and close at hand. All dental personnel should know how to use each item.

▌ AIRWAY OBSTRUCTION AND CPR PROTOCOL

One of the most feared emergency situations is an airway obstruction, which occurs when a blockage prevents the patient from receiving air into the lungs. Symptoms include an inability to speak or make a noise; fearful, opened eyes; clutching of the throat; and **cyanosis** (**sigh**-ah-**NO**-sis = *blue condition*), a bluish discoloration of the skin caused by a lack of oxygen.

abdominal thrust: quick, jabbing pressure and force at belt line to force air up the windpipe.

asphyxiation (ass-**fick**-see-**AY**-shun): not breathing, a result of oxygen imbalance.

chest thrusts: applying quick pressure on the chest to force air upward in the windpipe to dislodge the obstruction; may be used on pregnant women as a substitute for abdominal thrusts.

cricothyrotomy (**kry**-koh-thigh-**ROT**-oh-mee; crico = ring, thyreo = *shield*, tomy = *cut*): an insert or cut into the thyroid and cricoid cartilage to introduce an emergency air supply.

gastric distension: a condition resulting from air having been forced into the abdomen instead of the lungs.

Heimlich maneuver: procedure in which abdominal thrusts are applied to a choking patient, which forces air from the diaphragm upward to expel a blockage in the airway (see Figure 6-2).

hypoxia (high-**POCK**-see-ah = *lack of oxygen*): a lack of inspired oxygen

stoma (**STOH**-mah = *mouth*): an artificial opening into the windpipe that is placed between the mouth and lungs; the opening is at the frontal base of the neck into the windpipe for air intake.

tracheotomy (tray-kee-**AH**-toh-mee = *cutting into the trachea*): a cut and an insertion of a tube into the trachea for an emergency air supply.

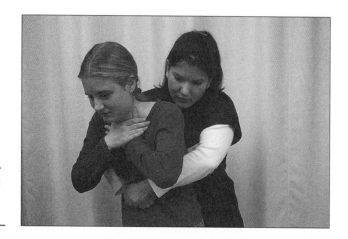

FIGURE 6-2
Heimlich maneuver being administered to a conscious victim.

Trendelenburg position: patient placed in a subsupine position with the feet higher than the head.

Cardiopulmonary Resuscitation

Occasionally an emergency requires **cardiopulmonary resuscitation**, commonly known as CPR, a life-saving measure that combines artificial respiration with external cardiac massage.

ABCDs: A = open airway; B = give breath (respiration); C = external compression to heart; D = **defibrillation** (**dee**-fib-rih-**LAY**-shun = *reversal of cardiac standstill*).

AED (automatic external defibrillation) unit: a mechanical/electrical device used to revive and stimulate the heart of a patient in a cardiac arrest.

airway device: tube inserted into the mouth and down the throat to provide air to the windpipe.

compression: force applied to the chest, providing pressure on the heart to imitate a heartbeat or pulsation.

finger sweep: using a finger in the mouth of an unconscious person to locate and wipe out any airway obstruction.

sternum (**STIR**-num): "breastbone," flat bone between the ribs.

xiphoid (**ZIF**-oyd) **process:** lowest portion of the sternum (breastbone) with no ribs attached.

▌CLASSIFICATION OF SHOCK

When a patient incurs a condition that alters the intake of oxygen and its passage and use, the body may react by the shutting down of any or all of its systems. The most common symptom of shock is **syncope** (**SIN**-koh-pee = *fainting*). The pulse may become weak, fast, or irregular, and blood pressure may drop. Breathing may increase, accompanied by pale skin, sweating, and possibly vomiting. Treatment includes finding the source of shock, providing suitable treatment, maintaining body functions, and obtaining assistance. The nine basic types of shock are.

anaphylactic (an-ah-fih-**LACK**-tick): shock arising from a reaction to a body allergen.
cardiogenic (**kar**-dee-oh-**JEN**-ick): shock arising from improper heart action.
hemorrhagic shock: shock arising from excessive blood loss.
metabolic (met-ah-**BAHL**-ick): shock arising from endocrine diseases and disorders, such as diabetes.
neurogenic (**new**-row-**JEN**-ick): shock arising from nervous impulses.
postural (**POSS**-chew-rahl): shock arising from a sudden change in body positions.
psychogenic (sign-koh-**JEN**-ick): shock with mental rather than physical origins.
respiratory (**RES**-purr-ah-tore-ee): shock arising from insufficient breathing.
septic (**SEP**-tick): shock arising from a microbial infection.

COMMON MEDICAL EMERGENCIES

During the course of treatment in the dental facility, an occasional medical emergency arises that complicates the handling and care of the patient. These include allergies, asthma, reactions related to diabetes, epilepsy, hyperventilation, and heart conditions.

Allergies

An allergic reaction is caused by a person's sensitivity to a specific antigen that can result in a variety of symptoms. Some are as mild as a slight rash, and others are quite involved, including death from severe anaphylactic shock.

anaphylaxis **(an-ah-fill-ACK-sis):** an allergic reaction of the body resulting in lowered blood pressure, swelling of the throat, shock, and can even result in death.
itching: a condition of irritation to the skin, scalp, or mucous membranes.
erythema (air-ih-**THEE**-mah = *skin redness*): a red rash or blotching of the skin.
edema (eh-**DEE**-mah): a tissue swelling, enlargement of a body area.
vesicle (**VES**-ih-kuhl = *small blister*): small, watery blisters.
urticaria (yur-tih-**CARE**-ee-ah = *vascular skin reaction*): commonly called hives or wheals.

Asthma

Asthma (**AZ**-mah = *panting*) is a chronic disorder characterized by shortness of breath, wheezing, and coughing caused by spasms of the bronchial tubes or swollen mucous membranes. Asthmatic conditions are classified as:

▶ extrinsic: resulting from allergens (animal, dust, foods) entering the body (usually affecting children).
▶ intrinsic: resulting from bronchial infection allergens (usually affecting older patients).
▶ status asthmaticus: severe attack that may be fatal.

Diabetes Mellitus

Diabetes mellitus (dye-ah-**BEE**-tus = *passing through*; mel-**EYE**-tis = *sugar in the urine*) is a disorder of the metabolism of carbohydrates. This disease has been divided into two types.

1. Type I, insulin-dependent diabetes (once termed juvenile diabetes), has an early onset and is more severe in course; treatment consists of insulin intake.
2. Type II, non-insulin-dependent diabetes, usually develops later in life and may be regulated by controlling the diet and /or taking oral medication.

Various terms related to diabetic emergencies are:

diabetic coma: loss of consciousness because of severe untreated or unregulated hyperglycemia, a condition termed diabetic acidosis.
glucose (GLUE-kose): sugar, an important carbohydrate in body metabolism.
hyperglycemia (high-purr-gly-SEE-mee-ah; hyper = *over*, glyco = *sweet*, emia = *blood*): a condition characterized by an increase in blood sugar.
hypoglycemia (high-poh-gly-SEE-me-ah; hypo = *under*; glyco = *sweet*; emia = *blood*): a condition in which the blood sugar is abnormally low.
insulin (IN-sue-lin): a hormone released by the pancreas that is essential for the proper metabolism of sugar (glucose).
insulin shock: a condition produced by an overdose of insulin resulting in a lowered blood sugar level (hypoglycemia).
juvenile diabetes: onset of diabetes in a person under 15 years of age.
keytone (KEY-tone): acidic substance resulting from metabolism.

Epilepsy

Epilepsy (**EP**-ih-**lep**-see = *a seizure*) is a disease characterized by recurrent seizures resulting from disturbed brain functioning. Symptoms can range from mild twitching to periods of unconsciousness accompanied by body movements and actions.

petit mal (PEH-tee-mahl) seizure: small seizures consisting of momentary unconsciousness with mild body movements or actions.
grand mal seizure: significant epileptic attack that may include an aura, unconsciousness, spasms, mouth frothing, incontinence, and coma.
status epilepticus: a rapid succession of epileptic attacks without the person's regaining consciousness between occurrences.
aura (AW-rah = *breeze*): a subtle sensation of oncoming physical or mental disorder.
clonic (KLON-ick = *turmoil*): seizure marked by alternating contraction and relaxation of muscles, producing jerking movements.
partial epilepsy: form of epilepsy consisting of convulsions, without loss of consciousness, that are restricted to certain areas, such as one side of the body.
tonic (tahn-ick) seizure: seizure marked by continuous muscular tension, producing rigidity or violent spasms.
incontinence (in-KAHN-tin-ense): loss of bladder control, which may occur during a seizure.

Hyperventilation

Hyperventilation (**high**-per-ven-tih-**LAY**-shun) is a condition of increased inspiration resulting in a decrease in carbon dioxide (*acapnia*) in the body. This may cause tingling of the fingers and/or toes, a drop in blood pressure, dizziness, and possible syncope. Treatment consists of calming the patient's fears and requesting him/her to breathe into a paper bag, or to cup the hands over the mouth and take deep breaths. This helps the body regain a carbon dioxide/oxygen balance.

Heart Conditions

Heart problems are cardiac diseases and conditions that are related to the heart, the muscular organ that powers the circulatory system. The heart, as seen in Figure 6-3, is encased in a sac called the **pericardium** (pair-ih-**KAR**-dee-um = *sac around the heart*), which has three layers:

1. **epicardium** (epp-ih-**KAR**-dee-um): outer serous layer.
2. **myocardium** (my-oh-**KAR**-dee-um): middle cardiac muscular layer.
3. **endocardium** (en-doh-**KAR**-dee-um): inner layer, lining the four heart chambers.

Various terms are used to describe heart structure, conditions, and diseases.

atrium (**AY**-tree-um = *corridor*; plural is **atria**): two upper chambers of the heart, right and left.

ventricle (**VEN**-trih-kul = *little belly*): two lower chambers of the heart, one on each side, beneath the atrium.

FIGURE 6-3
Interior of heart.
(1) right atrium
(2) right ventricle
(3) left atrium
(4) left ventricle
(5) septum
(6) superior vena cava
(7) inferior vena cava
(8) tricuspid valve
(9) pulmonary valve
(10) pulmonary artery
(11) pulmonary veins
(12) mitral valve
(13) aortic valve
(14) aorta

Note: The arrows indicate the flow of blood.

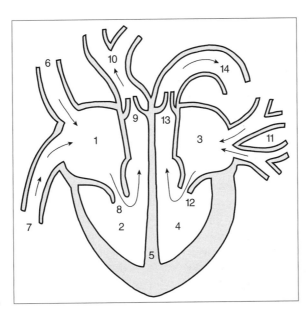

valve (*tiny fold*): a heart structure for temporary closing of the blood vessels; valves also control the flow of blood through the heart.

atrioventricular (**ay**-tree-oh-ven-**TRICK**-you-lar) orifice: an opening between the atrium and the ventricle where the valves are situated.

semilunar valves: heart valves. The aortic valve is found at the entrance of the aorta to the heart, and the pulmonary valve or tricuspid valve is situated between the right atrium and the right ventricle of the heart. The mitral, or bicuspid valve, is on the left side between the atrium and the ventricle.

aorta (ay-**ORE**-tah): main artery that exits from the heart.

murmur: abnormal sound heard over the heart or blood vessels; an indication of improper blood flow or valve action.

arteriosclerosis (ar-**teer**-ee-oh-skleh-**ROH**-siss): thickening and hardening of small arteries.

atherosclerosis (**ath**-er-oh-skleh-**ROH**-sis): blocking of larger artery, often from plaque buildup.

angina pectoris: a pain in the chest caused by a heart malfunction.

myocardial infarction (my-oh-**KAR**-dee-ahl in-**FARK**-shun) (MI): necrosis or death of the myocardium muscle tissue; a heart attack.

bacterial endocarditis: sometimes termed *infective endocarditis*, an inflammation of the heart lining of patients who have had rheumatic fever, open heart surgery, body part replacements, or implants. Although this is not an immediate emergency chairside threat, these patients require pre-treatment with antibiotic therapy to ward off future infections.

nitroglycerin: medication for the immediate relief of heart pains, particularly angina pectoris

Stroke

A common illness related to the blood supply and circulation is stroke. A stroke is technically termed a cerebrovascular (**sare**-ee-broh-**VASS**-kyou-lar = *pertaining to the blood vessels of the brain*) accident (abbreviated as CVA). A stroke is the result of insufficient blood supply to the brain because of a rupture or blockage.

embolism (**EM**-boh-lizm): a floating clot or air bubble that may lodge in a blood vessel.

hemorrhage (**HEM**-or-rij = blood burst): a rupture in a brain artery.

infarction (in-**FARK**-shun): a decreased blood supply causing necrosis or tissue death.

thrombosis (throm-**BOE**-siss): a clot forming in a blood vessel.

hemiplegia (hem-ih-**PLEE**-jee-ah = *paralysis on one side of the body*): may result from a brain lesion, thrombosis, hemorrhage, or tumor of the cerebrum.

transient ischemic attack (TIA): localized, temporary anemia resulting from an obstruction in blood circulation. Ischemia (iss-**KEE**-me-ah) means a holding back of blood. TIAs may be precursors of a stroke (CVA).

aneurysm (**AN**-you-rizm = *dilation or bulging of a blood vessel because of wall weakness*): a balloon-like enlargement of a cerebral artery or another vessel.

COMMON DENTAL EMERGENCIES

Some emergencies are specifically dental-related, occurring as a result of recent dental treatment or the need for dental treatment.

alveolitis (al-vee-oh-**LIGH**-tiss): inflammation of the alveolar area, commonly called "dry socket."

avulsed (ah-**VUL**-sed): describes a tooth or body part that has been knocked out, forced, or torn away.

epistaxis (ep-ih-**STACK**-sis): nosebleed.

hemorrhage: excessive bleeding; treatments for hemorrhage are:

astringent (ah-strin-**JENT**): agent that has a binding effect, constricts.

coagulant (koh-**AG**-you-lant): agent that causes blood to coagulate or congeal.

hemostatic (**hee**-moe-**STAT**-ick): agent that stops bleeding, such as vitamin K.

trismus (**TRIZ**-mus): tonic contraction of muscle, perhaps muscles of mastication (jaw).

postural hypotension: a decrease in blood pressure resulting from quickly raising the body after having been in a lowered position for a period of time; rapid sit-up resulting in dizziness.

sequestra (see-**KWESS**-trah): small bone pieces or spicules working to the surface after surgery, causing bleeding and soreness.

syncope fainting: the most common emergency in a dental facility.

REVIEW EXERCISES

MATCHING

Match the following word elements with their meaning:

1. _____hemorrhage
2. _____apnea
3. _____metabolic shock
4. _____ketone
5. _____axillary
6. _____tonic
7. _____insulin
8. _____sternum
9. _____nitroglycerin
10. _____bradycardia
11. _____septic shock
12. _____atrium
13. _____stoma
14. _____alveolitis
15. _____edema

a. pulse rate under 60 beats per minute
b. artificial neck opening for inspiration of air
c. breastbone
d. muscular tension
e. cessation of breathing
f. shock arising from microbial infection
g. excessive bleeding
h. dry socket
i. swelling
j. medicine for angina pain
k. acid substance resulting from body metabolism
l. reaction from disease of body metabolism
m. an upper chamber of the heart
n. pertaining to the armpit
o. hormone released from pancreas for metabolism

DEFINITIONS

Using the selection given in each sentence, choose the best term to complete the definition.

1. The machine that is exclusively used to determine arterial blood pressure is the:
   a. sphygmomanometer   b. arteriogram
   c. diaphragm   d. thermometer

2. Which of the following is not considered a vital sign?
   a. blood pressure   b. temperature
   c. pulse   d. weight

3. A pulse rate under 60 beats per minute is termed:
   a. tachycardia   b. bradycardia
   c. endocardia   d. arythrocardia

4. A pulse rate over 100 beats per minute is termed:
   a. tachycardia   b. bradycardia
   c. endocardia   d. arythrocardia

5. A body temperature exceeding 105 degrees F is termed:
   a. hypothermia   b. hyperthermia
   c. aurathermia   d. diathermia

6. A body temperature below 95 degrees F is termed:
   a. hypothermia   b. hyperthermia
   c. aurathermia   d. diathermia

7. The act of bringing an unconscious person back to consciousness is:
   a. asphyxiation   b. syncope
   c. fainting   d. resuscitation

8. Which device is placed over the nose and mouth to deliver oxygen?
   a. regulator   b. mask
   c. flowmeter   d. tank

9. What type of shock arises from improper heart action?
   a. anaphylactic   b. cardiogenic
   c. metabolic   d. psychogenic

10. What type of shock arises from the body's reaction to an allergen?
    a. anaphylactic   b. cardiogenic
    c. metabolic   d. psychogenic

11. What type of shock arises from fear or mental stress?
    a. anaphylactic   b. cardiogenic
    c. metabolic   d. psychogenic

12. A bluish cast to the skin resulting from a lack of oxygen is called:
    a. cyanamide   b. cyanosis
    c. aura   d. cryptitis

13. Small blisters that may form as a result of an allergy are called:
    a. edemas   b. rales
    c. foliciles   d. vesicles

14. Which type of asthmatic attacks results from an allergen and is usually seen in children?
    a. intrinsic   b. extrinsic
    c. spastic   d. status asthmaticus

15. The normal rate of respirations per minute for an adult is:
    a. 8–10   b. 10–15
    c. 15–20   d. 20–25

16. The outer serous layer of the heart muscle is the:
    a. epicardium   b. myocardium
    c. endocardium   d. mitral

17. The middle cardiac muscular layer of the heart is the:
    a. epicardium   b. myocardium
    c. endocardium   d. mitral

18. The inner layer of the heart, lining the four chambers, is the:
    a. epicardium   b. myocardium
    c. endocardium   d. mitral

19. Another term for the condition of hardening of the blood vessels is:
    a. arthroscope   b. atherosclerosis
    c. arteriovascular   d. arteriosclerosis

20. Another term for the condition of narrowing of the arteries, from plaque buildup, is:
    a. arthroscope
    b. atherosclerosis
    c. arteriovascular
    d. arteriosclerosis

BUILDING SKILLS

Locate and define the prefix, root/combining form, and suffix (if present) in the following words:

1. **cerebrovascular**
   prefix   _____
   root/combining form   _____
   suffix   _____

2. **hypothermia**
   prefix   _____
   root/combining form   _____
   suffix   _____

3. **cricothyreotomy**
   prefix   _____
   root/combining form   _____
   suffix   _____

4. **hyperglycemia**
   prefix   _____
   root/combining form   _____
   suffix   _____

5. **endocardium**
   prefix   _____
   root/combining form   _____
   suffix   _____

FILL-INS

Write the correct word in the blank space to complete each statement.

1. Small pieces of bone or bone spicules working to the surface after surgery are called _____.

2. A/an _____ _____ _____ is a written survey of a patient's past and present health condition.

3. A pulse indicating an occasional skipped beat is termed _____.

4. A/an _____ is an instrument used to intensify body sounds.

5. A balance of body heat loss and production is called body _____.

6. One method of removing airway obstructions is the _____ maneuver.

7. Another word for the breastbone, used in giving CPR is _____.

8. A sensitivity to an allergen present in the body is a/an _____.

9. _____ is commonly known as hives.

10. The most severe type of asthma attack is the _____ _____.

11. _____ is the hormone released by the pancreas for metabolism.

12. Awareness of oncoming physical or mental disorder is termed a/an _____.

13. _____ is a condition of increased inspirations resulting in a decrease in carbon dioxide.

14. The two upper chamber halves on each side of the heart are the _____.

15. The _____ is the main artery exiting the heart.

16. A/an _____ is a decreased blood supply causing necrosis of tissue.

17. A/an _____ is a tonic concentration of the mastication muscles.

18. _____, or fainting, is the most common emergency in the dental facility.

19. Another term for nosebleed is _____.

20. The inner elbow space used to obtain blood pressure readings is termed the _____ fossa.

WORD USE

Read the following sentences and give the meaning of the bolded words.

1. Taking and recording the patient's **vital signs** is standard office protocol for every patient.

_____

_____

2. Ever since her **cerebrovascular accident (CVA)**, Mrs. Brown's speech and motor skills have been limited.

_____

_____

3. The assistant noticed that the patient was showing signs of **erythema** and itching after the injection of a local anesthetic.

_____

_____

4. The receptionist noted that Mr. Harris included **hyperglycemia** as a medical condition on his health history.

_____

_____

5. The dentist offered a **nitroglycerin** tablet to Mr. Roberts to assist him in his distress.

_____

_____

AUDIO LIST

This list contains selected new, important, or difficult terms from this chapter. You may use the list to review these terms and to practice pronouncing them correctly. When you work with the audio for this chapter, listen to the word, repeat it, and then place a checkmark in the box. Proceed to the next boxed word and repeat the process.

- ❏ anaphylactic (an-ah-fih-**LACK**-tick)
- ❏ aneroid (**AN**-er-oyd)
- ❏ aneurysm (**AN**-you-rizm)
- ❏ aorta (ay-**ORE**-tah)
- ❏ apnea (**AP**-nee-ah)
- ❏ arrhythmia (ah-**RITH**-mee-ah)
- ❏ arteriosclerosis (ar-teer-ee-oh-skleh-**ROH**-siss)
- ❏ asphyxiation (ass-**fick**-see-**AY**-shun)
- ❏ atherosclerosis (**ath**-er-oh-skleh-**ROH**-sis)
- ❏ atrioventicular (**ay**-tree-oh-ven-**TRICK**-you-lar)
- ❏ atrium (**AY**-tree-um)
- ❏ aural (**ORE**-ahl)
- ❏ axillary (**ACK**-sih-lair-ee)
- ❏ bradycardia (bray-dee-**KAR**-dee-ah)
- ❏ cardiogenic (kar-dee-oh-**JEN**-ick)
- ❏ cerebrovascular (sare-ee-broh-**VAS**-kyou-lar)
- ❏ clonic (**KLAHN**-ick)
- ❏ cricothyrotomy (kry-koh-thigh-**ROT**-oh-mee)
- ❏ cyanosis (sigh-ah-**NO**-sis)
- ❏ defibrilation (dee-fib-rih-**LAY**-shun)
- ❏ deficit (**DEF**-ih-sit)

- ❏ diastolic (dye-ah-**STAHL**-ick)
- ❏ dyspnea (**DISP**-nee-ah)
- ❏ embolism (**EM**-boh-lizm)
- ❏ endocardium (en-doh-**KAR**-dee-um)
- ❏ epicardium (epp-ih-**KAR**-dee-um)
- ❏ epilepsy (**EP**-ih-lep-see)
- ❏ epistaxis (ep-ih-**STACK**-sis)
- ❏ erythema (air-ith-**EE**-mah)
- ❏ expiration (ecks-purr-**AY**-shun)
- ❏ febrile (**FEEB**-ril)
- ❏ hemiplegia (hem-ih-**PLEE**-jee-ah)
- ❏ hyperthermia (high-per-**THER**-mee-ah)
- ❏ hyperventilation (**high**-per-ven-tih-**LAY**-shun)
- ❏ hypoglycemia (**high**-poh-gly-**SEE**-me-ah)
- ❏ hypothermia (**high**-poh-**THER**-mee-ah)
- ❏ hypoxia (high-**POCK**-see-ah)
- ❏ incontinence (in-**KAHN**-tin-ense)
- ❏ inspiration (in-spur-**AY**-shun)
- ❏ ischemia (iss-**KEE**-me-ah)
- ❏ metabolic (met-ah-**BAHL**-ick)
- ❏ myocardial infarction (my-oh-**KAR**-dee-ahl in-**FARK**-shun)
- ❏ myocardium (my oh-**KAR**-dee-um)
- ❏ neurogenic (new-roh-**JEN**-ick)

- ❏ pericardium (pair-ih-**KAR**-dee-um)
- ❏ postural (**POSS**-chew-rahl)
- ❏ psychogenic (sigh-koh-**JEN**-ick)
- ❏ respiratory (**RESS**-purr-ah-tore-ee)
- ❏ septic (**SEP**-tick)
- ❏ sequestra (see-**KWESS**-trah)
- ❏ sphygmomanometer (**sfig**-moh-man-**AHM**-eh-ter)
- ❏ sternum (**STIR**-num)
- ❏ stethoscope (**STETH**-oh-scope)
- ❏ stetorous (**STARE**-toe-rus)

- ❏ stoma (**STOW**-mah)
- ❏ systolic (sis-**TAH**-lick)
- ❏ tachycardia (tack-ee-**KAR**-dee-ah)
- ❏ tracheotomy (tray-kee-**AH**-toh-mee)
- ❏ trismus (**TRIZ**-mus)
- ❏ tympanic (tim-**PAN**-ick)
- ❏ urticaria (yur-tih-**CARE**-ee-ah)
- ❏ ventricle (**VEN**-trih-kul)
- ❏ vesicle (**VES**-ih-kuhl)
- ❏ xiphoid (**ZIF**-oyd)

Examination and Prevention

Examination and Prevention

OBJECTIVES   Upon completion of this chapter, the reader should be able to identify and understand terms related to:

1. **Procedures involved in the initial examination.** Identify and list the various procedures necessary to complete an initial examination.

2. **Examination of the oral tissues.** Identify the methods used to examine the oral tissues and the diseases associated with them.

3. **Examination of the teeth.** Discuss the methods used to examine the teeth and detect the associated diseases.

4. **Charting methods.** List and explain the various types of tooth and mouth charting techniques.

5. **Alginate impression.** Explain alginate impression and the words related to the procedure.

6. **Home preventive techniques.** Define preventive education and identify the various methods of home dental care.

7. **Dental facility preventive practices.** Explain the various methods to prevent tooth decay that are used in the dental office.

PROCEDURES INVOLVED IN THE INITIAL EXAMINATION

One of the most important visits to the dental office is the initial examination. During this appointment the dentist assesses the patient's general and dental health. To complete a thorough evaluation, several procedures must be performed. These include taking a health history, checking vital signs, making a visual assessment and palpating the head structures and mouth conditions, and examining the oral cavity. The initial exam may require additional procedures including radiographs, alginate impressions, photography by intra- and extra-oral cameras and any other diagnostic test deemed necessary.

Health History

The health history, as reported by the patient and reviewed by the dentist, includes the chief complaint, general medical condition, allergies, medications taken, past history of surgeries and illnesses, medical doctor's name, and emergency contact numbers.

Vital Signs

As discussed in Chapter 6, Emergency Care, vital signs include blood pressure, respiration, temperature, pulse, and pain. These signs may not be taken and recorded at each visit, but during the first, or initial, examination, it is important to obtain these measurements. The initial findings, recorded as the *baseline vital signs*, may be used to determine the present condition and also as a comparison or standard for future visits by the patient.

Visual Assessment

During the initial visit, the dentist assesses the condition of the head structures, looking to determine if the face is **symmetric** (sim-**ET**-rick; sym = *together,* metric = *measurement*) or **asymmetric** (**ay**-sim-**ET**-rick = *without proportion or balance*). A facial imbalance may suggest various diseases.

trismus (**TRIZ**-mus = *grating*): tension or contraction of the mastication muscles; may result from mouth infection, inflamed glands, and some diseases such as tetanus (commonly called *lockjaw*).

dysphagia (dis-**FAY**-jee-ah; dys = *bad,* phagein = *to eat*): difficulty swallowing; another term for swallowing is **deglutition** (**dee**-glue-**TISH**-un).

sialoadenitis (**sigh**-al-oh-**add**-eh-**NIGH**-tis; sial = *saliva,* aden = *gland,* itis = *inflammation*): an inflamed condition of a salivary gland.

tic douloureux (**tic**-doo-loo-**ROO**): degeneration or pressure on the trigeminal (5th cranial) nerve that causes neuralgia and painful contraction of facial muscles; also known as trigeminal neuralgia.

Bell's palsy: a sudden but temporary unilateral facial paralysis from unknown cause but may involve swelling of the facial nerve from an immune or viral infection.

temporomandibular joint (TMJ): union of the joints of the temporal and the mandibular bones. Many problems can arise in this area for an assortment of reasons and or causes. TMJ treatment varies from bite adjustment to bone surgery.

Facial color is observed, and an evaluation of the external lip structure includes the condition of the:

philtrum (**FILL**-trum): median groove on the external edge of the upper lip to the base of the nose.

commissure (**KOM**-ih-shur): corners of the mouth where the lips meet.

vermillion (ver-**MILL**-yon) border: area where the pink-red lip tissue meets the facial skin.

These landmarks are shown in Figure 7-1.

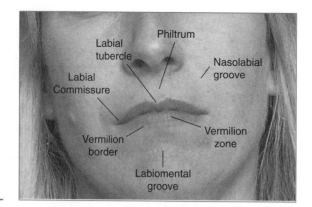

FIGURE 7-1
Landmarks of the face.

Palpation

One method of determining the condition of a tissue condition is to **palpate** (**PAL**-pate = *touch or feel*) an area. The dentist uses finger pressure to sense swellings, softness, irregularities, or movement in skin and mouth tissues. Lymph nodes and neck muscles are tested for lumps or swellings; and lip, cheek, tongue, and mouth tissues also are examined for irregularities. The temporomandibular joint (TMJ) area is palpated for movement and tenderness. The dentist may use a stethoscope to **ausculate** (awe-**SKUL**-ate = *listen to movement*) the joint area and blood flow in the carotid arteries in the neck.

EXAMINATION OF THE ORAL TISSUES

Before the dentist examines the teeth, an inspection of the oral tissues is done to determine the condition of the mouth. This usually is performed by visual observation using regular, dental, and halogen lighting with or without special dyes. The tongue is grasped by a gauze pad and extended to full length, and the gingiva and cheek areas are palpated. Among the variety of diseases that may be found in the oral cavity are:

oral lesion (**LEE**-zhun = *injury, wound*): altered inflammatory tissue or infected patch in the skin. Causes could be infection, hemorrhage, ulcerations, melanoma, fat deposits, amalgam tattoos, dilated veins, or other causes. Associated symptoms may be pain, swelling, or pus. Lesions that affect tooth tissue are called caries.

gingivitis (**jin**-jih-**VIE**-tis = *inflammation of gingiva*): redness and swelling of gingival tissues that may be caused by irritants, disease, improper hygiene, and/or poor general or nutritional health.

periodontitis (**pear**-ee-oh-don-**TIE**-tiss; peri = *around*, don = *tooth*, itis = *inflammation*): inflammation of the gingiva with involvement of deeper periosteal tissues indicated by formation of pockets and bone loss. A common name for this diseased condition is pyorrhea (**pie**-oh-**REE**-ah = *pus collection*).

periodontal (**pear**-ih-oh-**DON**-tal) abscess = (*abscess in periodontal tissues*): abscess originating in and progressing from inflammation of periodontal tissues; differs from periapical abscess, which originates in the pulp and progresses to the apical tip.

pericoronitis (**pear**-ih KOR-oh-**NIGH**-tiss; peri = *around*, corono = *tooth crown*, itis = *inflammation*): inflammation around the crown of a tooth. Pericoronitis happens quite often with erupting third molar teeth.

ANUG (*acute necrotic ulcerative gingivitis*): highly inflamed and dying gingival tissues; also called trench mouth or Vincent's infection.

cellulitis (sell-you-**LYE**-tiss = *inflammation of cellular or connective tissue*): infection and inflammation extending into adjacent connective tissues.

fistula (**FISS**-tyou-lah = *pathway for escape of pus; pipe*): tissue opening for pus drainage, providing some pain relief from buildup of pulpal pressure.

epulis (ep-**YOU**-liss = *gumboil*): fibrous tumor of oral tissue.

aphthous ulcer (**AF**-thuss **UHL**-sir; alpha = *little ulcer*): small, painful ulcer within the mouth; also called *canker sore*.

Fordyce granules: small, yellow spots on the mucous membrane, usually the soft palate and buccal mucosa; considered a developmental condition.

thrush: fungus infection of mouth and/or throat; appears as white patches or ulcers on tissues and is caused by *Candidiasis* infection of the oral mucosa.

candida albicans: sore, white plaque areas resulting from long-term antibiotic therapy permitting fungus buildup.

herpes (**HER**-peez) simplex virus (HSV): vesicles or watery pimples that burst and crust, caused by a virus; also called fever blisters or cold sores when on the lips, and gingivostomatitis when present on the oral mucosa. Types of herpes simplex are:

primary herpes: occurs in young children in the mouth or on the lips.

recurrent herpes: reappears on the lip area (*labialis*) throughout life.

herpes genitalis: lesions occurring on male/female genitalia; called HSV-2; sexually transmitted.

cheilosis (kee-**LOH**-sis; cheilo = *lips*, osis = *condition*): inflammation of the lip, particularly at the corners of the lips. Primary causes include candidiasis, vitamin B deficiency, or lack of vertical dimension at the commissures because of ill-fitting dentures.

mucocele (**MYOU**-koh-seal): soft nodule commonly found on the lower lip, caused by trauma to accessory salivary gland.

glossitis (glah-**SIGH**-tiss = *tongue inflammation*): inflammation of the tongue.

geographic tongue: flat, irregular, red lesions on the dorsum of the tongue.

hairy tongue: small black or dark brown projections resembling hairs, arising from the tongue dorsum; may be caused by medications or drug treatment.

fissured tongue: deep crack in center of tongue dorsum; considered a developmental cause.

circumvallate papillae: large, mushroom-shaped papillae on the posterior dorsum area of the tongue, considered to have developmental cause.

Oral Cancer

Some lesions of a suspicious nature can be detected in the mouth and examined more closely with excision and biopsy to determine if they are malignant or premalignant. A malignancy is a cancerous tumor with the ability to infiltrate and spread to other sites. Conditions that should be investigated include:

leukoplakia (**loo**-koh-**PLAY**-key-ah; leulos = *white*, plax = *plate*): white patches on oral tissues, particularly the tongue, that may become malignant.

neoplasm (**NEE**-oh-plazm = *new tissue*): all unusual or abnormal tissues, which should be tested to determine if the condition is benign or malignant. Some common neoplasms are:

> fibroma (fie-**BROH**-mah; fibr = *fiber*, oma = *tumor*): benign tumor of connective tissue.

> granuloma (gran-you-**LOH**-mah = *granular tumor*): benign tumor of lymph and skin cells.

> sarcoma (sar-**KOH**-mah = *tumor of flesh/tissues*): a malignant skin tumor arising from underlying tissues.

> hemangioma (heh-**man**-jee-**OH**-mah): benign tumor of dilated blood vessels.

> neurofibroma (new-roh-fie-**BROH**-mah): neoplasm of nerve sheath cell; may be single or multiple nodules.

> lymphoma (lim-**FOH**-mah): new tissue growth within the lymphatic system.

> carcinoma (kar-sih-**NO**-mah = *tumor of connective tissue*): malignant tumor of epithelial origin that may infiltrate and metastasize (meh-**TASS**-tah-size = *move*).

> nicotine stomatitis: malignant leukoplakia of the hard palate, caused by smoking.

AIDS: related symptoms include gingival lesions, thrush, swollen glands, and herpes lesions. There may be indications of Kaposi's sarcoma (skin lesion cancer).

▌ EXAMINATION OF THE TEETH

During the initial visit the dentist will exam and chart or record the present conditions of the teeth. Radiographs will be taken to determine the internal state of the teeth and other procedures (found in Chapter 13, Endodontics). After the tooth surfaces have been cleaned, a visual and physical tooth examination will be performed. The operator may use an explorer to detect carious lesions, defects, and tooth flaws, or may search for decay with a laser caries detector handpiece unit that measures the fluorescence level of undetected caries (see Figure 7-2).

Various diseases related to teeth include dental decay that takes various forms, periapical abscesses, and other maladies.

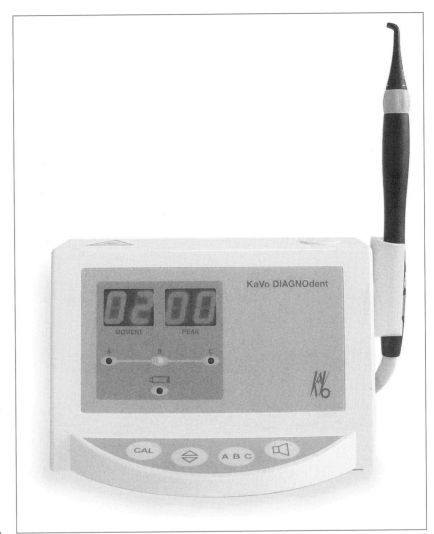

FIGURE 7-2
Laser probe.
(Courtesy of Kavo
Dental Corporation)
Note: Number
values of 10–15
require no care;
values of 15–30
require preventive
care; and values
over 30 need
restorative care.

Dental Caries

Dental **caries** (**CARE**-eez = *tooth decay*) are also known as decay or carious lesions. One cause of decay is the *Streptococcus mutans* bacteria, which produce acid that destroys tooth tissues through decalcification and demineralization of the enamel tissue and its matrix, and later moves into other tissue structures. Assorted types of dental decay include:

incipient caries: beginning decay.
rampant caries: widespread or growing decay.

recurrent caries: decay occurring under or near repaired margins of tooth restorations.
arrested caries: decay showing no progressive tendencies.

Destruction of tooth surfaces by dental decay varies according to the size and position of the decay. Dental caries are classified into three types.

1. **simple cavity:** decay involving one surface of the tooth, usually on the occlusal surface, the lingual surface of maxillary incisors, or fissured buccal surfaces of the mandibular posterior teeth.
2. **compound cavity:** decay involving two surfaces of a tooth, usually charted as mesioocclusal (MO), or distocclusal (DO), or any other two surfaces.
3. **complex cavity:** decay involving more than two surfaces, usually charted as mesiocclusodistal (MOD) or any other three or more surfaces.

In operative dentistry, caries are further classified as Class I through Class VI, in accordance with the operative needs, instrumentation, and procedures associated with the lesion. Figure 7-3 depicts this classification system.

FIGURE 7-3
Cavity classification according to Dr. G.V. Black's system.
(A) Class I caries on occlusal surface of molars and premolars
(B) Class II caries on proximal surfaces of a premolar and a molar
(C) Class III caries on proximal surfaces of a central incisor and a lateral incisor.
(D) Class IV fracture on proximal incisal surface of incisor
(E) Class V caries on gingival buccal areas of teeth
(F) Class VI caries on occlusal surface of mandibular incisor resulting from abrasion

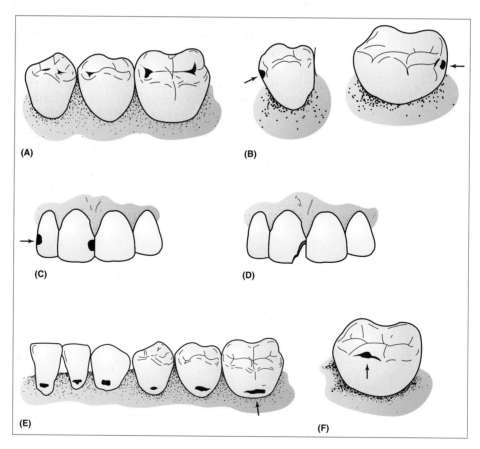

Periapical Abscess

A periapical (**pear**-ee-**APE**-ih-kahl = *around the tooth apex*) abscess is also called a *gum abscess*. An abscess results from necrosis (death) of pulp tissues. The three stages of pulp irritation are:

1. hyperemia (high-per-**EE**-mee-ah = *over, blood*): an increase in blood and lymph vessels as a result of irritation from decay.
2. pulpalgia (pul-**PAL**-jee-ah; pulp = *inner tooth tissue*, algia = *pain*): tooth pain or toothache resulting from irritation and infection in the pulp chamber.
3. pulpitis (pul-**PIE**-tis = *inflammation of the pulp*): inflammation and swelling of pulp tissue, leading to necrosis or death of the pulp.

Miscellaneous Maladies

In addition to dental caries and periapical abscesses or pulpal irritations, common dental maladies that may be observed during the dental examination are:

fistula (**FISS**-tyou-lah = *pathway for pus escape, pipe*): tissue opening for pus drainage, providing some pain relief from the buildup of pulpal pressure.

abrasion (ah-**BRAY**-zhun = *scraping from*): wearing away of tooth structure from abnormal causes such as malocclusion or bad habits.

attrition (ah-**TRISH**-un = *rubbing against*): wearing away of tooth structure from normal causes such as usual tooth chewing or mastication (mass-tih-**KAY**-shun = *the act of chewing*).

erosion (ee-**ROE**-zhun = *gnawing away*): wearing away or destruction of tooth structure as a result of disease or chemicals such as stomach acid from bulimia.

ankylosis (ang-kill-**OH**-sis = *stiff joint*): tooth fixation, retention of deciduous tooth past exfoliation time, or retention of permanent teeth that are fixed in the tooth socket because of an absence of periodontal ligaments; may be a result of heredity, disease, or constant trauma.

avulsion (ah-**VULL**-shun = *pulling away from*): tearing or knocking out; forcible removal of tooth.

bruxism (**BRUK**-sizm = *grinding of teeth*): grinding of teeth, especially during sleep or from bad habits.

malocclusion (**mal**-oh-**CLUE**-zhun; mal = *disorder*): imperfect occlusion, or irregular meeting of teeth, malposition of teeth.

abfraction (ab-**FRACK**-shun): loss of tooth surface in the cervical area, caused by tooth grinding and compression forces, resulting in hypersensitivity of the area.

acid etching: loss of enamel surfaces on the lingual side of anterior teeth caused by stomach acid fluids in reflux or purging by anorexic patients.

CHARTING METHODS

Tooth charting is a visual recording of existing oral conditions of the teeth and oral tissues. The graphic area representing the patient's teeth may be drawn in anatomical replication or shown in a geometric diagram, as illustrated in Figure 7-4.

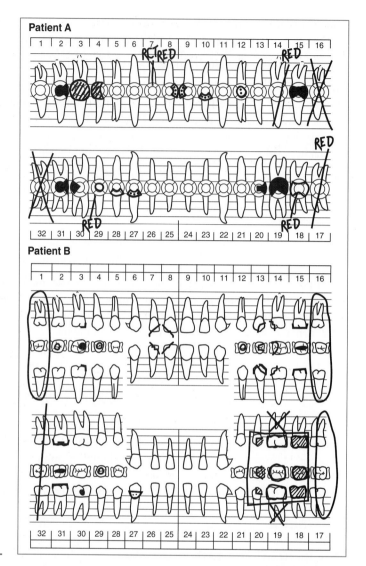

FIGURE 7-4
Examples of tooth-charting methods. Patient A: a geometrical reproduction of tooth charting Patient B: an anatomical reproduction of tooth charting

Each facility records or "charts" conditions in its own fashion, using coded letters and marks to designate areas of interest. Colors, particularly red and blue, often are used to note treated and untreated areas. The completed chart is a written and legal record.

Assorted styles of charts are used in this process. All charts number the teeth for abbreviation and organization. The three generally accepted methods of tooth numbering used in charting tooth conditions are:

1. *Universal.* Each adult tooth has a number from 1–32, and the deciduous teeth range from A to T. Assessment begins at the maxillary right third molar (#1), progresses along the arch to the maxillary left third molar (#17), and then down to the mandibular left third molar (#17) and back across to the mandibular right third molar (#32). The deciduous teeth follow the same pattern, using letters instead of numbers.

2. *Palmer.* Teeth are numbered 1–8 with a bracket indicating quadrant location. Each central incisor is tooth #1, and the quadrant signal indicates which quadrant. Deciduous teeth are lettered A (central incisor) to E (second molar) with a quadrant indicating bracket.

3. *Federation Dentaire Internationale (FDI).* Teeth are numbered in the same manner as the Palmer method but with no quadrant sign. Instead of brackets, a number prefix of 1 to 4 indicates the quadrant. The deciduous prefix quadrant numbers are 5 to 8.

Radiographs, commonly called x-rays, are normally taken at the initial appointment and are considered part of the patient's usual dental records. Radiology examination may discover maladies in the bone and hard tissues of the mouth, such as retained roots, unerupted teeth, missing tooth buds, cysts, and other difficulties. Radiographs are discussed in Chapter 9, Radiography.

ALIGINATE IMPRESSIONS

Impressions of the patient may be completed during the initial visit. The most common material used to make teeth impressions is **alginate** (**AL**-jih-nate = *seaweed, agar-based impression material*). Several terms are used to describe working with this material and the process of taking impressions.

negative reproduction: impression of the teeth in which each cusp or protrusion in the tooth is now a dent in the impression material.

positive cast: a gypsum reproduction of the patient's mouth; also called a **study model** (see Figure 7-5). This reproduction may be used for diagnosis or preparation of treatment plans. A reproduced cast has two parts:

anatomical portion: part of the cast that reproduces the teeth and gingiva.
art portion: part of cast that is added to make an esthetic base support.

bite registration: a piece of wax material or commercial pad that is placed into the patient's mouth; when the patient bites down on it, it registers the occlusion

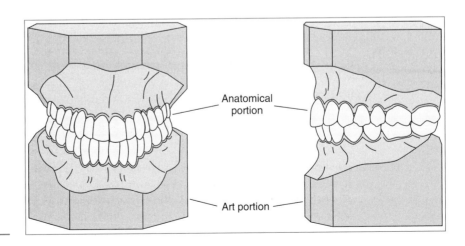

Anatomical portion

Art portion

FIGURE 7-5
Study models.

pattern that is used to put the models together to imitate the patient's normal bite position.

articulation (are-**tick**-you-**LAY**-shun; articulatus = *jointed*): placement of positive casts into the patient's bite or articulating position.

HOME PREVENTIVE TECHNIQUES

After examination and charting, dental personnel may instruct the patient in **prevention education,** including demonstrations of proper toothbrushing and flossing, information on diet correction, or whatever a specific existing problem indicates for home treatment. Preventive treatment also may be performed in the dental facility. Use of fluoride, a tooth strengthener, is encouraged. Terms related to fluoride use include:

regulated fluoride use: regular intake or use of fluorinated water and vitamins, and uses of mouthwashes and toothpastes containing fluoride.

fluorosis (floor-**OH**-sis = *excessive fluoride ingestion*): condition that can cause molting and discoloration of enamel tissue.

systemic fluoride: fluoride that is taken orally, in the water supply, in drops, or in vitamins.

ingestion (in-**JEST**-shun = *taking into gastrointestinal tract*): taking a substance into the gastrointestinal tract.

topical fluoride: fluoride that is placed upon the tooth surfaces, such as liquids, gels, and pastes.

Miscellaneous Prevention Aids

Dental personnel also may recommend the use of additional home prevention aids to eliminate decay and gingival problems.

rinse: anti-plaque mouth rinses containing therapeutic chemicals may reduce the amount of a thin covering on the teeth called plaque.

mouthwash: breath freshening rinses may reduce the **acquired pellicle** (**PELL**-ih-kal; pellicula = *little skin*) on the tooth surfaces.

disclosing dyes: red/blue food coloring or a sodium fluorescein solution that is placed upon tooth surfaces to disclose or stain the acquired pellicle or plaque.

powered toothbrushes: electric or battery-driven devices used to clean the teeth; may have single or double heads, with or without self-contained dentifrices.

dentifrice (**DEN**-tih-friss): tooth powder or toothpaste used to clean teeth and prevent **halitosis** (bad breath).

floss holders and **threaders:** devices used to hold or insert floss under bridgework and between teeth; floss may be waxed, unwaxed, colored, flavored, or plain, and available in thin, regular, and extra-thick rope or tape style.

interdental brushes and **picks:** handles that hold small brush tips to be inserted between the teeth and into sulcus areas. Small battery-powered floss and interdental appliances have been developed to perform this work.

wooden picks or flat balsam wedges: used to stimulate interproximal gingival tissue circulation.

water irrigation machines: electrically powered water spray devices with pulsating tips to power-rinse interproximal areas and bridgework gaps.

Diet Plans

Diet modification lessons may be presented after the patient completes a diet evaluation form, the patient's diet diary of food eaten over a few days. Meals and snacks with fewer cariogenic (care-ee-oh-JEN-ick; carie = *decay*, genic = *start*), or caries-forming, properties may be suggested, along with instructions in how to balance the diet, in keeping with a food pyramid of values.

▌ DENTAL FACILITY PREVENTIVE PRACTICES

The dental facility may provide some professional decay-prevention procedures throughout the patient's treatment. These include:

fluoride application: professional application of fluoride in the form of liquid, gel, foam, or varnish to tooth surfaces. The fluoride is placed on cleaned tooth surfaces, timed, and removed. After 30 minutes or more, the fluoride is rinsed off.

sealant application: placement of gel or liquid acrylic material on clean and prepared (acid-etched) occlusal surfaces of teeth to cover and protect tooth surfaces; sealant may be clear or tinted, auto- or self-cured, or may require ultraviolet light to set or become hard.

selective adjustment: deep occlusal pits or fissures eliminated by selective abrasive or grinding of some enamel surfaces, thereby lessening the chances of deep carious lesions; also called enamoplasty.

▌ REVIEW EXERCISES

MATCHING

Match the following word elements with their meaning:

1. _____incipient caries
2. _____fluorosis
3. _____cheilosis
4. _____pulpitis
5. _____cariogenic
6. _____erosion
7. _____complex cavity
8. _____ausculate
9. _____glossitis
10. _____lesion

a. decay of more than two surfaces
b. chemical wearing away of tooth surfaces
c. new tissue growth
d. inflammation of the tongue
e. mottled enamel
f. inflammation of pulp tissue
g. candidiasis of oral mucosa
h. beginning decay
i. listening to movement
j. abscess in tissues surrounding tooth

11. _____neoplasm

12. _____thrush

13. _____philtrum

14. _____periodontal abscess

15. _____bruxism

k. grinding of teeth, especially in sleep

l. inflammation of the lips

m. caries-forming foods

n. injury, wound, or altered tissue

o. median groove on external edge of upper lip

DEFINITIONS

Using the selection given for each sentence, choose the best term to complete the definition.

1. Foods that encourage the development of dental caries have been termed:
   a. sugar-coated
   b. dentocarious
   c. cariogenic
   d. caries

2. The system of tooth numbering associated with a different number from 1–32 for a tooth is:
   a. Universal
   b. Palmer
   c. Federation Dentaire
   d. National Internationale

3. Which of the following is not considered a decay-prevention procedure:
   a. tooth whitening
   b. sealant application
   c. selective adjustment
   d. enamoplasty

4. Which of the following is not considered an item for the health history:
   a. insurance coverage
   b. allergies
   c. past surgeries
   d. medical doctor's name

5. Which type of reproduction is an impression of the human dentition?
   a. positive
   b. negative
   c. neutral
   d. central

6. Another word for widespread decay is:
   a. rampant caries
   b. recurrent caries
   c. arrested caries
   d. incipient caries

7. Another term for gum abscess is:
   a. periapical calculus
   b. periapical abscess
   c. subgingival decay
   d. fibroma

8. Pus from an abscess may escape from the sub-gingival area into the mouth through a/an:
   a. abscess drain
   b. hypogingival fissure
   c. fistula
   d. transferral

9. Inflammation of the pulp tissue, leading to necrosis is called:
   a. hyperemia
   b. pulpalgia
   c. pulpitis
   d. septicemia

10. The tearing out or forcible removal of a tooth is:
    a. abrasion
    b. avulsion
    c. attrition
    d. alienation

11. The wearing away of tooth tissue through normal occlusion and wear is:
    a. abrasion
    b. avulsion
    c. attrition
    d. alienation

12. The wearing away of tooth structure from bad habits is:
    a. abrasion
    b. avulsion
    c. attrition
    d. alienation

13. Inflammation extending into connective tissue is:
    a. cellulitis
    b. gingivitis
    c. glossitis
    d. pulpititis

14. A viral disease that forms painful vesicles or watery pimples that burst and crust is:
    a. leukoplakia
    b. carcinoma
    c. herpes simplex
    d. thrush

15. Canker sores, occurring throughout the mouth, are also called:
    a. aphthous ulcers
    b. herpes simplex
    c. epulis
    d. fistulas

16. ANUG (acute necrotic ulcerative gingivitis) is also called:
    a. trench mouth
    b. periodontal abscess
    c. thrush
    d. trimus

17. Kaposi's sarcoma is a cancer disease linked with:
    a. tobacco rubbing   b. ANUG patients
    c. AIDS patients   d. cigar smoke

18. Tonic contraction of the muscles of mastication, caused by infection or inflammation, is:
    a. cellulitis   b. trismus
    c. epulis   d. tic

19. Which of the following tumors would be considered malignant?
    a. carcinoma   b. fibroma
    c. granuloma   d. neoplasm

20. Which of the following decay-prevention measures is *not* considered home therapy:
    a. brushing and flossing
    b. fluoride rinsing
    c. sealant application
    d. dyes

BUILDING SKILLS

Locate and define the prefix, root/combining form, and suffix (if present) in the following words:

1. **pulpalgia**
   prefix   _____
   root/combining form   _____
   suffix   _____

2. **pericoronitis**
   prefix   _____
   root/combining form   _____
   suffix   _____

3. **glossitis**
   prefix   _____
   root/combining form   _____
   suffix   _____

4. **cariogenic**
   prefix   _____
   root/combining form   _____
   suffix   _____

5. **asymmetric**
   prefix   _____
   root/combining form   _____
   suffix   _____

FILL-INS

Write the correct word in the blank space to complete each statement.

1. Decay that involves two surfaces of a tooth is called a/an _____cavity.

2. An increase in the pulp's blood, lymph vessels is called _____.

3. Decay occurring under or near the margins of a restoration is called a/an _____ cavity.

4. An aphthous ulcer is also called a/an _____ _____.

5. The disease, _____ is a degeneration of or a pressure on the fifth cranial nerve.

6. The disease, _____, appears as white patches on oral tissue and may become malignant.

7. Tooth fixation, due to heredity, disease, or constant trauma is called _____.

8. Inflammation and the degenerative breakdown of all periosteum tissues is called _____.

9. _____ is the imperfect meeting of teeth or improper occlusion.

10. An application of a/an _____ _____ is the placement of a clear or tinted acrylic material to the occlusal surfaces of newly erupted teeth.

11. Toothbrush, floss, floss threader, disclosing solution, water irrigation, perio picks, and the like are examples of _____ prevention aids.

12. A gumboil, or fibrous tumor of oral tissue is called a/an _____.

13. _____ herpes occurs in young children in the mouth or on the lips.

14. _____ is the loss of tooth surface in the cervical area caused by tooth grinding.

15. The term _____ is
    used when a cancerous tumor moves to
    another site and infiltrates the area.

16. Disorders in the joint union of the temporal
    and mandible bones is termed _____
    disorder.

17. A/an _____ is
    a connective tissue tumor.

18. The _____ portion of
    a study cast is the section that contains the
    teeth and gingival areas.

19. The charting system that numbers the teeth
    1-8 and uses brackets to designate quadrants
    is termed the _____
    method.

20. Red, blue, or fluorescent solutions used to
    dye or color plaque and acquired pellicle is
    called _____
    solutions or pills.

WORD USE

Read the following sentences and define the bold-faced words.

1. The **cellulitis** caused the patient's eye to swell
   so much that his eyes were almost totally
   closed.

   _____

2. **Dysphagia** may be one of the side effects
   when undergoing chemotherapy treatments.

   _____

3. Mrs. Sanchez asked the hygienist to
   recommend a new **dentifrice** for her.

   _____

4. The dentist advised Mrs. Jacobs to make an
   appointment for a **sealant application** for her
   son, Timmy.

   _____

5. The assistant took the laboratory report of the
   leukoplakia biopsy to the dentist
   and recorded the outcome on the patient's
   chart.

   _____

AUDIO LIST

This list contains selected new, important, or difficult terms from this chapter. You may use the list to review these terms and to practice pronouncing them correctly. When you work with the audio for this chapter, listen to the word, repeat it, and then place a checkmark in the box. Proceed to the next boxed word and repeat the process.

- ❏ abfraction (**ab-FRACK-shun**)
- ❏ abrasion (ah-**BRAY**-zhun)
- ❏ alginate (**AL**-jih-nate)
- ❏ ankylosis (ang-kill-**OH**-sis)
- ❏ aphthous (**AF**-thuss)
- ❏ articulation (are-**tick**-you-**LAY**-shun)
- ❏ asculate (awe-**SKUL**-ate)
- ❏ asymmetric (**ay**-sim-**ET**-rick)
- ❏ attrition (ah-**TRISH**-un)
- ❏ avulsion (ah-**VULL**-shun)
- ❏ bruxism (**BRUCK**-sizm)
- ❏ calculus (**KAL**-kyou-luss)
- ❏ carcinoma (kar-sih-**NO**-mah)
- ❏ caries (**CARE**-eez)
- ❏ cariogenic (care-ee-oh-**JEN**-ick)
- ❏ cellulitis (sell-you-**LYE**-tiss)
- ❏ cheilosis (kee-**LOH**-sis)
- ❏ commissure (**KOM**-ih-shur)
- ❏ dentifrice (**DEN**-tih-friss)
- ❏ dysphagia (dis-**FAY**-jee-ah)
- ❏ epulis (ep-**YOU**-liss)
- ❏ erosion (ee-**ROE**-zhun)
- ❏ fibroma (fie-**BROH**-mah)
- ❏ fistula (**FISS**-tyou-lah)

- ❏ fluorosis (floor-**OH**-sis)
- ❏ gingivitis (**jin**-jih-**VIE**-tis)
- ❏ glossitis (glah-**SIGH**-tiss)
- ❏ hemangioma (heh-**man**-jee-**OH**-mah)
- ❏ herpes (**HER**-peez)
- ❏ hyperemia (high-per-**EE**-mee-ah)
- ❏ injestion (**in-JEST-shun**)
- ❏ lesion (**LEE**-zhun)
- ❏ leukoplakia (loo-koh-**PLAY**-key-ah)
- ❏ lymphoma (lim-**FOH-**mah)
- ❏ metastasize (meh-**TASS**-tah-size)
- ❏ mucocele (**MYOU**-koh-seal)
- ❏ neoplasm (**NEE**-oh-plazm)
- ❏ neurofibroma (new-roh-fie-**BROH**-mah)
- ❏ palpate (**PAL-pate**)

- ❏ periapical (pear-ee-**APE**-ih-kahl)
- ❏ pericoronitis (pear-ih-kor-oh-**NIGH**-tiss)
- ❏ periodontitis (pear-ee-oh-don-**TIE**-siss)
- ❏ periodontosis (pear-ee-oh-don-**TOH**-sis)
- ❏ philtrum (**FILL**-trum)
- ❏ prophylaxis (pro-fih-**LACK**-sis)
- ❏ pulpalgia (pul-**PAL**-jee-ah)
- ❏ pulpitis (pul-**PIE**-tis)
- ❏ pyorrhea (pie-oh-**REE**-ah)
- ❏ sarcoma (sar-**KOH**-mah)
- ❏ sialoadenitis (**sigh**-al-oh-add-eh-**NIGH**-tis)
- ❏ symmetric (sim-**ET**-rick)
- ❏ tic douloureux (tic-**DOO**-loo-roo)
- ❏ trismus (**TRIZ**-mus)
- ❏ vermillion (ver-**MILL**-yon)

CHAPTER 8

Pain Management/ Pharmacology

Pain Management/ Pharmacology

OBJECTIVES   Upon completion of this chapter, the reader should be able to identify and understand terms related to:

1. **Description of pain and methods to relieve distress:** Discuss the meaning of pain and ways to relieve and control pain.

2. **Local anesthesia.** Explain the means of administering local anesthesia and identify the necessary equipment and injection sites.

3. **General anesthesia.** Explain the conditions for using general anesthesia, the methods used, stages of sedation, and the items used.

4. **Pharmacology and the science of drugs.** Define the study of drug agents, explain the difference between generic and brand names, and name the regulatory bodies that are concerned with drugs.

5. **Drug interactions with body functions.** Discuss how the body reacts when processing drugs and effects of drugs on the body systems.

6. **Drug forms and methods of distribution.** List and identify the various forms in which drugs are delivered.

7. **Routes for drug administration.** Identify the assorted routes, and give examples of drug administration.

8. **Drug prescription content.** Describe and explain the different parts of a drug prescription and the federal drug regulatory bodies that control drugs.

9. **Classifications and types of drug agents.** List and explain the assortment and classification or families of the common drugs.

DESCRIPTION OF PAIN AND METHODS TO RELIEVE DISTRESS

Pain has been described as physical or mental suffering or distress with a variety of sources. Pain may come from emotional factors, or it may be a reaction to injury, illness, or body sickness. Each person has an individual threshold of pain (ability to withstand pain) that is either **hypokinetic** (**high**-poh-kih-**NET**-ick; hypo = *under*, kinetic = *energy*), which is associated with high tolerance for pain, or **hyperkinetic** (**high**-per-kih-**NET**-ick; hyper = *over*; kinetic = energy), low tolerance for pain. The patient's concept of the intensity of pain is so important that it has been termed the **fifth vital sign**. Patients are requested to describe their pain in levels from 1 to 10 to determine a mean level.

Pain and anxiety are controlled and managed applying our current knowledge of medicine and techniques. The two main ways to control pain are:

anxiety abatement: control of emotional and stress factors through psychological methods such as hypnosis, relaxation management, distraction methods, vocal calming, and manners needed for dental treatment.

conscious sedation (see-**DAY**-shun): relaxation of mental and physical distress without loss of consciousness.

Relief of pain without the loss of consciousness is accomplished through:

pre-medication: medicine to depress the central nervous system (CNS) administered prior to treatment by mouth or by intramuscular or intravenous injection. Some anti-anxiety classifications of medications, with examples, are:

- ▶ **benzodiazepines** (ben-zoh-dye-**AZ**-eh-peens): *Xanax, Ativan, Librium, Valium, Halcion, Serax.*
- ▶ **barbiturates** (bar-**BIT**-you-rates): *Nembutal, Surital, Seconal, Amytal, Luminal, Mbaral.*
- ▶ **hypnotic:** *chloral hydrate, Equanil.*

T.E.N.S. (trancutaneous electrical nerve stimulations): device to send small electrical impulses to nerve endings to block pain signals.

analgesia (an-al-**JEE**-zee-ah): relaxation and sedation without loss of consciousness by inhalation of a combination of nitrous oxide and oxygen gas. A smaller-concentration formula will permit sedation, and the same gases in stronger concentrations will cause loss of consciousness and general anesthesia. Analgesic drugs are classified according to:

nonnarcotic drugs or nonopiod drugs: substances that have an effect on the peripheral nerve endings:

- ▶ **acetaminophens** (ah-seat-ah-**MIN**-oh-fens): used as an aspirin replacement for young children; has analgesic and **anti-pyretic** (an-tee-pye-**RET**-ick = *lower fever*) qualities (e.g. *Tylenol*).
- ▶ **salicylates** (sah-**LIH**-sil-ates): used as an analgesic, anti-pyretic, and anti-inflammatory; may be helpful in preventing myocardial infarction (**MI**). Supplied as regular aspirin (*Bayor, Empirin*), **enteric-coated** (en-**TARE**-ick = *to the intestinal tract*; *Ecotrin*), or with buffer chemicals added to reduce stomach upset (*Alka-Seltzer, Ascriptin*).
- ▶ **non-steroid anti-inflammatory:** analgesic, anti-pyretic, and anti-inflammatory: **ibuprofen** (eye-byou-**PROH**-efin) group (*Advil. Motrin*); or **naproxen** (nah-**PROX**-en) family (*Naprosyn, Anaprox*).

narcotic drugs or opiods (**OH**-pee-oyds): substances that depress the central nervous system (**CNS**), providing an altered perception of pain.

- ▶ Morphine (**MORE**-feen)
- ▶ Methadone (**METH**-ah-doughn; *Dolophine*)
- ▶ Meperidine (**MEP**-er-ah-dine; *Demerol*)
- ▶ Hydromorphine (high-droh-**MORE**-feen; *Dilaudid*)
- ▶ Oxycodone (ox-ee-**KOH**-done; *Percodan, Percocet, Roxipin, Tylox*)
- ▶ Pentazocine (pen-**TAZ**-oh-seen; *Talwin*)
- ▶ Codeine (**KOH**-deen; *Tylenol #3, Empirin #3*)
- ▶ Propoxyphene (pro-**POX**-eh-feen; *Darvocet*)

LOCAL ANESTHESIA

Local anesthesia (**an**-ess-**THEE**-zee-ah) (derived from two Greek words: an = *without* and athesia = *feeling*) is given while the patient is fully conscious. It blocks nerve endings from transporting pain messages to the brain. It can be differentiated as:

1. topical (*in a specific place*) analgesia: application of topical anesthetics to pain sites, to minor operative-procedure areas, and to places about to receive injections. Anesthetics in the form of cream, liquids, sprays, gels, and ointments are used to desensitize nerve endings and work only on mucous tissue. Two topical sprays used on skin tissue are *benzocaine* and *lidocaine*.
2. local (*limited to one place*) anesthesia: loss of sensation in a selected area.

Methods of Administration of Local Anesthesia

Local anesthesia is administered in several different ways:

infiltration (**inn**-fill-**TRAY**-shun = *passing into*) anesthesia: directed into the tissue near the nerve ending of the operative site, used for minor treatment, root planning, gingivectomy, and some tissue surgery.

regional or field anesthesia: around the nerve ending for anesthesia of a block of two or three teeth apices.

block anesthesia: injection into a nerve bundle to enable anesthesia to a wider area, such as the mandibular quadrant of teeth.

intraosseous (in-trah-**OSS**-ee-us = *into the bone structure*): directly into the spongy bone for a single tooth or multiple teeth in the same quadrant. It may be used for a patient who does not desire a fat lip or tongue. The perforation for the injection is made with a needle in the slow hand piece and placed directly into the cortical plate of the bone.

interpulpal (inter-**PUHL**-pahl): injecting directly into the pulp chamber using a long needle.

intraligamentory (in-trah-ligg-ah-**MEN**-tah-ree = intra = *within*, ligamentory = *ligament*), also called periodontal ligament injection: done mainly in the mandibular arch for one or two teeth in the same quadrant. The needle is

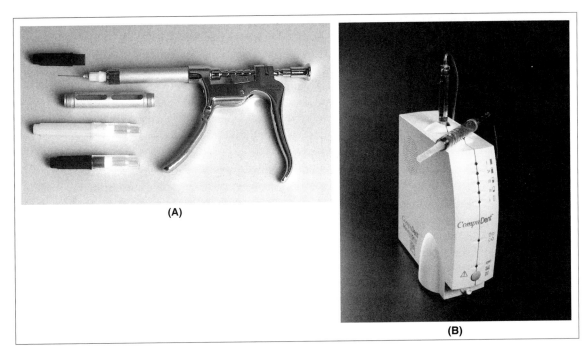

(A)

(B)

FIGURE 8-1

Two additional methods for delivering local anesthesia. (A) A Periodontal Ligament Injection Syringe. (B) Electronic-controlled Unit with a Local Anesthesia Injector ("The Wand").

placed into the sulcus along the long axis of the tooth using a pressure syringe (see Figure 8-1 A).

electronic controlled local anesthesia ("The Wand"): computer-controlled anesthetic-delivery system for subcutaneous or intramuscular local anesthetic and nerve blocks, consisting of a sterile disposable handpiece component and a computer control unit. The solution is delivered through a small needle in the connected handpiece and is controlled by an operator's foot pump. The computer regulates the amount and flow of the solution at a precise pressure dependent upon the tissue thickness and resistance. It is effective for all standard types of anesthetic injections plus dense palatal and periodontal ligament injection sites, see Figure 8-1 B.

Equipment Used for Local Anesthesia

Most local anesthetic injections are delivered using the basic equipment listed below:

anesthetic syringe: two types—plain and aspirating. The aspirating syringe has a harpoon on the plunger end to penetrate the rubber plunger in the carpule and provide suction to draw back the solution. It is the syringe of choice, as it is used to determine if the needle penetration has been placed in the proper site.

needle: size gauges 25, 27, and 30; the higher the number, the thinner the needle. The length of the needle typically is 1 inch for infiltration, or 1-⅝ inch for deeper penetration, as for a block injection. The **bevel** of the needle is the slant at the entry tip, and the **lumen** of the needle is the hole in the needle's shaft for the solution to pass through.

carpule (**CAR**-pule), also called cartridge: glass vial containing the anesthetic solution to be placed by the syringe; it is labeled with contents and has an aluminum cap, rubber plunger, and a diaphragm for puncture.

anesthetic solution: either of two types:

> ester: alcohol-based solution, such as procaine or propoxycaine.
> amide: water-based solution, such as lidocaine, prilocaine, articaine.

A **vasoconstrictor** (vas-oh-kahn-**STRICK**-tore), (vaso = *vessel*, constrictor = *tightener*) is a chemical (epinephrine) that is added to the anesthetic solution to constrict blood vessels, which allows less bleeding and longer anesthesia through **hemostasis** (hee-moh-**STAY**-sis) (hemo = *blood*, stasis = *stationary*). Epinephrine is added in various intensities from 1 drop of epinephrine to 50,000 drops of anesthetic solution (1:50,000), 1:20,000, 1: 100,000, 1: 200,000, or none added at all.

Complications with Local Anesthesia

Complications arising with local anesthesia include:

allergy: a reaction to the anesthesia.
anaphylactic shock: a reaction to the medication, delivery, or amount of anesthesia.
hematoma (he-mah-**TOE**-mah): blood swelling or bruise.
trismus (**TRIZ**-mus): grating or tonic contracting of the jaw, or muscle rigidity.
paresthesia (**pare**-ah-**THEE**-zee-ah): abnormal feeling occurring after anesthesia has worn off.

Common Local Anesthetics

Some local anesthetics commonly used in the dental office are:

▶ Benzocaine (topicals—**BEN**-zoh-kane; *Hurricane, Solarcaine*)
▶ Tetracaine (**TEH**-trah-kane; *Pontocaine*)
▶ Procaine (**PROH**-kane; *Novocain*)
▶ Propoxycaine (proh-**POCKS**-ih-kane; *Ravocaine*)
▶ Lidocaine (**LYE**-doh-kane; *Xylocaine, Octocaine*)
▶ Mepivacine (meh-**PIV**-ah-kane; *Carbocaine, Polocaine, Isocaine*)
▶ Bupivacaine (boo-**PIV**-ah-kane; *Marcaine*)
▶ Prilocaine (**PRIL**-oh-kane; *Citanest*)

Injection Sites for Local Anesthetics

Because anesthetic solution is to be placed into the oral tissues to produce a loss of sensation, the dental professional has to be aware of the location of these sites for

TABLE 8-1   Maxillary Arch Injections

TEETH OR TISSUE TO RECEIVE LOCAL ANESTHESIA	NERVE BRANCH INVOLVED	INJECTION SITE LOCATION
Individual teeth	Infiltration areas	Apex of tooth, near the mucobuccal fold.
Maxillary quadrant	Maxillary nerve block	Over the distal root of the maxillary molar. View U-1.
Centrals, laterals, and canines	Anterior superior alveolar	In mucobuccal fold between the canine and first premolar. View U-2.
Premolars, and mesial root of the maxillary first molar	Middle superior alveolar	In mucobuccal fold at the apex of the second premolar. View U-3.
Remaining maxillary molars and buccal molar tissues	Posterior superior alveolar	In mucobuccal fold at the apex of the second molar. View U-4.
Anterior block from canine to canine	Nasopalatine block	On palate near the incisive papilla. View U-5.
Hard palate	Greater anterior palatine	Palate near the second molar and greater palatine foramen. View U-6.

placement of topical anesthetic material. Proper placement provides for better anesthesia and less solution to be used. Injection sites are named after the specific nerve area that provides sensation. See Tables 8-1 and 8-2, as well as Figure 8-2, for these nerve sites.

TABLE 8-2   Mandibular Arch Injections

TEETH OR TISSUE TO RECEIVE LOCAL ANESTHESIA	NERVE BRANCH INVOLVED	INJECTION SITE LOCATION
Individual teeth	Infiltration areas	Near apex of individual teeth.
Mandibular quadrant	Inferior alveolar nerve	Posterior to the retromolar pad inside the mandibular ramus. View L-1.
Molar buccal tissues	Buccal nerve block	On the buccal side, distal to most posterior tooth. View L-2
Lingual tissue, side of tongue, molars to mid-quadrant	Lingual nerve block	Mandibular posterior lingual area, near mandibular ramus. View L-3.
Premolars, canine in quadrant	Mental nerve block	Between apices of mandibular premolars in mucobuccal fold. View L-4.
Premolars, canine, laterals, and centrals, lips, mucous membranes	Incisive nerve block	Anterior to the mental foramen in the mucobuccal fold. View L-5.

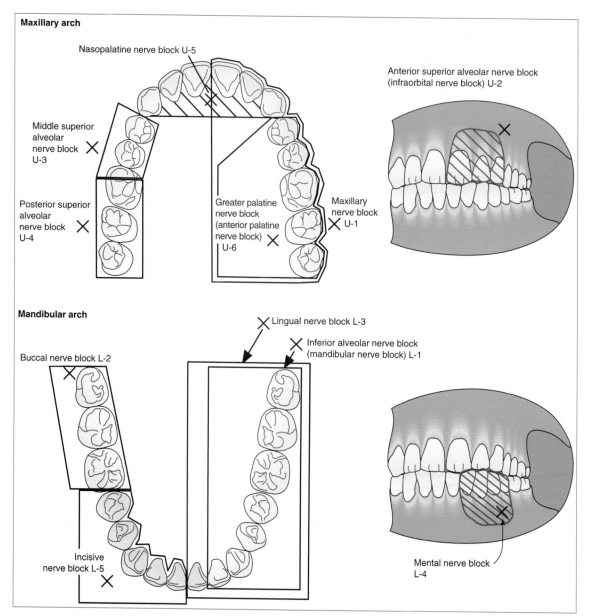

Maxillary arch

Nasopalatine nerve block U-5

Anterior superior alveolar nerve block
(infraorbital nerve block) U-2

Middle superior
alveolar
nerve block
U-3

Posterior superior
alveolar
nerve block
U-4

Greater palatine
nerve block
(anterior palatine
nerve block)
U-6

Maxillary
nerve block
U-1

Mandibular arch

Lingual nerve block L-3

Inferior alveolar nerve block
(mandibular nerve block) L-1

Buccal nerve block L-2

Incisive
nerve block L-5

Mental nerve block
L-4

FIGURE 8-2
Injection sites for
local anesthesia.

GENERAL ANESTHESIA

General anesthesia is the lack of pain and sensation in which the patient loses consciousness. Although the patient is capable of performing the auto-reflexes, the central nervous system has been temporarily depressed and does not respond to pain or sensations. General anesthesia may be administered by injection or by inhalation methods. The method used most commonly in the dental office is the inhalation of nitrous oxide and oxygen gas sedation.

Stages of Sedation

The four stages of anesthesia are:

Stage I—analgesia: a loss of sensation but conscious and able to carry on a conversation.

Stage II—excitement: loss of consciousness; the patient may experience delirium or become violent; blood pressure may rise and/or become irregular, breathing increases, and muscle tone heightens.

Stage III—surgical anesthesia: skeletal muscles relax, breathing becomes regular, eye movement stops. This stage has four planes or levels:

Plane I: light surgery stage
Plane II: moderate stage of surgery
Plane III: deep surgery
Plane IV: respiratory and circulatory dysfunction

Stage IV—medullary paralysis: not desired; breathing center and vital function stop working; death may ensue if patient is not revived immediately.

Other complications occurring with general anesthesia may be nausea, temporary dizziness from hypoxia (high-**POCK**-see-ah = *oxygen insufficiency in lungs and tissues*), drug interaction, organ dysfunction, and malignant hyperthermia, a reaction that may cause high fever, muscle rigidity, and fluctuations in heart and blood pressure rates.

Equipment Needed for Administration of General Anesthesia

Most facilities that administer general anesthesia have large tanks of nitrous oxide (blue) and oxygen (green) gases in a centrally located area, used with equipment to provide anesthesia. Relevant terminology is as follows.

anesthesia unit: equipment that receives and delivers gases by means of tubing and regulation devices to control anesthetic flow (see Figure 8-3).

pressure gauges: indicate the amount of gas pressure present within the cylinder tanks.

regulators: control the amount of gases coming from the central supply to the anesthesia stand.

flowmeters: control the amount of gas from the anesthesia unit to the patient.

nasal mask: placed over patient's nose to present gas into the body.

reservoir bag: may be used for hand-forced induction pressure of monitor to observe patient's breathing rate and force.

During the administration of general anesthesia, the operatory contains some important items:

emergency tray: a tray or box containing syringes and equipment necessary to deliver drugs or medicines for medical emergencies, such as vasodilators, anticonvulsives, stimulants, antihistamine, and so forth. An assortment of airway devices, such as endotracheal and nasopharyngeal tubes, a laryngoscope for viewing the larynx area, and suction equipment also are needed.

emergency plans and numbers: emergency transportation and phone numbers.

defibrillator: mechanical device to restore heart contractions.

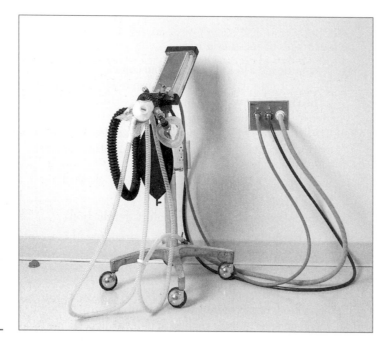

FIGURE 8-3
Portable anesthetic unit connected to wall ports for oxygen and nitrous oxide gases.

oximeter: monitoring equipment used to determine oxygen saturation in the blood.
patient records and history: current records of patient with history and condition.

If nitrous oxide and oxygen gases are not used to obtain general anesthesia, other available volatile liquids include ether, chloroform, **halothane** (**HAL**-oh-thane; Fluothane), **enflurane** (**EN**-floh-rane; Ethrane), and **isoflurane** (eye-soh-**FLUR**-ane; Forane).

General anesthesia agents given intravenously include opioids (Sublimaze, Sufenta, Alfenta), barbiturates (Pentothal, Brevital, Surital), and benzodiazepines (Valium, Versed), which are primarily used for sedation and preanesthesia. An intramuscular general anesthetic is **Ketamine** (**KEET**-ah-meen; Ketalar).

PHARMACOLOGY AND THE SCIENCE OF DRUGS

The use of drugs and medicines in operative treatment and care of the patients requires knowledge of drug agents and body reactions. The study of drugs and their effects is termed **pharmacology** (**far**-mah-**KAHL**-oh-jee). Each drug has a registered U.S. patented name, called the **brand** or **proprietary name**, and a **generic name**, the official name given by the U.S. Adopted Name Council. Drugs are regulated by the Food and Drug Administration (FDA), Drug Enforcement Administration (DEA), and the Federal Trade Commission (FTC).

Several books are excellent sources of information regarding drugs and medicinal products. These include the *Physician's Desk Reference*, commonly called the **PDR**, *United States Pharmacopedia*, *The Pill Book*, and *The Dental Therapeutic Digest*.

DRUG INTERACTIONS WITH BODY FUNCTIONS

Although drugs enter the body by various methods, each undergoes the same processing of the body organs and systems. Effectiveness of a drug depends on bodily processes involved in taking in (absorbing), distributing, using (metabolizing), and removing drugs from the body.

absorption: process in which fluids are transferred from the administration site by the circulating body fluids.

distribution: process of dividing and delivering the absorbed drug to the desired site.

metabolism (meh-**TAB**-oh-lizm): process of physical and chemical changes that enable the body to use the drug.

excretion (ecks-**KREE**-shun): process of elimination of waste products from the body.

Effects of Drugs on the Body

Drugs produce a variety of effects on the body, defined as follows:

adverse effect: response to a drug that is not desired because it is too intense, too weak, toxic, possibly allergic, or other effect. Also called a *side effect*.

addiction (ah-**DICK**-shun): compulsive, uncontrollable dependence on a drug to the extent that cessation causes severe physiological and emotional reactions.

allergy: specific body reaction to a drug, also termed *hypersensitivity*; can be the result of an antibody harbored in the patient's body.

anaphylaxis (an-ah-fill-**ACK**-sis): a life-threatening allergic reaction to a drug that may produce an immediate or a delayed body reaction; called anaphylactic shock.

antagonism (an-**TAG**-oh-nizm): opposite or contrary action of a drug.

dependence: physical (chemical) or psychological (desire) need to use a drug despite problems that may accompany it.

drug interaction: effect resulting from the combination of two or more drugs at one time.

idiosyncrasy (**id**-ee-oh-**SIN**-krah-see): unusual and abnormal drug response that may be genetic in nature or a result of an immune disorder.

intolerance (inn-**TAHL**-er-anse): inability of the body to endure a drug or the incapacity of a drug to achieve a desired effect because of long-term use.

overdose: effect from excessive drug dosage. A toxic dose resulting in systemic poisoning; and a lethal dose results in death.

side effect: reaction from a drug that is not the desired treatment outcome.

secondary effect: an indirect effect or consequence resulting from drug action.

synergism (**SIN**-er-jizm): harmonious action of two drugs to produce a desired effect. A drug may be added the original drug to enhance the properties of the original drug.

teratogenic (**tare**-ah-toh-**JEN**-ick; terato = *monster*; genesis = *production*): drug effects on a fetus—for example, thalidomide producing short limbs; tetracycline affecting tooth color.

┃FORMS OF DRUGS AND METHODS OF DISTRIBUTION

Drugs are supplied in various forms. Some medicines are prepared in more than one shape or form, and other drugs are available in only one specific preparation. A drug may be given in an injection to begin immediate protection and then have its action sustained by the ingestion of the same drug in pill form. The various methods of distribution of drug preparations are given in Table 8-3.

TABLE 8-3   Methods of Distribution of Drug Preparations

FORM	METHOD OF DISTRIBUTION	EXAMPLE
aerosol spray	drug solution suspended in and delivered by a propellant	inhaler, nasal spray
capsule	drug encased in gelatin shell, dissolved in the stomach	antibiotic (e.g., Ampicillin)
cream, balm	oil- and water-suspended emulsion	hydrocortisone, lip balm
elixir	sweetened, aromatic, hydroalcoholic solutions	phenobarbital elixir
emulsion	mixture of two liquids that are not mutually soluble	laxative preparations
intradermal implant	pellets or drug pack implanted under the skin for sustained slow release	estrogen (e.g., Norplant)
lozenge or troche	solid medicinal mass of drug, flavored for holding in mouth and slow dissolving of mass	cough, irritated throat
micropump	implanted device with timed release of drug	insulin
ointment	medicine suspended in fatty substance, cream	topical anesthetic (e.g., Betadine)
pill	compressed mass of drug powder	analgesic (e.g., Tylenol caplet)
solution	liquid containing dissolved drug	otic solution
spirit	volatile substance solution in alcohol	camphor, ammonia
suppository	medicated disc- or cone-shaped, wax-based form to be inserted into rectum or vagina for release	glycerin suppository
suspension	solution of liquid drug mixed with but not dissolved in	fluoride solution
syrup	drug mixed in sugary solution	cough syrup
tablet	small, disc-like mass of medicine powder	antibiotic (e.g., Ceclor)
tincture	diluted alcoholic solution of drug	Iodine tincture
transdermal patch	membrane backed patch containing drug dose, applied to skin for slow release	tobacco cease (e.g., Nicoderm)

ROUTES FOR DRUG ADMINISTRATION

The route and method of drug administration affect the action of a medication. The onset, or start, of the drug effect and the length of its effect—its duration—depend on its method of entry into the body. Intravenous (IV) is the quickest method, and rectal entry is the most ineffective method.

The potency (**POH**-ten-see = *strength*) and efficacy (**EFF**-ih-kah-see = *intensity*) of a drug also are affected by the route of administration. Drugs may be taken into the gastrointestinal tract by the oral or rectal route. These methods are termed enteral (**EN**-ter-ahl = *into the intestines*), and other methods, such as injections, bypass the GI system and are called parenteral (pair-**EN**-ter-ahl = *opposite the intestines*).

Methods of Drug Administration

The various ways to administer drugs are presented in Table 8-4.

DRUG PRESCRIPTION CONTENT

Some drugs can be purchased at the corner drugstore or the health and beauty section of the supermarket. The drugs are termed over-the-counter (OTC). Other drugs require a prescription to obtain and are carefully monitored by local, state, and federal governments.

TABLE 8-4   Methods of Drug Administration

ABBREVIATION	ROUTE OF ADMINISTRATION	METHOD OF ADMINISTRATION
PO	oral route	swallowing, ingesting medication
IV	intravenous	injection within a blood vessel
IM	intramuscular	injection into a muscle
SC, SQ	subcutaneous	injection into subcutaneous tissue
ID	intradermal	injection into the skin epidermis
IH	inhalation	breathing in of drugs, NO_2 gas
SUPPOS	rectal	insertion into rectum, suppository
IT	intrathecal (**in**-trah-**THEE**-kal)	within the spinal canal
	intraperitoneal (in-trah-**pare**-ih-toh-**NEE**-ahl)	within the peritoneal cavity
	topical	on the surface
	sublingual, buccal	under the tongue or side of cheek
	transdermal patch	applied to skin
	drug implant	surgical implant under skin

Government Control of Drugs

Various federal drug laws regulate how drugs are dispensed. These include:

Food, Drug, and Cosmetic Act (1906): FDC regulation of interstate drug business.
Harrison Narcotic Act (1914): control over narcotics and those prescribing narcotics.
Food, Drug and Cosmetic Act (1938): control of drug safety and effectiveness.
Durham-Humphrey Law (1952): labeling of drugs.
Drug Amendments (1962): changed **FDC** laws to require testing, reporting of adverse effects, use of generic names, and effects of drug.
Drug Abuse Control Amendments (1965): control of potential abuse drugs such as barbiturates and amphetamines.
Controlled Substance Act (1970): replaced former control acts and set the schedule for drugs.

The Controlled Substance Act in 1970 designated certain drugs as substances that require special oversight in their handling and distribution Table 8-5 gives the schedules or classifications of controlled substances.

The Drug Prescription

Most drug prescriptions look alike (see Figure 8-4). They may differ in the color or type of stationery and the type style, but the standard drug prescription must contain the following:

Heading   Name, address, and telephone number of the prescriber
Name, address, telephone number, and age of the patient
Date

TABLE 8-5   Schedules of Controlled Substances Act 1970

I	heroin, marijuana, LSD, hallucinogens	High potential for abuse No accepted medical use Experimental use, research
II	morphine, amphetamine, secobarbital, codeine, methadone, opium	High potential for abuse By prescription only, no refill
III	stimulants, sedatives	Moderate potential for abuse Prescription may be phoned No more than 5 refills in 6 months.
IV	depressants, diazepam (Valium, Darvon)	Less potential for abuse Same prescription requirements as Schedule III drugs
V	mixtures with limited opiates, cough syrups	Least potential for abuse; may include a few over-the-counter drugs (OTC)
All	Prescriptions for controlled substances require prescriber's DEA number (Drug Enforcement Administration identification number assigned to the prescriber)	

Superscription	Lester Payne, D.D.S.
	1000 Central Avenue
	Anytown, US 12345
	1-867-555-5667

For _____ Date _____

Address _____ Age _____

Rx

Inscription	Name and amount of drug =	Drug X tabs xx mg.
Subscription	Directions to the pharmacist =	Dispense xx tabs.
Transcription	Directions to the patient =	sig: 1 tab. as needed

_____ D.D.S.

D.E.A. #12345

FIGURE 8-4
Example of a standard drug prescription.

Body	Rx symbol
	Name, dose, size, or concentration of drug
	Amount to be dispensed
	Instructions to patient
Closing	Signature of prescriber
	DEA number (if required)
	Refill instructions

The prescription blank is further divided into four separate parts:

Superscription	Name, address, age of patient, date, and Rx symbol
Inscription	Drug name, dose form, and amount of drug
Subscription	Directions to the pharmacist
Transcription or Signature	Directions to the patient

CLASSIFICATIONS AND TYPES OF DRUG AGENTS

Drugs are classified according to their chemical content, drug manufacturer, and their intended effect or purpose. Listed below are some drug families that have not been mentioned but are concerned with or related to dental health.

Anti-Infective Drugs

An **anti-infective drug** is an agent that combats or destroys infections. These substances include antibiotic, antimicrobial, antifungal, and antiviral agents. There are two classes of anti-infectives, **prophylactic** (proh-fih-**LACK**-tick = *warding off disease*) and **therapeutic** (thair-ah-**PYOU**-tick = *healing agent*). The **spectrum** is the range of the drug's activity, and **resistance** is the ability of microorganisms to be unaffected by the drug. Both characteristics help to determine the choice of drug. The major anti-infective drugs are:

▶ **penicillin** (pen-ih-**SILL**-in): family of antibiotic drugs, such as penicillin G and V groups.
▶ **ampicillin** (am-pih-**SILL**-in; *Polycillin, Omnipen*).
▶ **amoxicillin** (ah-mocks-ih-**SILL**-in; *Amoxil. Larotid*).
▶ **erythromycin** (eh-rith-roe-**MYE**-sin; *E-mycin, ERYC, Erycette*).
▶ **tetracycline** (teh-trah-**SIGH**-klean; *Achromycin V, Sumycin*).
▶ **cephalosporin** (sef-ah-low-**SPORE**-in; *Keflex, Anspor, Cecelor, Ceftin, Suprax*).
▶ **topical antibiotics:** applied to the skin at the infection site (*Neosporin, Bacitracin*).
▶ **antiviral drugs:** agents that destroy or suppress the growth of viruses, such as herpes simplex, AIDS, influenza, and other viral diseases; supplied for oral, topical, IV or IM injection, cream, and aerosol use. Some dental-related antivirals are *Zovirax, IDU, Herplex*, as well as *AZT* and *Retrovir* in treatment of HIV.
▶ **antifungal drugs:** agents that destroy or hamper the growth or multiplication of fungi, such as *Mycostatin, Nilstat, Diflucan, Nizoral, Tinactin, Desenex*.

Cardiovascular Drugs

Cardiovascular drugs are agents employed for treatment of a variety of diseases of the heart and blood vessels. These include:

▶ **anticoagulants** (an-tie-koh-**AGG**-you-lants): delay or prevention of blood clots, coagulation. (*Heparin, Coumadin, Dicumarol*).
▶ **antihyperlipids** (an-tie-high-per-**LIP**-ids): decrease or prevent high blood plasma lipid, cholesterol (*Questran, Lipid, Colestid, Lopid, Zocor, Lipitor*).
▶ **antihypertensives** (an-tie-**high**-per-**TEN**-sivs): lower or decrease high tension (*Lopressor, Inderal, Capoten, Vasotec, Tenex, Apresoline, Prinvil, Procardia*).
▶ **antihypertensives with diuretic** (dye-you-**RET**-ick): drugs to increase secretion of urine (*Aldactone, Dyazide, Ser-Ap-Es, Lasix*).
▶ **angina pectoris** (an-**JYE**-nah **PECK**-tore-iss = *condition of pain or pressure around the heart*): treated with nitroglycerin, amyl nitrate (*Cardizem*).
▶ **arrhythmia** (ah-**RITH**-mee-ah = *absence of rhythm*: treated with *Rythmol, Inderal, Tonocard, Enkaid*.

Allergy Drugs

Drugs are used to treat allergies and other maladies related to the immune system are classified as:

adrenocorticosteroids (ah-dren-oh-**kor**-tih-koh-**STARE**-oyds = *byproducts secreted from the adrenal cortex*): drugs to treat inflamed conditions, allergies, and emergencies (examples: *Kenalog, Kenacort, Valisone*, and *Hexadrol*).

antihistamines (**an**-tie-**HISS**-tah-means = *drugs that counteract the effects of histamine*): (examples: *Benadryl, Dramamine, Chlor-Trimeton, Dimetane, Vistaril, Claritin*).

Anti-inflammatory Agents

Anti-inflammatory drug agents are used to relieve inflammation from arthritis and inflammatory conditions. They include *Celebrex, Clindoril, Feldene, Tolectin, Nalfon,* and *Indocin.*

Antidepressant Agents

Antidepressant drugs, used to treat depression, include SSRIs (Selective Serotonin Reuptake Inhibitors) such as *Prozac, Zoloft, Paxil, Luvox,* and *Celexa.*

Anticonvulsant Agents

Drugs used to control convulsions and seizures include *Phenobarbital, Dilantin, Zarontin, Valium,* and *Ativan.*

REVIEW EXERCISES

MATCHING
Match the following word elements with their meanings.

1. _____drug potency
2. _____quadrant
3. _____arrhythmia
4. _____hypokenetic
5. _____bevel
6. _____carpule
7. _____PO
8. _____IV
9. _____anesthesia
10. _____Rx
11. _____elixer
12. _____lumen
13. _____vaso-constrictor
14. _____analgesia
15. _____drug side effect

a. hole or opening in the anesthetic needle
b. underactive pain threshold—may withstand pain well
c. glass vial holding anesthetic solution
d. strength of a drug
e. slant of needle at the tip
f. oral route for drug administration
g. one-fourth area of the mouth
h. absence of rhythm
i. relaxation and sedation without loss of consciousness
j. recipe
k. without feeling
l. sweetened, aromatic water or alcohol solution
m. intravenous delivery of a drug
n. undesirable reaction from a drug
o. added to anesthetic to prolong effects

DEFINITIONS
Using the selection given for each sentence, choose the best term to complete the definition.

1. Which stage of general anesthesia is termed the excitement stage?
   a. Stage I   b. Stage II
   c. Stage III   d. Stage IV

2. The name, address, and age of the patient appears in which part of the prescription?
   a. heading   b. body
   c. salutation   d. closing

3. If a patient is able to easily withstand pain, it is said that patient has a:
   a. hyperkinetic threshold of pain
   b. hypokinetic threshold of pain
   c. sedation threshold of pain
   d. no threshold of pain

4. Which of the following anesthetic needles is thinnest?
   a. 25 gauge
   b. 26 gauge
   c. 27 gauge
   d. 30 gauge

5. An anesthetic solution that is water-based, such as lidocaine, is a member of which family?
   a. amide
   b. ester
   c. opiate
   d. petroleum

6. Morphine, opium, methadone, amphetamine, and secobarbital are examples of which schedule of controlled substances?
   a. I
   b. II
   c. III
   d. IV

7. A drug used to lower or decrease blood pressure is termed a/an:
   a. antihistamine
   b. anticoagulant
   c. antibiotic
   d. antihypertensive

8. A monitoring device that indicates the amount of oxygen level in the blood is called a/an:
   a. oximeter
   b. defibrillator
   c. sphygmomanometer
   d. thermometer

9. An injection into a nerve bundle to enable anesthesia to a wider area is called:
   a. block anesthesia
   b. field anesthesia
   c. topical anesthesia
   d. general anesthesia

10. A vasoconstrictor is added to an anesthetic solution to obtain which result?
    a. dilation of blood vessels
    b. increased blood supply to the area
    c. maintenance of current blood temperature
    d. decreased blood flow in the area

11. Medication given prior to surgery is termed:
    a. pre-medication
    b. post-medication
    c. surface medication
    d. surgery medication

12. Local anesthesia that is administered by placing a needle into the tooth sulcus with a pressure syringe is which type of anesthesia?
    a. intrapulpal
    b. intraosseous
    c. intraligamentory
    d. infiltration

13. Which of the following is not found in a dental anesthetic carpule?
    a. diaphragm
    b. aluminum cap
    c. harpoon
    d. rubber plunger

14. Anesthetic injections at the apex of the individual tooth are which type of anesthesia?
    a. infiltration
    b. block
    c. general
    d. intrapulpal

15. The process of dividing and circulating a drug throughout the body is termed:
    a. healing
    b. distribution
    c. metabolism
    d. absorption

16. Which drug preparation is used as an aspirin substitute for young children?
    a. histamine
    b. salicylate
    c. acetaminophen
    d. morphine

17. The loss of sensation but conscious and able to carry on a conversation describe the effects of a/an:
    a. local anesthetic
    b. general anesthetic
    c. analgesia
    d. antibiotic

18. If anesthesia of the side of the tongue is desired, which of the following nerves would be injected?
    a. maxillary middle superior alveolar
    b. maxillary greater palatine nerve
    c. mandibular mental nerve block
    d. mandibular lingual nerve block

19. The study of drugs and their effects is called:
    a. pharmacology
    b. pharmacopedia
    c. formulary
    d. therapeutics

20. A reaction to general anesthesia that causes high fever, muscle rigidity, fluctuations of the heart, and irregular blood pressure rates is called:
    a. malignant hypothermia
    b. malignant hyperthermia
    c. medullary paralysis
    d. delirium majoris

BUILDING SKILLS

Locate and define the prefix, root/combining form, and suffix (if present) in the following words.

1. **antihypertensive**
   prefix _____
   root/combining form _____
   suffix _____

2. **teratogenic**
   prefix _____
   root/combining form _____
   suffix _____

3. **pharmacokinetics**
   prefix _____
   root/combining form _____
   suffix _____

4. **intraligamentary**
   prefix _____
   root/combining form _____
   suffix _____

5. **infiltration**
   prefix _____
   root/combining form _____
   suffix _____

FILL-INS

Write the correct word in the blank space to complete each sentence.

1. Anesthesia that is placed in a specific area, prior to injection is called _____ anesthesia.

2. The mechanical device that sends electrical impulses to nerve endings to block pain signals is termed: _____.

3. A/an _____ anesthetic injection is placed directly into the pulp.

4. The anesthetic syringe that contains a harpoon in the barrel is called a/an _____ syringe.

5. The _____ is a drug's range of strength.

6. The symbol for intradermal applications of a drug is _____.

7. A blood swelling or bruise that may be a complication of local anesthesia is called a/an _____.

8. The process of eliminating waste products from the body is _____.

9. A periodontal ligament injection is also called a/an _____ injection.

10. _____ is an abnormal feeling that occurs after anesthesia has worn off.

11. Injection of local anesthetic to the anterior superior alveolar nerve branch will result in lack of sensation to the canines, laterals, and _____.

12. The surgical anesthesia plane is the Stage _____ degree of anesthesia.

13. An indirect effect or consequence from drug action is a/an _____.

14. The _____ is a part of the anesthesia unit that may be squeezed to provide positive pressure for gases to enter the lungs.

15. To anesthetize the mandibular premolars and canine in the same quadrant, the operator must inject near the _____ block area.

16. The physical or psychological need or desire for a drug is termed _____.

17. The _____ anesthetic syringe is considered the syringe of choice to enable the dentist to draw back during the injection to test the proper site penetration.

18. A/an _____ is placed over the patient's nose during the application of general anesthesia.

19. _____ is considered by many to be the fifth vital body sign.

20. An injection placed around the nerve ending that will desensitize two or three teeth apices is termed a/an _____ anesthetic injection.

WORD USE
Read the following sentences and define the bold-faced words.

1. When placing drugs in storage, the assistant must take precautions to ensure that the **potency** of the drug will not be affected.

   _____

2. The recently ordered **defibrillator** has been delivered and is being readied for use.

   _____

3. One of the most dreaded emergencies in the dental office is **anaphylactic shock.**

   _____

4. The dental personnel make it a practice to use **anxiety abatement** in dealing with every patient. _____.

5. Prior to surgery, the doctor prescribed an antibiotic as a **prophylatic** medicine for the patient. _____.

AUDIO LIST

This list contains selected new, important, or difficult terms from this chapter. You may use the list to review these terms and to practice pronouncing them correctly. When you work with the audio for this chapter, listen to the word, repeat it, and then place a checkmark in the box. Proceed to the next boxed word and repeat the process.

❑ acetaminophen (ah-seat-ah-**MIN**-oh-fen)
❑ addiction (ah-**DICK**-shun)
❑ adrenocorticosteroids (ah-dren-oh-**kor**-tih-koh-**STARE**-oyds)
❑ analgesia (an-al-**JEE**-zee-ah)
❑ anaphylaxis (an-ah-fill-**ACK**-sis)
❑ anesthesia (an-ess-**THEE**-zee-ah)
❑ angina pectoris (an-**JYE**-nah **PECK**-tore-iss)
❑ antagonism (an-**TAG**-oh-nizm)
❑ anticoagulants (an-tie-koh-**AGG**-you-lants)
❑ antihistamines (an-tie-**HISS**-tah-means)
❑ antihyperlipid (an-tie-high-per-**LIP**-ids)
❑ antihypertensives (an-tie-high-per-**TEN**-sivs)
❑ arrhythmia (ah-**RITH**-mee-ah)
❑ carpule (**CAR**-pule)
❑ diuretics (dye-you-**RET**-icks)
❑ efficacy (**EFF**-ih-kah-see)
❑ enflurane (**EN**-floh-rane)
❑ enteral (**EN**-ter-ahl)
❑ enteric (en-**TARE**-ick)

❑ excretion (ecks-**KREE**-shun)
❑ halothane (**HAL**-oh-thane)
❑ hematoma (hee-mah-**TOE**-mah)
❑ hemostasis (hee-moh-**STAY**-sis)
❑ hyperkinetic (**high**-per-kih-**NET**-ick)
❑ hyperthermia (high-per-**THER**-mee-ah)
❑ hypokinetic (**high**-poh-kih-**NET**-ick)
❑ hypoxia (high-**POCK**-see-ah)
❑ ibuprofen (eye-byou-**PROH**-fen)
❑ idiosyncrasy (**id**-ee-oh-**SIN**-krah-see)
❑ infiltration (in-fill-**TRAY**-shun)
❑ interpulpal (inter-**PUHL**-pahl)
❑ intolerance (inn-**TAHL**-er-anse)
❑ intraligamentary (in-trah-**ligg**-ah-**MEN**-tah-ree)
❑ intraosseous (in-trah-**OSS**-ee-us)
❑ intraperitoneal (**in**-trah-**pare**-ih-toh-**NEE**-ahl)
❑ intrathecal (**in**-trah-**THEE**-kal)
❑ isoflurane (eye-soh-**FLUR**-ane)
❑ metabolism (meh-**TAB**-oh-lizm)
❑ naproxen (nah-**PROX**-en)

- ❑ opiod (**OH**-pee-oyd)
- ❑ parenteral (pair-**EN**-ter-al)
- ❑ paresthesia (**pare**-ah-**THEE**-zee-ah)
- ❑ pharmacokinetics (**far**-mah-koh-kih-**NEH**-ticks)
- ❑ pharmacology (**far**-mah-**KAHL**-oh-jee)
- ❑ potency (**POH**-ten-see)
- ❑ prophylactic (proh-fih-**LACK**-tick)
- ❑ proprietary (pro-**PRY**-eh-tare-ee)

- ❑ salicylates (sah-**LIH**-sil-ates)
- ❑ sedation (see-**DAY**-shun)
- ❑ synergism (**SIN**-er-jizm)
- ❑ teratogenic (**tare**-ah-toh-**JEN**-ick)
- ❑ therapeutic (thair-ah-**PYOU**-tick)
- ❑ topical (**TAH**-pih-kahl)
- ❑ trismus (**TRIZ**-mus)
- ❑ vasoconstrictor (vas-oh-kahn-**STRICK**-tore)

Radiography

OBJECTIVES

Upon completion of this chapter, the reader should be able to identify and understand terms related to:

1. **Definition and production of x-rays.** Define the principle of radiant energy and discuss how these x-rays, or Roentgen rays, are generated.

2. **Properties of Roentgen rays.** Identify the perils of radiation and describe the various effects on the body.

3. **Radiation protection.** List and give examples of acceptable methods for radiation protection in the dental facility.

4. **Composition, types, and qualities of dental radiographs.** Discuss the composition of film packets. Describe the various types of dental radiographs available and the qualities necessary for diagnosis.

5. **Techniques for exposing radiographs.** Identify the methods used to expose various dental radiographs.

6. **Radiographic film processing.** Describe the methods used to produce a processed dental radiograph.

7. **Mounting radiographs.** Discuss the types of radiograph mounts and the system used to place processed films.

8. **Assorted radiographic errors.** List and describe common radiographic errors and the causes of each.

DEFINITION AND PRODUCTION OF X-RAYS

X-rays are **radiant** (**RAY**-dee-ant) energy waves that are produced, charged, and emitted from a common center in the dental radiation tube. These highly active, penetrating waves of charged electrons are tiny energy bundles or waves of photons with extremely short wavelengths that are able to penetrate matter and expose photographic film surfaces. When first discovered by Wilhelm Conrad Roentgen

(**RENT**-gen) in 1895, they were termed x-rays, but in many places today they are called *Roentgen rays* in his honor. The resulting film image is called an x-ray or a radiograph. This type of radiant energy is considered "hard" radiation, as contrasted with "soft" radiation, such as microwaves, luminous dials on clocks, and so forth.

How X-rays Are Generated

The **x-ray tube**, also known as a *vacuum tube*, produces x-rays (see Figure 9-1). The vacuum tube contains these seven elements of note.

cathode (**KATH**-ode = *negative pole*): electrode in the vacuum tube that serves as the electron source.

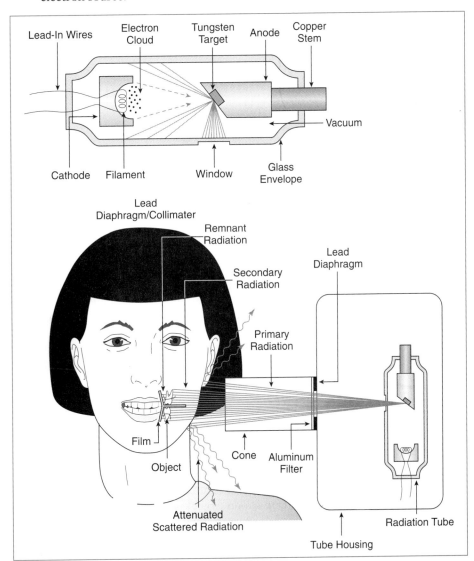

FIGURE 9-1

Internal view of a typical x-ray tube and examples of radiation.

filament (**FILL**-ah-ment = *fine thread*): tungsten coil in the cathode focusing cup that generates the electrons.

anode (**ANN**-ode = *positive pole*): the target for the electron barrage to convert the electron force into photons.

focal spot: target area where rays are projected to make the primary beam, or *central beam*; the smaller focal spot produces a better image.

collimator (**KAHL**-ih-**may**-tore = *to align*): a device used to regulate the beam's exit from the tube into parallel rays and to avoid stray radiation; usually made in a lead washer on the connecting end of the **PID** (*position indicating device*) that also has lined walls to assist collimation.

aperture (**AP**-er-**chur** = *opening* or *port*): opening in the lead collimator disk that regulates the size of the primary beam.

filter: aluminum disks that are placed between the collimator attachment and the exit window of the tube to absorb weak radiation. The types of filtration are:

> inherent filtration: all filtration (tube wall, insulating oil, aluminum disks) devices that filter weak, longer-wavelength x-rays.
>
> added filtration: filtration placed outside the tube head to meet safety standards.
>
> total filtration: sum of inherent and added filtration, expressed in mm of aluminum equivalent.

Control Factors in X-ray Generation

The production and the generation of x-rays in the tube head are affected by regulating conditions that are set on the control panel. Each of the following factors affects the outcome of the radiation.

milliampere control (**mil**-ee-**AM**-peer = *one-thousand of an ampere* [electric current]), abbreviated as mA): also known as *milliameter*; an increase in milliamperage increases the amount of electrons available and darkens the radiograph.

kilovolt power (**KILL**-oh-volt = *1000- volt unit*, abbreviated as kVp): controls the force that attracts the electrons to the anode; helps to determine the penetrating power and the quality/energy of the radiation rays.

exposure time: duration of the interval during which current will pass through the x-ray tube; this period may be stated as fractions of a second or *impulses* (60 pulses to a second). The amount of exposure that a patient actually receives is measured in milliampere seconds (mAs) (mA × exposure time = mAs).

target-film distance (source-film distance, or focus-film distance): distance of the film surface from the source of radiation (target or focal spot).

target-object distance (source-object distance, or focus-object distance): distance between the anode target and the object to be radiographed.

film speed: A (slowest) to F (fastest) speed; faster film requires less radiation exposure time for the patient.

Types of X-ray Radiation

Different types of x-ray radiation are generated during radiography (see Figure 9-1).

primary radiation: central ray of radiation emitting from the tube head and PID. Primary radiation is the desired radiation and is used to expose radiographic film.

secondary radiation: radiation given off from other matter that is exposed to the primary beam.

scattered radiation: radiation deflected from its path during its passage through matter; may be deflected or defused in all directions, becoming attenuated (weakened) or another form of secondary radiation.

stray radiation: also called *leakage*, any radiation other than the useful beam produced from the tube head. A faulty or broken tube head may be the source of stray radiation.

remnant radiation: radiation rays that reach the film target after passing through the subject part being radiographed. These rays form the latent image on the film emulsion.

PROPERTIES OF ROENTGEN RAYS

Roentgen rays are considered hazardous and dangerous to the body tissues. x-radiation is made possible by producing ions. An **ion** (**EYE**-on = *going*) is a particle that carries an electrical charge. This unbalanced atom particle may attempt union with body cell atoms, causing *ionizing radiation*, or a change in cell structure that has a variety of effects.

sensitivity: ability of x-rays to penetrate and possibly ionize. The reproductive cells (*genetic*) are more radiosensitive than the radioresistant body tissues (*somatic* cells). Younger cells are more sensitive than older, thicker cells.

cumulative effect: long-term outcome of radiation. Repetition increases and intensifies the ionizing effect on cells for a buildup of damage. The latent period of exposure is the time interval between the exposure and the effect or its detection.

mutation (**myou-TAY-shun**) effect: abnormal growth or development as a result of radiation causing a genetic change.

Types of Exposure

The two types of x-radiation exposure that will damage the body cells are:

1. acute radiation exposure: radiation occurring from a massive, short-term ionizing dose, such as accidental exposure or explosion of radiation material.
2. chronic radiation exposure: accumulated radiation effects from continual or frequent small exposures absorbed over a period of time (thus the need for questioning the patient as to when the last x-ray was taken).

RADIATION PROTECTION

Among the methods of protection against overexposure of x-radiation are:

ALARA (*as low as reasonably achievable*): a policy of using the lowest amount of radiation exposure possible. Measures to accomplish this include proper exposure-protection aids, good techniques, and the proper calculations or control settings.

maximum permissible dose (MPD): highest rate of exposure permissible for the occupationally exposed person. The formula for calculating this factor is (5 rem per year) – [age −18] × 5 rem per year = MPD.

Roentgen (R) (international unit is *coulomb per kilogram* [C/kg]): the basic unit of exposure to radiation; the amount of x-radiation or gamma radiation needed to ionize 1 cc of air at standard pressure and temperature conditions.

rad (radiation absorbed dose) (international unit is *gray* [*Gy*]): the unit of absorbed radiation dose equal to 100 ergs (energy units) per gram of tissue.

rem (roentgen equivalent measure) (international unit is *sievert* [*Sv*]): the unit of ionizing radiation needed to produce the same biological effect as one roentgen (R) of radiation.

erythema (air-ih-**THEE**-mah = *redness*) dose—radiation overdose that produces temporary redness of the skin.

Safety Precaution Items

When exposing x-rays, the use of radiation safety apparel and devices is critical. These items include:

dosimeter (doh-**SIH**-meh-ter = *giving measure*): radiation-monitoring device with ionizing chamber or a device to indicate exposure and measure accumulated doses of radiation; available in the form of a film badge, pen, ring, etc.

lead apron/thyrocervical collar: patient apparel with lead protection for genetic (sex) cells in the torso and the thyroid glands in the cervical area (see Figure 9-2).

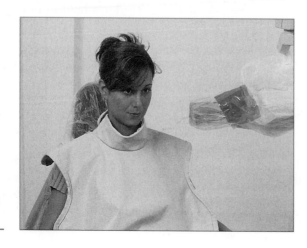

FIGURE 9-2
Lead apron /
thyrocervical collar
for protection from
radiation.

lead barriers, shields: devices used by operators to block out scattered radiation.

phantom (**FAN**-tum): practice manikin containing tooth and head structures to imitate actual condition. A popular model is DXTTR, affectionately called Dexter.

▌COMPOSITION, TYPES, AND QUALITIES OF DENTAL RADIOGRAPHS

Dental radiographs are composed of a celluloid base that supports an emulsion containing silver bromide, silver sulfide, and silver halide crystals. This emulsion is sensitive to light and x-rays and will record the radiographic image. Radiographs may be exposed within the oral cavity (intraoral) or outside the mouth (extraoral). Most intraoral dental film packets contain one film, but they also are supplied in double film packets. There are several basic kinds of dental films.

periapical film packet: size 0 (pedodontic size), 1 (adult anterior), or 2 (adult posterior); used for the intraoral periapical view of the entire tooth or teeth in a given area along with adjacent tissues and oral structures. This film also may be placed in a device to expose an intraoral bitewing view and may be ordered in a double film packet, if desired.

bitewing film packet (also known as interproximal radiograph, size 3): film used to record the crown and interproximal views of both arches while in occlusion; used intraorally. Other films sizes may be adapted to accomplish this task.

occlusal film packet, size 4: film that may be used intraorally or extraorally to expose large areas (2¼″ × 3″). These film packets may contain more than one film and are marked and color-coded to identify the amount of film enclosed.

extraoral films: radiographs exposed outside the oral cavity; larger in size and loaded in a film cassette or wrapped for protection from light rays.

cephalometric (**seff**-ah-low-**MEH**-trick; cephal = *head*, metric = *measure*): also called headplates. These extraoral radiographs of the head are used in orthodontic, oral surgery, and sometimes in prosthodontic dentistry.

cephalostat (**SEFF**-ah-loh-stat): a device used to stabilize the patient's head in a plane parallel to the film and at right angles to the central ray of the x-ray beam. It is used for large radiographs of the head.

panoramic radiograph: a special radiograph producing the entire dentition with surrounding structures on one film. The extraoral film is placed in the machine's cassette and rotates around the patient at the same speed as the tubehead rotation, providing a panorama view. It is in popular use in orthodontics and oral surgery.

intensifying screen: a layer of fluorescent crystals or calcium tunstate within the cassette that gives off a bluish light when exposed to radiation. This light and radiation form latent images on the film faster, thereby reducing exposure time.

Diagnostic Qualities for Dental Radiographs

Dental radiographs must exhibit certain qualities to be effective. Relevant terminology is defined and explained in the following:

contrast: variations in shades from black to white. A radiograph exhibiting many variations in shades is said to possess "long-scale contrast." Increased kilovoltage helps to produce this effect.

density: amount of film blackening associated with the percentage of light transmitted through a film. An increase or decrease in density is easily accomplished by an increase or decrease in milliamperage and exposure time (mA/second).

detail: point-to-point delineation or view of tiny structures in a radiograph image. Proper exposure, handling factors, and kVp selection provide good detail.

definition: outline sharpness and clarity of image exhibited on a radiograph. Movement of the film, patient, or tube head is the most common cause of poor definition or fuzzy outline, called **penumbra**.

radiolucent (**RAY**-dee-oh-**LOO**-sent; radius = *ray*, lucent = *shine*): describes a radiograph that appears dark; or the ability of a substance to permit passage of x-rays, thereby cause the radiographic film to darken.

radiopaque (**RAY**-dee-oh-**payk**; radius = *ray*, pacus = *dark*): the portion of the radiograph that appears light, or the ability of a substance to resist x-ray penetration, thereby causing a light area on the film.

TECHNIQUES FOR EXPOSING RADIOGRAPHS

The two basic methods used to expose intraoral radiographs are shown in Figure 9-3.

1. bisecting angle: The central x-ray beam is directly perpendicular with an imaginary bisecting line of the angle formed by the plane of the film and the long axis of the tooth. This technique is also called the *short cone technique*.
2. paralleling: The film packet is placed parallel to the long axis of the tooth and at a right (90-degree) angle to the central x-ray beam. This technique also is called the *extension cone* or *right angle technique*.

Two systems are used to acquire a direct digital dental image:

1. CCD (charged coupled device): a solid-state sensor that may or may not be wired to the computer work station, barrier-wrapped and inserted into a positioning device for placement and exposure in the mouth. Once the surface is exposed, the information is transported to the work station and an image is viewable.
2. PSP (photostimulable phosphor device): an indirect sensor storage plate that absorbs radiation to complete a latent image. The plate is placed in a barrier, a positioning device, and exposed. Instead of processing the plate like x-ray film, the plate is put through a processor that is placed into the scanner to transfer the image into the patient's dental records.

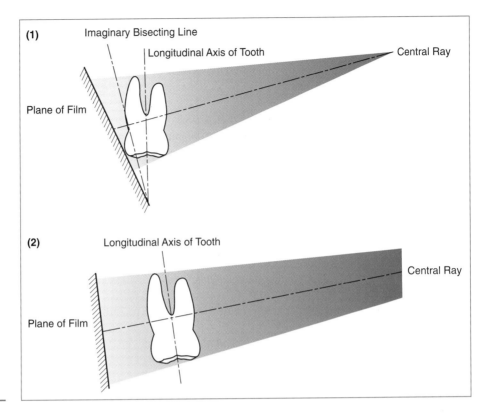

FIGURE 9-3
Two common methods of dental radiographic exposures. (1) bisecting angle technique (2) paralleling technique

Both methods reduce the patient's radiation exposure time. Also, the technology can be used for extraoral views.

Additional terminology includes:

indirect dental radiography digital image: x-ray image already processed by the usual method, scanned by an adapter in the database; or a digital camera can record a picture of the film and transfer the image to the database.

electronic image processing: operator's manipulation of the digital image, consisting of contrast, brightness, image reversal, embossing, and grayness to enhance, measure, compare, or obtain information.

digital subtraction radiography: digital comparison of the image to a previous radiograph, subtracting all that is the same and analyzing or comparing the remainder.

Positioning Terms for X-ray Exposure

Various positioning methods and angulations that affect the outcome of exposure are.

sagittal plane: also called midsaggital plane; imaginary vertical line bisecting the face into a right half and a left half; important during exposure to determine positioning of the patient.

ala tragus (ah-la-**TRAY**-gus) **line:** imaginary line from the ala (wing) of the nose to the tragus (skin projection anterior to acoustic meatus) center of the ear. This line is important for positioning the patient in the bisecting angle technique.

The angulation or positioning of the PID and the direction of the central beam are vital to the exposure technique.

horizontal angulation: direction of the central x-ray beam in a horizontal plane. The central beam must be placed perpendicular to the film front and teeth alignment. The error observed with improper horizontal angulation is called *overlapping* or *cone cutting*.

vertical angulation: direction of the central x-ray beam in an up or down position. Improper vertical angulation results in *foreshortening* or *elongation* errors.

negative angulation: angulation achieved by positioning the PID upward; also called *minus angulation*. Mandibular exposures are made with the PID in a negative or minus angulation.

positive angulation: angulation achieved by positioning the PID downward; also called *plus angulation*. Maxillary exposures are made with the PID in a positive angulation.

zero angulation: angulation achieved by positioning the PID parallel with floor.

Positioning Devices

Positioning devices are employed to help produce a good radiograph.

PID: position indicating device formerly called a *cone*; may be a *long cone* (12–16 inches) or a *short cone* (8 inches); may be a round or rectangular open-ended tube. It is used to collimate and direct the central beam, and determines the target-surface distance.

Film-holding instrument: device used to place and retain the film during exposure. Common sets are the *VIP (Versatile Intraoral Positioner)* by UpRad and the *Rinn BAI* for the bisecting angle technique; *XCP (extension cone paralleling device)*; *Rinn XCP-DS* for sensor use; and *Rinn XCP* for endodontic views (see Figure 9-4, View A). Locator or aiming rings are color-coded to designate area placement, as follows:

blue = anterior,
yellow = posterior,
red = bitewing,
green = endodontic

There are universal film holders for digital imaging. One system, Total Care, has been developed to maintain the digital sensors for x-ray exposure. It is composed of five holders: Kwik Bite Senso for bite wings; Super Bite Senso for anterior and Super Bite Senso posterior periapicals; Endo Bite Senso for anterior and Endo Bite Senso for posterior endodontic images (see Figure 9-4 View B for examples of this system).

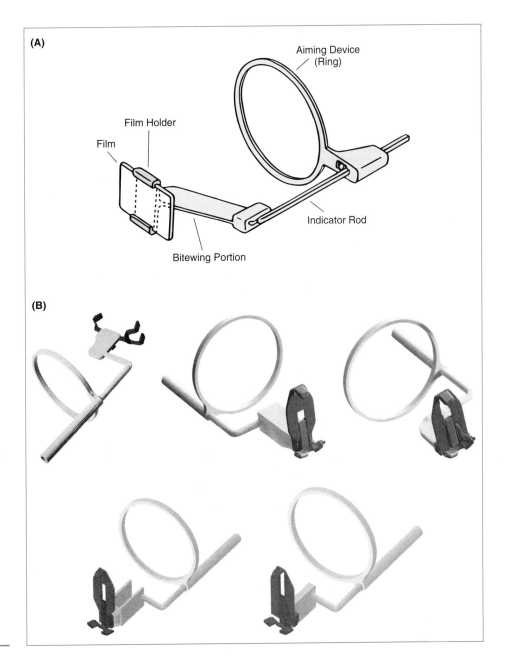

FIGURE 9-4
Examples of radiographic exposure holders. (A) film holder for parallel exposure (B) Total Care universal digital sensor holder system.

biteblock: a device inserted between the teeth to hold the film during exposure; made of foam, wood, or plastic.

bite loop/tab: paper tab or a celluloid circle placed around periapical film, enabling the film to be used in a bitewing position. This combination is used in place of a commercially manufactured interproximal film.

film safe container: a lead-lined container used to hold exposed films until processing; protects the film from exposure to scattered or secondary rays during exposure of films.

X-ray Surveys

Although x-rays may be taken to diagnose a specific tooth, most radiographs are taken in a survey or a combination of exposures. When placed in a mount, side by side, these multiple exposures reveal the condition of a large area. The amount and placement of a survey of exposures depends upon the nature of the dental visit and the problems encountered.

full mouth survey (FMX): multiple exposures of the oral cavity showing crown and root area in a series of radiographic views. When arranged in mounts these films give a survey or view of the condition of the entire mouth.

bitewing survey (BWX): two or four film exposures of posterior view to observe the crowns of maxillary and mandibular posterior teeth. Anterior bitewing exposure is also possible.

edentulous (ee-**DENT**-you-lus = *without teeth*) **survey:** radiographic survey of a patient without teeth.

▌ RADIOGRAPHIC FILM PROCESSING

After exposure of the dental film to radiation, the film must be processed or developed to present a picture of the existing conditions. **Radiograph processing** is a procedure for bringing out the latent image on a film and making the exposure permanent. The procedure involves developing, rinsing, fixing, washing, and drying. Processing may be completed in an automatic film processor or by manual methods in a processing tank.

developing: chemical process using the chemical elon to bring out contrast and another chemical, hydroquinone, to show contrast in films. Developing brings out the latent image on the film's silver halines that were affected or darkened by radiation.

accelerator: solution used to swell the film emulsion during the processing.

activator: solution used to aid other chemicals in the processing activity.

replenisher solution: super-concentrated developing solution that is added to the developing tank to restore fluid levels.

underdeveloping: insufficient processing with weak chemicals or incorrect time or temperature that results in light, difficult-to-view films.

overdeveloping: overprocessing that results in radiographs that are too dark and difficult to interpret.

rinsing: water bath used to remove chemical liquids from films during solution exchanges.

fixing: chemical process that stops the developer action and "fixes" the image, making it permanently visible.

hyposulfite or **hyposulfite of sodium:** chemical that removes exposed and unexposed silver grains from the film.

drying: procedure to dry films after the chemical and water baths.

safelight: special light or filtered light that can remain during the developing procedure.

duplicating radiograph: procedure utilizing a cabinet-like unit and special duplicating films to make a duplicate exposure of a processed radiograph for purposes of insurance, referral, or records.

MOUNTING RADIOGRAPHS

Once the dental films have been processed, they must be viewed and stored. To hold the films in place for viewing and later for patient records, the films are mounted. **Mounting,** also called *carding*, of radiographs is a procedure to arrange the processed radiographs in a cardboard, plastic, or stiff carrier to present a view of the oral cavity. Mounts have preset window openings, horizontal for posterior views and vertical for anterior shots. A mount may be obtained with various window arrangement.

horizontal window: preset window in the mount, used to place posterior films.

vertical window: preset window in the mount, used for placement of anterior films.

bitewing window: also called *interproximal* window, used to place bitewing exposures.

identification dot: preset pressed or raised area on the surface of the film. The rounded or convex view indicates the surface of film that faced the radiation source (facial side). The convex or inward dot view on the film indicates that the film surface was placed away from the tubehead or radiation source (lingual side).

viewbox: a box or wall-mounted frame with fluorescent lights behind a frosted glass plate; used to view x-rays.

ASSORTED RADIOGRAPHIC ERRORS

When dental radiographs have not been exposed properly or handled in a clean manner, a faulty film will result. This may cause the radiograph to be unreadable and require additional radiation exposure for a patient in a makeup film. Included among the various radiographic errors seen in the dental facility are:

elongation (ee-lon-**GAY**-shun): image of the tooth structure appearing longer than the actual size; caused by insufficient vertical angulation of the central ray (see Figure 9-5A).

foreshortening (fore-**SHORE**-ten-ing): tooth structures appearing shorter than their actual anatomical size; caused by excessive vertical angulation of the central ray (see Figure 9-5B).

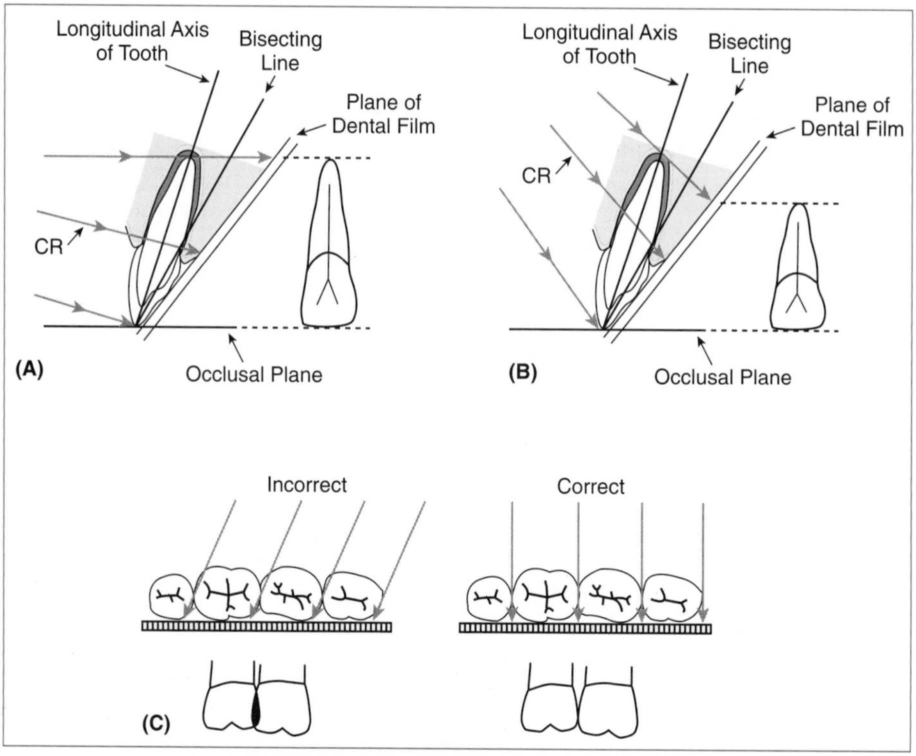

FIGURE 9-5
Examples of errors caused from improper angulation during exposure. (A) elongation of tooth image from too-low central ray angulation (B) foreshortening of tooth image from too-high central ray angulation (C) overlapping of tooth tissue caused by improper central ray angulation

overlapping: distortion of the film showing an overlap of the crowns of adjacent teeth superimposed on neighboring teeth; caused by improper horizontal angulation of the central ray (see Figure 9-5C).

cone cutting: improper placement of the central beam, which produces a blank area or unexposed area on the film surface caused by lack of exposure to radiation, such as when the PID is not centered properly on the film. A totally clear film indicates that no radiation has affected or exposed the film.

reticulation (ree-**tick**-you-**LAY**-shun): crackling of film emulsion caused by wide temperature differences between processing solutions. Reticulation gives a stained glass effect.

fog: darkening of or blemish on film that may be caused by old film, old or contaminated solutions, faulty safelight, scattered radiation, or improper storage of films.

penumbra: poor definition or fuzzy outline of forms, caused by movement.

herringbone effect: fish-bone effect on the film surface resulting from improper placement of the film. Radiographs placed in the mouth in a backward position exhibit a shadow impression of the lead foil backing in the visual image.

REVIEW EXERCISES

MATCHING
Match the following word elements with their meanings:

1. _____cathode
2. _____sensitivity of rays
3. _____indirect digital x-ray
4. _____detail
5. _____radiolucent
6. _____cephalometric
7. _____definition
8. _____sagittal plane
9. _____ala-tragus line
10. _____edentulous survey
11. _____aperture or port
12. _____reticulation
13. _____ion
14. _____elongation
15. _____biteblock

a. conversion of a processed radiograph to a digital work station
b. radiograph of head, used in orthodontics, prosthodontics
c. opening in lead collimator to regulate beam size
d. sharpness and clarity of image outline on radiograph
e. ability of substance to permit ray passage, making film dark
f. tooth structure appearing longer than anatomical size
g. point-to-point delineation or view of tiny x-ray structures
h. imaginary line dividing head into right and left sides
i. negative pole in tube, source of electrons
j. particle carrying electric charge
k. crackling of film emulsion surface caused by temperature change
l. device used to maintain films in the mouth during exposure
m. radiographs of patient without teeth
n. imaginary line to direct placement of PID during exposures
o. ability of rays to penetrate and possibly ionize tissues

DEFINITIONS
Using the selection given for each sentence, choose the best term to complete the definition.

1. The controlling factor in the production of electrons available for radiographs is:
   a. kilovolt power
   b. milliampere control
   c. timer switch
   d. timer

2. Aluminum disks placed between the collimator and the tube window to remove weak radiation are:
   a. collimators
   b. anodes
   c. filters
   d. cathodes

3. The tubehead area where the central beam or primary ray is projected is the:
   a. target plane
   b. focal spot
   c. primary target
   d. filament

4. The positive pole in the tubehead that serves as a target for electron barrage is the:
   a. filter
   b. filament
   c. anode
   d. PID

5. The abbreviation for the term milliampere is:
   a. MA
   b. mA
   c. Ma
   d. MilA

6. The central ray or beam of radiation emitting from the tubehead or PID is:
   a. primary radiation
   b. secondary radiation
   c. stray radiation
   d. soft radiation

7. The time or duration of interval when the current will pass through the x-ray tube is the:
   a. processing time
   b. count-up time
   c. exposure time
   d. latent time

8. The distance between the anode target and the object to be radiographed is called the:
   a. target–film distance
   b. target–object distance
   c. film–PID distance
   d. focal spot distance

9. Cumulative effect is the:
   a. effect required to expose film emulsion to radiation.
   b. effect required to process the radiograph.
   c. effect of continual exposure to radiation

10. The color of a Rinn positioning device used for endodontic work is:
    a. blue   b. green
    c. red   d. yellow

11. The ability of x-rays to penetrate and possibly ionize body tissues is called:
    a. mutation effect
    b. cumulative effect
    c. sensitivity
    d. ionization concentration

12. Radiation overdose that causes temporary redness of the skin is:
    a. rad   b. erythema dose
    c. Roentgen dose   d. Ma dose

13. Which type of film would be used to view the tooth crown, roots, and surrounding tissues:
    a. interproximal   b. periapical
    c. occlusal   d. panoramic

14. Another term for a bitewing exposure is:
    a. interproximal   b. periapical
    c. occlusal   d. panoramic

15. A size 4 radiograph packet would contain which film?
    a. interproximal   b. periapical
    c. occlusal   d. panoramic

16. Which of the following is not considered a basic safety precaution in exposure of radiographs?
    a. dosimeter
    b. safelight
    c. lead apron/thyrocervical collar
    d. lead barrier or screen

17. Which of the following radiographic films is of particular use in orthodontics?
    a. periapical
    b. occlusal
    c. cephalometric
    d. edentulous

18. Variations of black and white colors on a radiograph are considered an example of:
    a. contrast   b. detail
    c. definition   d. fog

19. Another name for the paralleling technique for radiographic exposures is:
    a. right angle technique
    b. short cone technique
    c. wide angle technique

20. If the PID is aimed in an upward position, it is considered to be which angulation?
    a. negative   b. positive
    c. zero   d. vertical

BUILDING SKILLS

Locate and define the prefix, root/combining form, and suffix (if present) in the following words:

1. **radiolucent**
   prefix   _____
   root word/combining form   _____
   suffix   _____

2. **cephalometric**
   prefix   _____
   root word/combining form   _____
   suffix   _____

3. **pedodontic**
   prefix   _____
   root word/combining form   _____
   suffix   _____

4. **milliampere**

   prefix _____

   root word/combining form _____

   suffix _____

5. **thyrocervical**

   prefix _____

   root word/combining form _____

   suffix _____

FILL-INS

Write the correct word in the blank space to complete each statement.

1. X-rays, also known as Roentgen rays, are a source of _____ energy.

2. A/an _____ is a device to regulate the x-ray beam exiting from the tubehead.

3. The tungsten coil in the cathode-focusing cup that generates the electrons is called the _____.

4. Another word for 1000 volts is _____.

5. Radiation that leaks from a faulty tubehead is called _____ radiation.

6. Abnormal growth or development in which radiation causes genetic changes is called the _____ effect.

7. A digital radiographic image obtained from the CCP sensor and immediately incorporated in the work station is consider to be a/an _____ acquired image.

8. A/an _____ film is used to expose large areas in the oral cavity.

9. A lead apron with thyrocervial collar is considered protection for the _____.

10. Another word for a bitewing packet is a/an _____ x-ray film.

11. Radiographs exposed outside the oral cavity are called _____ films.

12. A special rotating radiograph producing the entire dentition and surrounding structures and exposed outside the oral cavity is called a/an _____ radiograph.

13. A substance that resists radiation penetration and produces a light area on the exposed film is said to be _____.

14. The imaginary line down the middle of the face, bisecting the head into right and left is called the _____ plane.

15. An error in the horizontal angulation during exposure may cause cone cutting and _____.

16. An error in the vertical angulation during exposure may cause foreshortening or _____.

17. Placing the film in the oral cavity in a backward position may cause an error termed the _____ effect.

18. Extreme changes in temperature of processing solutions used in the procedure may produce a crackle film surface appearance called _____.

19. Improper storage, handling, or overdue or expired solutions may produce processed films with a cloudy appearance, called _____.

20. Poor definition or fuzzy outline of form caused by movement is known as _____.

WORD USE

Read the following sentences and define the meaning of the boldfaced word.

1. The orthodontic and prosthodontic offices require use of the **cephalometric** radiograph.

   _____

2. When positioning the patient for the exposure of a radiograph, imagine an **ala tragus line** on the patient's face.

_____

3. Metallic objects, such as restorations or crowns, appear as **radiopaque** areas on the patient's radiograph

_____

4. An **edentulous survey** may require more attention and effort than other types of radiographic surveys.

_____

5. One of the errors that can occur with incorrect positioning during radiographic exposure is **elongation**.

_____

AUDIO LIST 💿

This list contains selected new, important, or difficult terms from this chapter. You may use the list to review these terms and to practice pronouncing them correctly. When you work with the audio for this chapter, listen to the word, repeat it, and then place a checkmark in the box. Proceed to the next boxed word and repeat the process.

❑ anode (**ANN**-ode)
❑ aperture (**AP**-er-chur)
❑ cathode (**KATH**-ode)
❑ cephalometric (**seff**-ah-loh-**MEH**-trick)
❑ cephalostat (**SEFF**-ah-loh-stat)
❑ collimator (**KAHL**-ih-may-tore)
❑ dosimeter (doh-**SIH**-meh-ter)
❑ edentulous (ee-**DENT**-you-lus)
❑ elongation (ee-lon-**GAY**-shun)
❑ erythema (air-ih-**THEE**-mah)

❑ filament (**FILL**-ah-ment)
❑ foreshortening (fore-**SHORE**-ten-ing)
❑ kilovolt (**KILL**-oh-volt)
❑ milliampere (**mill**-ee-**AM**-peer)
❑ panoramic (pan-oh-**RAM**-ick)
❑ phantom (**FAN**-tum)
❑ radiant (**RAY**-dee-ant)
❑ radioluscent (**RAY**-dee-oh-**LOO**-sent)
❑ radiopaque (**RAY**-dee-oh-payk)

CHAPTER 10

Tooth Restorations

Tooth Restorations

OBJECTIVES   Upon completion of this chapter, the reader should be able to identify and understand terms related to:

1.   **Patient preparation and procedure area.** Discuss the purpose of dental restorations and their classifications, and identify the steps of the dental restoration procedure.

2.   **Isolation of the operative site.** List the various methods employed to maintain a dry mouth area during dental preparations.

3.   **Preparation of the restorative site.** List the steps in preparing a restorative site prior to placing the restorative materials.

4.   **Matrix placement.** Discuss the necessity for matrix placement, and identify the various types of matrix retainers and their uses.

5.   **Cement, liners, and base materials.** Identify and describe the assorted dental cements, liners, and base materials used in tooth restorations.

6.   **Restorative materials.** Discuss the various types and properties of dental restorative materials used in tooth restorations.

7.   **Finishing methods.** Identify the methods used to complete, finish, and refine the tooth restoration.

PATIENT PREPARATION AND PROCEDURE AREA

Perhaps the most common dental visit is the appointment for examination and prevention, but the restoration of teeth is the most popular treatment associated with the dental office. The purpose of a dental restoration is to:

◗ remove the **carious lesion** (**CARE**-ee-us, **LEE**-zhun = *decay area*);
◗ prepare the site for a restorative material of choice with the needed bases and liners; and
◗ restore the tooth to its normal function and **esthetic** (ehs-**THET**-ick = *pertaining to beauty*) appearance.

TABLE 10-1   Classification of Caries

CLASSIFICATION	TYPE OF CARIOUS LESION	GENERAL SURFACES INVOLVED
Class I	Pits and fissures	Occlusal surfaces of posterior teeth Posterior buccal and lingual fissures Lingual fissure (cingulum pit) of maxillary incisors
Class II	Interproximal of posteriors	Proximal walls and some occlusal surfaces of posterior teeth
Class III	Interproximal of anteriors	Proximal surfaces, walls of anterior teeth
Class IV	Interproximal of anteriors with incisal edge involved	Anterior proximal walls including incisal edges or surfaces
Class V	Smooth surfaces	Gingival third of tooth, common in canines
Class VI	Decay or abrasions of chewing surfaces	Decay or abrasion of anterior teeth incisal edges or occlusal edges of posteriors

Choice of the procedure and the materials used depend on the condition and site of the tooth involved. Dental caries are classified according to their position and degree of decay, as shown in Table 10-1.

Regardless of the type of restoration needed, the procedure or routine is the same. Anesthesia or pain control for the dental treatment precedes the restoration and varies according to the patient's individual need and type of treatment required. Pain management associated with dental treatment is explained in detail in Chapter 8.

ISOLATION OF THE OPERATIVE SITE

The operative site must be isolated throughout the restoring process, from before tooth preparation through the final polishing stage. Site isolation provides for better viewing and a drier climate for the proper use of dental materials. Oral evacuation by saliva ejectors and the assistant's evacuation tip remove saliva and cooling water from handpieces. Cotton rolls in various lengths or those placed in cotton-roll holders may be applied to strategic sites to control fluids. Absorbent pads may be situated over the parotid gland in the cheek to absorb the flow of saliva.

Isolation helps to control the tongue interference that is common among young and nervous patients, and also helps prevent an aspiration or swallowing of small dental items such as crowns, clamps, and amalgam debris. To assure total tooth isolation, a dental dam may be applied.

Dental Dam

A dental dam (also called rubber dam) is a material placed upon the teeth for certain dental procedures (see Figure 10-1). The dental dam serves two main functions:

1. isolation (**eye**-so-**LAY**-shun = *separate or detach from others*). The tooth or teeth to receive treatment are isolated and exposed for the procedure, presenting better viewing and access.
2. barrier (**BARE**-ee-er = *an obstacle or impediment*) control. The dam material protects against infection, damage from caustic materials, accidents to adjacent tissues, swallowing of small objects, and contamination of the site.

Items needed for placement of the dental dam are noted and explained in Chapter 13, Endodontics. Three steps are involved in preparing the dental dam material and positioning it in the mouth:

1. Place the ligature (**LIG**-ah-tchur = *banding or tying off*). Small pieces of floss or dam material are placed into the proximal areas to assist with control and retention of the dam material in the mouth

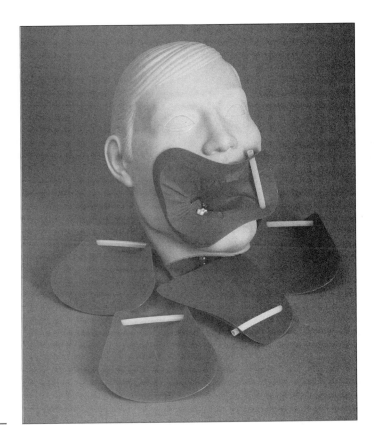

FIGURE 10-1
Quick dam, for minor procedures or when asepsis is not required. (Courtesy of Aseptico, Inc.)

2. **Invert** (in-**VERT** = *turn inward or reverse*) the material. This seals the edges of the dam material to the tooth surface and prevents moisture from escaping into the work area.
3. **Stabilize** (**STAY**-bill-ize = *condition of fixing, steadying, or firming*) the dam clamp. Ligatures, softened wax, or other materials may be placed about the dam clamp to help maintain a firm seating.

Also, quick dams are available to the dentist for isolating a site that does not require controlling moisture and maintaining a sterile field, such as endodontic preparations. These dams are smaller, with or without a frame, and are set into the mouth. They are used mostly for a single tooth prep or for general isolation (see Figure 10-1).

PREPARATION OF THE RESTORATIVE SITE

Each caries-affected tooth requires special attention, and the method, procedure, and choice of restorative materials for this tooth must be custom-planned and adapted. The basic **protocol** (**PROH**-toe-kahl = *steps or method to follow*) for returning a decayed tooth to a restorative level involves three steps:

1. Remove caries, and **debridement** (deh-**BREED**-ment = *removal of damaged tissue*), by the use of rotary burs or diamonds in handpieces, abrasion, laser or mechanical methods, and with hand **instrumentation** (in-strew-men-**TAY**-shun = *use of instruments*).
2. Prepare tooth forms to receive and retain restorative materials. To obtain the proper forms, preparations must be made in the **axial** (**AX**-ee-al = *pertaining to the long line*) wall, which receives its name from the surface wall involved. Examples are distal, buccal, lingual, mesial, labial, gingival, and pulpal. When two walls meet, they form a **line angle**, such as a distoocclusal (DO) restoration. If the pulpal wall is involved with the two axial walls, a **point angle** is formed and three surfaces are involved, such as a distobuccopulpal restoration. Tooth preparations include several prep forms.
   ◗ **outline form:** tooth cuts used to prepare the size, shape, and placement of restoration.
   ◗ **convenience form:** the cut of tooth material necessary for access to complete the cavity preparation.
   ◗ **retention form:** undercut of the walls to provide a mechanical hold of the restorative material.
   ◗ **resistance form:** preparation cuts to ensure that the restored natural tooth can withstand trauma and pressure use of the tooth.
3. Finish and **refine** (ree-**FINE** = *finish again*) of tooth walls and surfaces in preparation to receive the restorative material. Extensive loss of tooth surface may require placement of a matrix to restore the original shape, and a combination of materials may be used to fill the preparation. When filled, the tooth is carved, burnished, smoothed, polished, and checked for occlusion.

▎MATRIX PLACEMENT

Once a tooth wall has been removed in a tooth preparation, it must be replaced. To hold the shape and form of the original wall, and to prevent an **overhang** of restorative material, the dentist may use a **matrix** (**MAY**-tricks = *mold or shaping*), such as Tofflemire, AutoMatrix , T-strip, Ivory, or a customized copper band.

Tofflemire matrix: a retainer device and assorted stainless steel bands to fit and be tightened around the tooth. Wedges made of wood, resin, or celluloid for passage of ultraviolet light are placed at the base of the matrix to stabilize and provide **embrasure** (em-**BRAY**-zhur = *opening*) areas with nearby teeth (see Figure 10-2).

AutoMatrix: pre-sized, cone-shaped circle band with locking ends that are tightened and locked after being placed on the tooth; visibility may be better because no retainer is necessary to hold the band.

T-strips: stainless steel strips that are shaped like a T. The strip is circled with the T ends flapped over to retain the shape and hold the band on the tooth. Wedges are used to provide embrasure space and stabilization. T-strips are commonly used in pediatric dentistry.

ivory retainer and **sectional matrix:** system used mostly on posterior teeth. The strip does not circle the tooth but only replaces a wall. The retainer holds a stainless steel strip that is placed between the prep and the contact wall of the adjacent tooth. The strip is tightened and a wedge is used for space and to assist with retention.

mylar (**MY**-lar = *celluloid*) matrix strips and crown forms: used with anterior or tooth-shaded materials. The strips are placed around the tooth restoration and held in place by a clip or finger pressure until the restoration is set or light-cured. Crown forms are filled with restorative material and placed upon the prep until the material has set.

FIGURE 10-2
Example of Tofflemire matrix retainer with matrix and wedges in place.

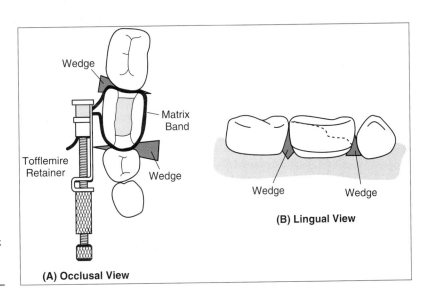

(A) Occlusal View

(B) Lingual View

CEMENTS, LINERS, AND BASE MATERIALS

Each dental material is chosen for its unique characteristic. The selection of a specific material is determined by the preparation site, involvement, and physical makeup of the prepared tooth. Among several popular choices for protecting or preparing materials are.

varnish: copal or resin gum in a suspension of organic solvents (acetone, ether, or chloroform); used to seal the cut edges of tooth surfaces and seal against leakage under all restorations except composites and resins. Universal varnish that does not contain the organic solvents may be used under all restorations.

liner: thin coating that provides a barrier against chemical irritation; usually a varnish material or a liquid suspension of calcium hydroxide or glass **ionomer** (eye-**AHN**-oh-mer) cement.

acid etchant: phosphoric acid solution used to prepare the cavity margins to provide retention for the bonding and restorative materials. Etching makes the enamel surface more porous, creating enamel tags, and removes the **smear layer** of bacterial and tooth debris matter. When prepared, the enamel looks chalky white.

bonding agent: material used to unite some restorative agents to the tooth surface and underlying materials; may be self-curing liquid or light-cured.

base: barrier against chemical irritation. Bases also provide thermal isolation, resist condensation forces, and are able to be contoured and shaped. A base may be zinc oxide eugenol (ZOE) or ZOE with ethoxybenzoic acid (EBA) added for strength, zinc phosphate, polycarboxylate, or glass ionomer. Each has its own characteristics.

cement: a thicker material that can be used as a temporary or permanent restorative material; for example, glass ionomer cement may serve as a cement or a restoration material. Cements also may be used to retain pins or posts in a deep preparation.

retention pin: metallic pin that is cemented into a drilled hole in the tooth prep. The exposed end of the pin will be incorporated into the restorative material.

core post: titanium / stainless steel posts of various sizes that are cemented into the pulpal canal of an endodonticly treated tooth. A core buildup of restorative material placed over the extending post end. All pin placements are drilled and cemented into place before applying a matrix. Figure 10-3 illustrates a pin and post.

Purposes of Submaterials

Some materials are placed into cavity preparations prior to the restorative material of choice. These liners, bases, and cements are chosen to serve a specific purpose, such as:

insulation (in-sue-**LAY**-shun = *to set apart*): prevents transfer of heat, stress force, and **galvanic** shock (gal-**VAN**-ick = *electrical charge from chemical reaction of two dissimilar metals meeting through biting forces*).

palliative (**PAL**-ee-**ah**-tiv = *relieves or alleviate pain*): encourages growth or reparative dentin; also called **tertiary** (**TERR**-shee-air-ee = *later stage*) dentin.

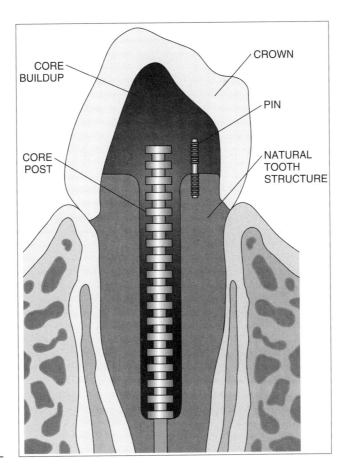

FIGURE 10-3
Example of
restoration buildup
using retention pin
and core post.

protective (proh-**TECK**-tiv = *shielding*): seal or temporary restoration between treatment visits.

luting (**LOO**-ting = *holding together*): retaining items in union; usually a temporary measure between treatments.

cementation (see-men-**TAY**-shun = *bonding or uniting of two or more items*): used to permanently unite or restore shape and purpose; also may be used to cement retention pins into the preparation.

laminate (**LAM**-in-**ate** = *thin plate or layer*): material applied in thin layers to the tooth surface; may be cemented or light-activated for permanency.

Restoration Placement Terminology

Terms specific to the preparation, handling, and insertion or use of cementing and restorative agents include:

manipulation (mah-**nip**-you-**LAY**-shun = *skillful operation or handling and use*): preparation and handling during use; each material requires a different method.

homogenous (hoe-**MAH**-jeh-nus = *same or alike in development*): describes a uniform mixture; some materials, such as cements, have to be blended.

trituration (**try**-chur-**AY**-shun = *pulverize*): the mechanical blending and mixing of the mercury and alloy materials; also called amalgamation (ah-**mal**-gah-**MAY**-shun), the chemical act of blending the alloy and mercury mix for an amalgam restoration. This procedure usually is accomplished in a machine called an amalgamator.

mulling: the further act of blending the amalgam material while it is in plastic form; performed in the amalgamator with the pestle removed from the mixing capsule.

dissipate (**DISS**-ih-pate = *to scatter or spread out*): to spread out over a larger area; some materials have to be mixed in a large area to allow escape from the exothermic (ecks-oh-**THER**-mick = *giving off heat*) reaction produced by the chemical union of some materials.

polymerization (pahl-ih-**mer**-ih-**ZAY**-shun = *change of compound elements into another shape*): transforming material from a plastic (movable) shape to a hard substance through a curing process, either automatically (self-curing) or using a light-source method.

bonding (**BON**-ding = *uniting through microscopic cementation*): using acid materials called etchants to prepare a tooth surface for attaching to another material.

RESTORATIVE MATERIALS

A variety of materials and procedures are used in restoring the affected tooth to normal function, use, and beauty. An amalgam (ah-**MAL**-gum = *soft alloy mass containing mercury*), a blend of various powdered metals and liquid mercury mixed into a plastic (movable) form that soon hardens. Amalgam may be supplied as spherical (**SFEAR**-ih-kul = *in the form of a sphere*) for better mixing or amalgamation and material flow, or the alloy may be supplied as lathe filings, which are small, irregular, metal grains. Amalgam is available in color-coded, single-, double-, or triple-dose premeasured capsules. Some capsules include a pestle, a small metal or hard plastic cylinder that aids mixing. When speaking of amalgam, the alloy proportion is mentioned before the mercury amount, such as 5:8 (five parts alloy to eight parts mercury).

Other relevant terms are:

cement: plastic material that can unite or bond materials. The choice of cement depends on the solubility (**sahl**-you-**BILL**-ih-tee = *capability of being dissolved*), viscosity (**viss**-**KAHS**-ih-tee = *sticky or gummy*), and adhesive (ad-**HEE**-siv = *sticky or adhering*) quality of the material.

composite (cahm-**PAH**-zit): resin material used in dental restorations; supplied in macrofilled (*large particles*), microfilled (*small particles*), and hybrid (*mixed particles*) and may be purchased in paste, syringe, or single-dose capsules (see Figure 10-4). Composites may be self- (auto) or light-cured.

gold foil: foil sheet of gold material that is annealed (placed in flame for a heat treatment to purify) to a clean and prepared surface for condensation into the

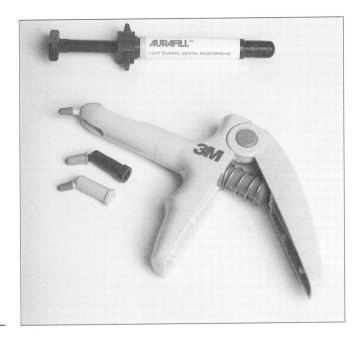

FIGURE 10-4
Example of a composite syringe and cartridge system.

prepared restorative site. Gold also is also supplied in mat or powder form for direct insertion into tooth prep.

veneer (veh-**NEAR** = *tooth shaped layer*): thin resin composite or porcelain surface shields that are cemented or bonded onto the facial surface of a tooth. Veneer also refers to the thin surface facial covering on the porcelain veneer (PV) crown.

FINISHING METHODS

After the tooth has been prepared and has received the liner and bases as needed, the restorative material has to be inserted, finished, and perhaps polished. Several terms are specific to this procedure:

increment (**IN**-kreh-ment = *increase or addition*): small amounts or doses of the materials that are placed into the preparation.

condensation (kon-den-**SAY**-shun = *to make thick*): the changed preparation as a result of the condenser or plugger instruments packing down the material into the preparation.

burnish (**BURR**-nish = *to smooth or rub*): to smooth the restoration surfaces toward the margins. Matrix strips may be burnished or rubbed into the proper shape. Burnishing also provides a shiny surface to gold.

articulating (are-**TICK**-you-lay-ting) paper: colored strip of paper used to test results of the bite. The articulating paper is placed on the occusal surfaces and the patient bites down. When the paper is removed, the high spots are

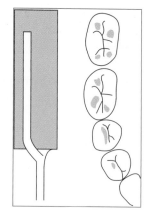

FIGURE 10-5
Articulating paper revealing high spots.

indicated by the marks that appear with carbon or colored traces to indicate where refinement is needed (see Figure 10-5).

laminate (**LAM**-inate = *thin plate or layer*): material applied in thin layers to the tooth surface; may be cemented or light-activated for permanency.

HVE (high velocity evacuation): fluid-removal system used to maintain a clear, dry field of operation.

When completed, finishing burs, diamonds, wheels, abrasive strips, and polishes are used to smooth and refine the restoration. Amalgam material may not be polished for 48 hours, but many composite and resin materials are completely refined at the insertion appointment.

REVIEW EXERCISES

MATCHING
Match the following word elements with their meanings:

1. _____ HVE
2. _____ embrasure
3. _____ dissipate
4. _____ insolate
5. _____ manipulation
6. _____ invert
7. _____ cementation

8. _____ laminate
9. _____ veneer
10. _____ burnish
11. _____ composite
12. _____ condense
13. _____ tertiary
14. _____ ligature
15. _____ debridement

a. to turn inward or reverse
b. to make thick or compact
c. to smooth or rub out
d. thin, resin, tooth-shaped layer
e. thin plate or layer
f. high velocity evacuation
g. open space between contact point and gingiva
h. binding or tying off material
i removing damaged tissue
j. later or third stage
k. bonding or uniting of two or more items
l. to scatter or spread out
m. skillful operation or handling and use
n. to set apart
o. resin material used in dental restorations

DEFINITIONS

Using the selection given in each sentence, choose the best term to complete the definition.

1. An example of a restorative material supplied in mat or powder form and annealed before use is:
   a. composite
   b. gold foil
   c. amalgam
   d. zinc oxide

2. Which of the following bases would not be placed under a composite restoration?
   a. copal varnish
   b. universal varnish
   c. calcium hydroxide
   d. acid etchant

3. A mylar matrix strip is used for which type of restoration?
   a. Class II amalgam
   b. Class I amalgam
   c. Class V composite
   d. Class III composite

4. "Beauty" or the condition related to looking attractive is:
   a. veneer
   b. viscosity
   c. galvanics
   d. esthetics

5. Which of the following matrix devices is commonly used in Pediatric Dentistry?
   a. T-band
   b. Tofflemire
   c. Ivory
   d. AutoMatrix

6. Tooth cuts used to prepare the size, shape, and placement of a restoration are which form of cavity preparation?
   a. outline form
   b. retention form
   c. resistance form
   d. convenience form

7. The removal of damaged or dead tissue is termed:
   a. condensation
   b. debridement
   c. manipulation
   d. instrumentation

8. The ability or the capacity of being dissolved is:
   a. viscosity
   b. solubility
   c. malleability
   d. adhesive

9. To ready the tooth for a restoration, preparations may be made to which type of wall?
   a. resistance
   b. outline
   c. axial
   d. retention

10. The use of small dental instruments in operative dentistry is called:
    a. instrumentation
    b. manipulation
    c. handling
    d. transfer

11. During some dental procedures, a tooth area may have to be set apart. This is called:
    a. injection
    b. infiltration
    c. inverting
    d. isolation

12. One of the important factors concerned with the use of cement is its holding power, called:
    a. adhesiveness
    b. viscosity
    c. solubility
    d. translucency

13. During an amalgam restoration, the material is placed into the prep in small loads called:
    a. macrofill
    b. increments
    c. injections
    d. barriers

14. A temporary cement that may be used as a shield between treatments is called:
    a. protective
    b. palliative
    c. homogeneous
    d. permanent

15. A base that may be used to sedate and provide pain relief may be called:
    a. protective
    b. palliative
    c. homogeneous
    d. permanent

16. A permanent restoration containing powdered metal alloy and mercury is called a/an:
    a. composite
    b. resin
    c. amalgam
    d. ZOE

17. The process of using a special mix to unite two or more separate items is called:
    a. polymerization
    b. cementation
    c. trituration
    d. burnishing

18. The process of two compound element materials changing into another shape is called:
    a. polymerization
    b. cementation
    c. trituration
    d. burnishing

19. The mixing of amalgam material in an amalgamator after the pestle has been removed is termed:
    a. tituration
    b. manipulation
    c. instrumentation
    d. mulling

20. Scattering or spreading out a mixture, which allows heat to be given off, is termed:
    a. dissipation
    b. bonding
    c. mulling
    d. inverting

BUILDING SKILLS

Locate and define the prefix, root/combining form, and suffix (if present) in the following words.

1. **stabilization**
   prefix   _____
   root/combining form   _____
   suffix   _____

2. **debridement**
   prefix   _____
   root/combining form   _____
   suffix   _____

3. **homogeneous**
   prefix   _____
   root/combining form   _____
   suffix   _____

4. **refinement**
   prefix   _____
   root/combining form   _____
   suffix   _____

5. **exothermic**
   prefix   _____
   root/combining form   _____
   suffix   _____

FILL-INS

Write the correct word in the blank space to complete each statement.

1. A carious lesion involving the interproximal of posterior teeth is Class _____.

2. The band or tie-off used in placing and retaining a dental dam is called a/an _____.

3. Placing wax or a compound around the wing of a dental dam clamp to fix or make steady is called _____.

4. A/an _____ anesthetic is placed at the injection site to lessen the feeling of pain during an infiltration injection.

5. An electrical shock caused by the chemical reaction of two dissimilar metals meeting in a biting force is called _____ shock.

6. _____ paper is used to mark or indicate high areas on the surface of the restoration.

7. The skillful operation or handling and use of dental materials is called
_____.

8. A thin, resin, tooth-shaped layer that is placed on the tooth surface is called a/an
_____.

9. The instrument used to pack down or make restorative material thick in the prep involves a process called
_____.

10. The family of plastic materials that can unite or bond materials is _____.

11. Restorative materials that are placed into the prep in a thin plate or layer are said to be
_____.

12. The act of uniting through microscopic cementation of material and tooth is called
_____.

13. A cavity-base material that relieves or alleviates pain is called _____.

14. The basic term for the steps or methods used in a procedure is: _____.

15. Spherical amalgam material is supplied in _____ form.

16. The small metal or hard plastic cylinder that is inside an amalgamator capsule is called a
_____.

17. A metallic pin that is cemented in a large restoration preparation and used to help support that restoration is a
_____ pin.

18. _____ is the term used to describe the capability of a material to be dissolved.

19. The blending of two materials into one uniform mixture is called _____.

20. During the chemical setup or curing, some cements give off heat called _____ action.

WORD USE

Read the following sentences and define the meaning of the boldfaced words.

1. The assistant frequently passes the amalgam carrier to the dentist so the tooth preparation may be filled in small **increments.**

2. The patient requested an **esthetic** restoration for her maxillary central incisor.

3. The dental assistant mixed a **palliative** material for the dentist to place in the temporary restoration.

4. The **trituration** is an important factor in the preparation of an amalgam restoration.

5. The dentist requested more **viscosity** in the preparation of restorative cement.

AUDIO LIST

This list contains selected new, important, or difficult terms from this chapter. You may use the list to review these terms and to practice pronouncing them correctly. When you work with the audio for this chapter, listen to the word, repeat it, and then place a checkmark in the box. Proceed to the next boxed word and repeat the process.

- ❏ adhesive (ad-**HEE**-siv)
- ❏ amalgam (ah-**MAL**-gum)
- ❏ amalgamation (ah-**mal**-gah-MAY-shun)
- ❏ articulating (are-**TICK**-you-lay-ting)
- ❏ burnish (**BURR**-nish)
- ❏ composite (cahm-**PAH**-zit)
- ❏ condensation (kon-den-**SAY**-shun)
- ❏ debridement (deh-**BREED**-ment)
- ❏ dissipate (**DISS**-ih-pate)
- ❏ embrasure (em-**BRAY**-zhur)
- ❏ esthetic (ehs-**THET**-ick)
- ❏ homogenous (hoh-**MAH**-jeh-nus)
- ❏ increment (**IN**-kreh-ment)
- ❏ instrumentation (in-strew-men-TAY-shun)
- ❏ insulation (in-sue-**LAY**-shun)
- ❏ isolation (eye-so-**LAY**-shun)
- ❏ laminate (**LAM**-inate)
- ❏ ligature (**LIG**-ah-tchur)
- ❏ luting (**LOO**-ting)
- ❏ manipulation (mah-**nip**-you-LAY-shun)
- ❏ matrix (**MAY**-tricks)
- ❏ mylar (**MY**-lar)
- ❏ palliative (**PAL**-ee-ah-tiv)
- ❏ polymerization (pahl-ih-mer-ih-**ZAY**-shun)
- ❏ protective (proh-**TECK**-tiv)
- ❏ solubility (sahl-you-**BILL**-ih-tee)
- ❏ spherical (**SFEAR**-ih-kul)
- ❏ trituration (try-chur-**AY**-shun)
- ❏ veneer (veh-**NEAR**)
- ❏ viscosity (viss-**KAHS**-ih-tee)

CHAPTER 11

Cosmetic Dentistry

Upon completion of this chapter, the reader should be able to identify and understand terms related to:

1. **Definition of cosmetic dentistry and related areas.** Define the meaning of cosmetic dentistry and discuss its various applications in dentistry.

2. **Tooth whitening.** Cite reasons for tooth whitening and methods used to lighten tooth surfaces.

3. **Tooth bonding and veneer application.** Discuss the procedures used to repair or alter size, shape, and color of teeth by bonding and veneer applications.

4. **Cosmetic tooth restorations.** Discuss the various types of cosmetic restoration including inlays, onlays, and crowns.

5. **Periodontal tissue surgery.** Identify the various techniques used to correct damaged tissue and make an esthetic gum presentation.

6. **Dental implants.** Describe the assortment of dental implants and the use and necessity of implant dentistry.

7. **Accelerated orthodontics.** Discuss accelerated orthodontics to improve the adult smile and mouth occlusion.

DEFINITION OF COSMETIC DENTISTRY AND RELATED AREAS

Beyond maintenance and reconstruction of the oral cavity, the modern dental patient desires an esthetic appearance. People seek dental care to improve their looks and turn to their dentist for cosmetic restorations and esthetic correction of diseased tissues, stains, genetic imperfections, accidents, and other maladies of the mouth.

Although most cosmetic dentistry procedures can be completed by the dentist, some require a team consisting of the dentist and other dental personnel such as a prosthodontist, oral surgeon, periodontist, and the dental laboratory technician.

Cosmetic techniques offered to improve patients' esthetic appearance and restore or provide functional use include tooth whitening, bonding, veneer application, cosmetic restorations, periodontal adjustment, implants, and tooth movement. Major repair and reconstruction of the mouth and facial structures are covered in Chapter 14, Oral and Maxillofacial Surgery.

TOOTH WHITENING

The most common cosmetic procedure is the whitening or lightening of tooth surfaces. Aging, chemically stained teeth, such as the tetracycline brown band line, and genetic disposition are causes of **intrinsic** (in-**TRIN**-sick, *from within*) stain. Personal diet may cause teeth to look dark and unattractive with **extrinsic** (ex-**TRIN**-sick, *from without*) stain. Whitening of teeth surfaces can be completed in the dental office, at home, or a combination. At the start of the procedure, the patient's present shade of tooth is recorded and will be compared to the new shade after the lightening. Relevant terms are:

shade guide: hand-held device with assorted numbered tooth-shade forms that are compared to the incisal two-thirds of the patients incisors. Color types and levels include:

    A. reddish brown: up to five variant levels
    B. reddish yellow: up to four variant levels
    C. gray: up to four variant levels
    D. reddish gray: up to four variant levels.

model impression: a positive reproduction of the patient's teeth that is made into a study model

tray fabrication: a plastic or celluloid tray made to fit the study model cast and used to hold chemicals for lightening.

gingival isolation: painting or covering the patient's gingiva with a liquid dam (mask) material to isolate the tissues from chemical damage; some systems also use face drapes for patients' protection.

tooth bleaching: techniques and equipment vary according to the degree of lightening desired and the manufacturer's recommendations and instructions. Some techniques are:

    acid brush: 35% phosphoric acid solution applied to surfaces, particularly to tetracycline band line on surfaces; remains on surface 15 seconds and then rinsed off.

    tray method: gel, or paste-filled tray placed into the mouth over cleaned tooth surfaces; gel may be activated by a diode laser handpiece or activating curing light.

    gel application: whitening gel containing a hydrogen peroxide or carbamide peroxide formula applied directly to cleaned, isolated tooth surfaces; may or may not be activated by bleaching, laser, or curing lights, as specified by the manufacturer.

tooth desensitization: following bleaching, a desensitizing liquid, paste, or gel applied to tooth surfaces that seal dentin tubules, to minimize discomfort and reduce shade relapse. Some formulas to remineralize the tooth include fluoride, calcium, and phosphate.

Following office lightening, the patient may be given a home tray and chemicals to complete the bleaching process. Assorted home bleach kits, strips, and gels are available, some from the dentist and others (OTC) at a local drugstore. Most contain a hydrogen peroxide or carbamide peroxide gel base that is placed in a tray, inserted in the mouth, and worn for a specified time, such as 2–3 hours or overnight, as directed. Professional whitening usually lasts a year provided that the patient does not use coffee or tea and does not smoke, all of which would darken the tooth surfaces.

TOOTH BONDING AND VENEER APPLICATION

Tooth bonding and veneer application are alternatives to tooth whitening, particularly if the tooth surfaces are excessively stained or have other irregularities such as open spaces, broken edges, pitted surfaces, or misshapen teeth.

Tooth Bonding

Tooth bonding involves applying a composite material that is mixed to a pliable dough then applied to a prepared tooth surface and sculpted into the tooth shape. The composite shade is chosen to match the existing tooth surface. The tooth is prepared by removing any decay, if present, and an abrasive roughening followed by a gel etch. The surface is primed and the composite material is applied in layers and activated by a curing light. When shaped and finished, the composite is smoothed and polished.

Veneer

In a **veneer** (veh-**NEAR**) application, a thin, fabricated resin or porcelain cover is applied to the prepared tooth surface. Along with covering stained and affected teeth, the shape or color of the tooth may be altered. Veneers, also called laminates, can be applied using either of two methods:

1. **Direct veneer application.** Similar to tooth bonding, a resin material is applied to tooth surfaces that have been roughened by air-abrasion or rotary burs and wheels. The plastic material is cemented directly onto the surface, smoothed, and polished.
2. **Indirect veneer application** (requires two visits). At the first visit, the teeth are prepared by removing a small amount (0.5 mm to 1.0 mm) of enamel tissue. An impression is taken for fabrication of the porcelain veneers or laminates. The dentist may or may not apply a temporary cover to last between visits. At the second

visit, the teeth are cleaned, acid-etched, and primed to receive the new laminates that are cemented on the tooth surface and light-cured to set up. Finally, the porcelain veneers are cleaned and polished.

COSMETIC TOOTH RESTORATIONS

Tooth restorations are completed using materials that resemble enamel tissue. Older amalgam fillings can be replaced using composite material to give the whole mouth a natural look. Restorative procedures include:

tooth restoration: prepared tooth receiving white composite restorative material instead of metallic amalgam or gold.

inlay: a solid casted or milled restoration involving some occlusal and proximal surfaces that is cemented into a tooth preparation.

onlay: a solid casted or milled restoration that covers some occlusal tooth cusp and side wall area that is cemented onto the prepared site.

tooth crowns: covering the crown surfaces of the tooth with artificial coverings. Figure 11-1 illlustrates some crowns. The type of crown depends upon the extent of the crown repair and is named by the area involved.

> **three-quarter crown:** cast restoration covering all surfaces except the facial view.
>
> **full crown:** cast restoration covering the entire crown area of a tooth.
>
> **porcelain fused to metal crown (PFM):** full cast crown restoration with porcelain facing for cosmetic appearance.
>
> **jacket crown:** thin metal cover with a porcelain facing for an anterior tooth.

The construction of cast restorations is covered in Chapter 18, Dental Laboratory Materials. Although most cast restorations are made with gold or precious metals and covered with porcelain to present an esthetic appearance, a new system of chairside ceramic restoration construction has been developed for immediate cosmetic restorations. **CEREC** (CEramic REConstruction) and **EVEREST** systems provide a ceramic, non-metallic, biocompatible veneer, inlay, onlay, or crown construction method.

The CEREC CAD/CAM system is made up of three parts: an acquisition unit, a milling machine, and a software system. The acquisition camera surveys the preparation that has been covered by a reflective powder and converts the picture to a 3-D figure on which the dentist designs the restoration (approximately 30 minutes). The milling machine then uses the information from the acquisition unit to carve the restoration out of a ceramic block (approximately 15 minutes) that the dentist polishes, then bonds into the preparation. The completed restoration is a solid ceramic block instead of a metal inlay, onlay, or crown with a porcelain esthetic covering. This method allows a one-trip restoration of tooth structure compared to other methods, when a provisional or temporary restoration must be prepared while the laboratory is fabricating the restoration. The EVEREST system produces a lab reproduction in zirconium, glass ceramic, or titanium materials.

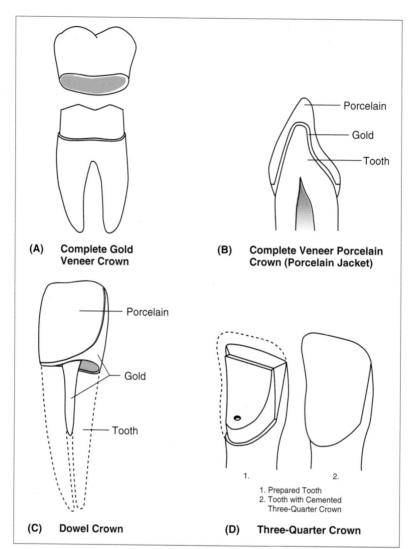

FIGURE 11-1
Examples of crowns.

(A) **Complete Gold Veneer Crown**

(B) **Complete Veneer Porcelain Crown (Porcelain Jacket)**

Porcelain
Gold
Tooth

(C) **Dowel Crown**

Porcelain
Gold
Tooth

(D) **Three-Quarter Crown**

1.   2.
1. Prepared Tooth
2. Tooth with Cemented Three-Quarter Crown

▌PERIODONTAL TISSUE SURGERY

Periodontal plastic surgery, also termed **mucogingival surgery**, can be performed as a treatment for diseased tissue and also as a means to enhance the patient's smile. Periodontal treatment is discussed in the chapters dealing with periodontic and oral surgery.

Gingival tissue surgery in cosmetic dentistry is used to either reduce or augment the gingiva as needed. Some examples of gingival cosmetic maladies are illustrated in Figure 11-2.

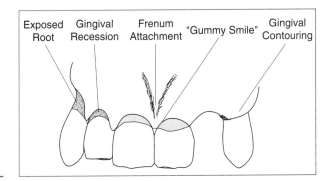

FIGURE 11-2
Some periodontal maladies.

Gingival Reduction

In gingival reduction, excessive gingival tissue is removed by laser, periodontal knives, or bipolar electrosurgery. Reduction is used for:

"crown lengthening": exposing more tooth surface to eliminate a "gummy smile."
gingival contouring: removing excessive tissue to obtain symmetry of the gingival crest.
exposing unerupted teeth: removing coronal tissue to expose the tooth surface.

Gingival Augmentation

Gingival augmentation is done to build up or reconstruct the gingiva to repair or replace tissue where needed. It involves:

soft tissue grafting: transplanting mouth tissue, from nearby gingival tissue or from the palate area, to other sites.
interdental papilla regeneration: replacing papilla tissue in intradental spaces.
gingival recession: restoring the gingival crest to a natural height.
pocket depth reduction: eliminating the pocket area and restoring the gingiva.
exposed roots covering: replacing gingival tissue over exposed roots.
ridge augumentation: building up gingiva and bone tissue in collapsed areas resulting from tooth extraction.

DENTAL IMPLANTS

Dental implants are titanium fixtures that are surgically installed in the jaw bone and used to stabilize or serve as an anchor for a tooth, an appliance, or a denture. They may be used as an alternative to a fixed bridge or in areas where tooth replacement requires stability. Placing an implant usually requires a team of several specialists, such as an oral surgeon, a prosthodontist, and perhaps a periodontist.

Implants are surgically installed and remain in place for three to six months while the appliance and bone unite in a process called **osseointegration** (**oss**-ee-oh-inn-teh-**GRAY**-shun = *union of the bone with the implant device*). Then they are uncovered and the artificial device is attached. An example of an implant is illustrated in the Figure 11-3.

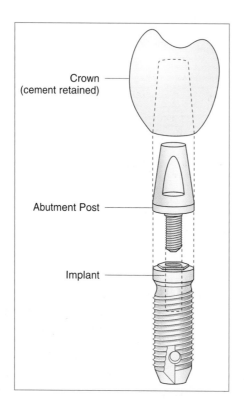

Crown
(cement retained)

Abutment Post

Implant

FIGURE 11-3
Parts of endosseous
implant with
prosthesis.

root form implant—endosseous (**en**-doe-**OSS**-ee-us = *within the alveolar bone*):
screw-type device that is screwed or cemented into the mandibular bone; used
for a single tooth or post implant.

plate form implant: used for the narrow jaw bone; flat plate style.

subperiosteal (**sub**-pear-ee-**OSS**-tee-ahl) implant: implant plate or frame placed
under the periodontium and stabilized on the mandibular bone. It is used when
bone height or width is insufficient; rests on top of the bone.

transosteal (trans-**OSS**-tee-ahl) implant: larger plate stabilized on the lower border
of the mandibular bone with posts extending through the gingiva; used to
anchor prostheses in difficult situations.

ACCELERATED ORTHODONTICS

Malocclusion can present an unattractive smile, and the desire for a better cosmetic appearance may cause a patient to seek accelerated orthodontic treatment.
Most orthodontic treatments require two years or more to complete, and many
adults desire a quicker treatment method. With accelerated orthodontics, the task
can be accomplished in three to nine months, with retainers to be worn another six
months.

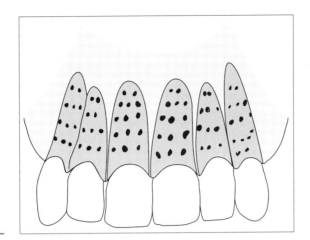

FIGURE 11-4
AOO surgery technique with holes drilled into the alveolar bone to cause "demineralization."

Accelerated Osteogenic Orthodontic (AOO)^tm treatment, also called Wilck-odontics^tm, is a surgical orthodontic approach requiring a team of specialists consisting of an oral surgeon, a periodontist, and an orthodontist, to permit faster and easier tooth movement. The gingiva is incised to expose the alveolar bone. Then a surgical drill is used to place holes in the alveolar bone to demineralize the bone, causing a condition called osteopenia (ahs-tee-oh-**PEE**-nee-ah = *lack of bone tissue*) (see Figure 11-4). A bone graft mixed with an antibiotic is placed on the site, and the gingiva is replaced and sutured into place.

While the bone is in a weakened stage, the bands are attached to the teeth and movement progresses rapidly while the alveolar bone remineralizes. Return visits are more frequent than with the normal orthodontic treatment, and retainers are worn for six months after the bands have been removed.

Other cosmetic applications for orthodontic treatment include:

orthodontic enamoplasty: removing small amounts of enamel walls to acquire enough room to cause a slight correction movement; usually performed in a small area or trouble spot.

lingual banding: placing brackets and bands on the lingual tooth surfaces, so they are not easily viewed.

Invisalign^tm: an orthodontic method for tooth alignment using a series of clear, pre-formed, custom trays that apply pressure for tooth movement.

REVIEW EXERCISES

MATCHING
Match the following words with their meanings.

1. _____ gingival contouring
2. _____ inlay
3. _____ transosteal implant
4. _____ crown lengthening

a. tooth stain from internal sources
b. thin resin or porcelain shell covering
c. protective gingival tissue covering when tooth bleaching
d. tooth stain from external sources

5. _____jacket crown   e. gingival reduction to acquire symmetry in the smile

6. _____osseo-integration   f. cast restoration for a tooth cusp and proximal walls

7. _____gingival reduction   g. implant placed through the jaw bone

8. _____onlay   h. removal of gummy tissue to expose tooth crowns

9. _____intrinsic stain   i. periodontal plastic surgery

10. _____root form implant   j. anterior tooth metal covering with porcelain covering

11. _____mucogingival surgery   k. cast restoration for some occlusal surface and side walls

12. _____gingival augmentation   l. union of bone with implant device

13. _____veneer   m. surgical removal of excessive gingival tissue

14. _____extrinsic stain   n. buildup of gingiva to replace tissue where needed

15. _____gingival isolation   o. screw-type device inserted into the jaw bone

DEFINITIONS

Using the selection given for each sentence, choose the best term to complete the definition.

1. A prepared restoration that is placed upon a tooth prep involving some occlusal cusps and proximal wall is a/an:
   a. full crown   b. jacket crown
   c. onlay   d. inlay

2. Tooth whitening completed by the application of phosphoric acid is which method?
   a. acid brush   b. tray application
   c. gel rub   d. air polish

3. Which procedure is considered gingival augmentation?
   a. gingival contouring
   b. crown lengthening
   c. exposing root surfaces
   d. interdental papilla regeneration

4. Tooth stain from genetic causes, aging, or chemical enamel reactions is which type of stain?
   a. intrinsic   b. extrinsic
   c. environmental   d. regional

5. Tooth stain resulting from diet, personal tooth care, and smoking is which type of stain?
   a. intrinsic   b. extrinsic
   c. environmental   d. regional

6. A tooth crown that covers all surfaces except the facial surface is termed:
   a. full crown   b. PFM crown
   c. jacket crown   d. three quarters crown

7. The last step in office power tooth bleaching is:
   a. gel application
   b. desensitizing
   c. tray fabrication
   d. model impression

8. A tooth diastema (open gap) can be corrected using which technique?
   a. tooth bonding
   b. gingival augmentation
   c. acid etching
   d. tooth restoration

9. Invisalign is the term applied to which orthodontic procedure method?
   a. lingual banding
   b. clear bracket use
   c. customized tray
   d. metal braces

10. The removal of a "gummy smile" is accomplished by which technique?
    a. gingival augmentation
    b. crown lengthening
    c. tooth bonding
    d. restorations

11. A cast restoration involving some occlusal and proximal walls and cemented into the tooth preparation is called:
    a. inlay   b. onlay
    c. full crown   d. jacket crown

12. Which of the following shades is not normally included in a dental shade guide?
    a. reddish orange b. reddish yellow
    c. gray   d. reddish gray

13. The method of applying gel whitening material directly to the tooth surfaces is termed:
    a. acid wash   b. tray coverage
    c. strip placement d. gel application

14. Gingival tissue is protected during application of chemicals in power bleaching by which method?
    a. liquid dam mask
    b. cotton roll application
    c. oral evacuation
    d. tooth bonding

15. Tooth veneers are thin porcelain covers measuring approximately how thick?
    a. 0.1–1.5 mm   b. 0.5–1.0 cm
    c. 1.0–1.5 mm   d. 1.0–1.5 cm

16. Soft tissue grafting is considered which type of periodontal surgery?
    a. gingival stabilization
    b. gingival reduction
    c. gingival desensitizing
    d. gingival augmentation

17. Which of the following implant devices is placed through the jaw bone?
    a. root form implant
    b. plate form implant
    c. subperiosteal implant
    d. transosteal implant

18. Which of the following implant devices is a screw-type device used mainly for a solitary tooth?
    a. root form implant
    b. plate form implant
    c. subperiosteal implant
    d. transosteal implant

19. The demineralization and lessening of the alveolar bone in accelerated orthodontics creates a condition termed:
    a. osteogenesis   b. osseointegration
    c. osteopenia   d. osteoporitis

20. Which type of crown is used mainly on anterior teeth?
    a. bracket crown
    b. jacket crown
    c. three quarters crown
    d. full crown

BUILDING SKILLS

Locate and define the prefix, root/combining form, and suffix (if present) in the following words.

1. **mucogingival**
   prefix   _____
   root/combining form   _____
   suffix   _____

2. **osseointegration**
   prefix   _____
   root/combining form   _____
   suffix   _____

3. **subperiosteal**
   prefix   _____
   root/combining form   _____
   suffix   _____

4. **osteopenia**
   prefix   _____
   root/combining form   _____
   suffix   _____

5. **extrinsic**
   prefix   _____
   root/combining form   _____
   suffix   _____

FILL-IN

Write the correct word in the blank space to complete each sentence.

1. The procedure in which small amounts of enamel wall are removed to permit orthodontic tooth movement is known as

   _____.

2. The union of bone with the titanium dental implant device is known as

   _____.

3. A/an _____ crown is a thin metal casted restoration with a porcelain covering and is placed on an anterior tooth.

4. The orthodontic treatment method of moving teeth by using customized activation trays is known as _____.

5. _____ is the term given to the surgical removal of gingiva to expose more enamel surface and reduce a "gummy smile."

6. When power-bleaching teeth with chemicals, the gingiva is protected by

   _____.

7. A/an _____ is taken to prepare a study model for fabrication of a bleaching tray.

8. A/an _____ is used to compare tooth colors and obtain the restoration color for a patient.

9. A dental implant is usually constructed using _____ metal.

10. Another term for periodontal plastic surgery is _____ surgery.

11. AOO or the Wilckodontic method is the technique used for _____ orthodontics.

12. The white or tooth-colored material of choice used for an anterior restoration is

    _____.

13. A/an _____ implant is used for a patient with a narrow jaw bone.

14. The placement of orthodontic bands on the back surfaces of the tooth is termed _____ banding.

15. _____ may be used to change the color and shape of the anterior teeth or to cover badly stained teeth.

16. A full casted crown that is covered by a porcelain covering is known as a/an _____ crown.

17. Repairing a chipped tooth by using a composite material in a dough consistency to restore the tooth is a process called tooth

    _____.

18. Another name for a dental veneer is a dental

    _____.

19. _____ stain is tooth stain caused by diet including coffee and tea, as well as smoking.

20. _____ is a term applied to the condition of the alveolar bone after receiving the surgical bur treatment in advanced orthodontics.

WORD USE

Read the following sentences and define the boldfaced words.

1. The dentist advised Mr. Sheller that there would be a few weeks between the inserting of the implant and the placement of the denture to allow for **osseointegration.**

   _____

2. Certain medicines can cause **intrinsic** staining of newly forming teeth.

   _____

3. Mrs. Swartz chose **veneers** to enhance the color and shape of her teeth.

   _____

4. When matching tooth colors to a **shade guide,** the guide should be moist so it reflects light like the natural tooth surfaces.

   _____

5. The assistant made an appointment for **gingival augmentation** for Mr. Peterson's gum recession.

   _____.

AUDIO LIST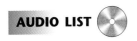

This list contains selected new, important, or difficult terms from this chapter. You may use the list to review these terms and to practice pronouncing them correctly. When you work with the audio for this chapter, listen to the word, repeat it, and then place a checkmark in the box. Proceed to the next boxed word and repeat the process.

- ❏ augmentation (awg-men-**TAY**-shun)
- ❏ extrinsic (ex-**TRIN**-sick)
- ❏ intrinsic (in-**TRIN**-sick)
- ❏ mucogingival (**myou**-koh-**JIN**-jih-**vahl**)
- ❏ osseointegration (**oss**-ee-oh-inn-teh-**GRAY**-shun)
- ❏ osteogenic (oss-tee-oh-**JEN**-ick)
- ❏ osteopenia (ahs-tee-oh-**PEE**-nee-ah)
- ❏ subperiosteal (**sub**-pear-ee-**OSS**-tee-ahl)
- ❏ transosteal (trans-**OSS**-tee-ahl)
- ❏ veneer (veh-**NEAR**)

CHAPTER 12

Prosthodontics

OBJECTIVES   Upon completion of this chapter, the reader should be able to identify and understand terms related to:

1. **Divisions in the field of prosthodontics.** Define the terms *prosthesis* and discuss fixed and removable prosthodontic appliances.

2. **Types and characteristics of prosthodontic materials.** List the assorted materials used in the construction of prostheses and describe their characteristics.

3. **Fixed prosthodontics.** List and describe the function or purpose of the various types of fixed prosthodontics.

4. **Removable dental prostheses.** List and describe the function or purpose of the various components used in removable dental prostheses.

5. **Procedures and methods used in prosthodontic practice.** List and describe the various procedural steps and methods used to complete construction of fixed and removable dental prostheses.

6. **Use of implants in prosthodontics.** Describe the various types of dental implants and their necessity in application of dental prostheses.

DIVISIONS IN THE FIELD OF PROSTHODONTICS

A prosthesis (prahs-**THEE**-sis; *plural* = prostheses) is a replacement for a missing body part. In the dental field, it may be a fixed or removable appliance that replaces removed or non-erupted tooth or teeth. A fixed appliance, such as a cemented crown, is one that is placed in the mouth and is not intended for removal. A removable appliance is one that is placed in and out of the mouth at the patient's will. Implantology, *the science of dental implants,* involves the use of both fixed appliances and removable appliances in some instances.

TYPES AND CHARACTERISTICS OF PROSTHODONTIC MATERIALS

Assorted materials are used in the construction of prostheses. Among the synthetic and precious or semi-precious metals used in appliance fabrication are:

noble metals: the valuable alloys—gold (Au), palladium (Pd), and platinum (Pt).

base metals: chromium-cobalt or chromium nickel, which may be used alone or in a mixture with noble alloys.

porcelain (**PORE**-silh-lin = *hard, translucent ceramic ware*): shells, veneer covers, or facings fused to the surface of a metal crown to give the appearance of natural tooth surface; often abbreviated PFM (porcelain fused to metal).

composite: resin material used for tooth-colored replacement.

acrylic (ah-**KRIL**-ick): synthetic resin material used in fabrication of appliance parts, as coverings for the metal frameworks, or as natural tissue replacement.

ceramic: a hard brittle material produced from non-metallic substances fired at high temperatures; supplied in block shape for milling into crown and tooth forms.

titanium: corrosion-resistant, lightweight, strong bio-compatible metal used in dental implants and posts.

The choice of which material to use for an appliance depends upon the characteristics of that material relevant to prostheses construction. Associated terms are:

hardness: ability of a material to withstand penetration.

tensile (**TEN**-sill) strength: capability of a material to be stretched.

elasticity (ee-las-**tiss**-ih-tee): ability of a material to be stretched and then resume its original shape.

ductility (duck-**TILL**-ih-tee): ability of a material to be drawn or hammered out, as into a fine wire, without breaking.

malleability (**mal**-ee-ah-**BILL**-ih-tee): ability of a material to be pressed or hammered out into various forms and shapes.

elongation (**ee**-lon-**GAY**-shun): ability of a material to stretch before permanent deformation begins.

▌FIXED PROSTHODONTICS

Various fixed prosthodontic appliances are used in mouth restoration, from the singular crown to a full arched bridge.

inlay: a solid casted or milled restoration involving some occlusal and proximal surfaces that is cemented into a tooth preparation.

onlay: a solid casted or milled restoration that covers some occlusal tooth cusp and side wall area that is cemented onto the prepared site.

crown: a fabricated, tooth-shaped cover replacement for a missing crown area that is cemented onto the remaining prepared crown surfaces. Some of the types of crowns are shown in Cosmetic Dentistry, Chapter 11, Figure 11-1.

full crown: cast metal, tooth-shaped cover that replaces the entire crown area. Acrylic resin crowns may be used as a temporary crown cover during treatment.

jacket crown: thin, preformed, metal shield used to cover a large area of anterior crowns; can be gold metal or metal covered with porcelain material to resemble tooth enamel.

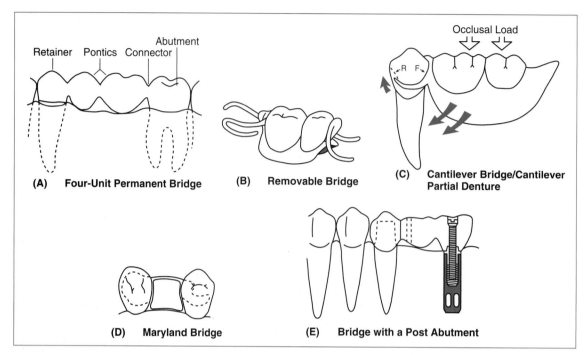

Retainer Pontics Connector Abutment

(A) Four-Unit Permanent Bridge

(B) Removable Bridge

Occlusal Load

R F

(C) Cantilever Bridge/Cantilever Partial Denture

(D) Maryland Bridge

(E) Bridge with a Post Abutment

FIGURE 12-1
Examples of bridges.

dowel crown: full crown cover with dowel pin extending into the root canal of a pulpless tooth, usually positioned on anterior teeth.

three-quarter crown: similar to full crown, covering all of the crown except the facial surface of the tooth that remains intact, to present an esthetic, natural appearance.

porcelain-fused-to-gold (PFM): crown that has a complete capping of metal base with fused porcelain to metal, giving tooth contour, shape, and cover.

veneer: A **direct veneer** is placed and cured directly on the tooth surface to build up the area or replace missing tooth structure. For **indirect veneer**, tooth material is prepared in the lab and later cemented onto the tooth structure.

Crown replacement also may be part of different fixed bridgework. A **bridge** is a prosthesis used to replace one or more teeth. Dental bridgework may be of a fixed or removable nature. Figure 12-1 gives examples of bridges.

fixed bridge: cemented into the oral cavity and not removed by the patient; the number of teeth involved in the appliance determines the number of units.

Maryland bridge: replaces anterior or posterior tooth and is cemented directly to the adjacent or abutting teeth; also called resin-bonded bridge.

cantilever (**KAN**-tih-**lee**-ver) **bridge**: bridge with unsupported end, usually saddled.

A bridge has three components or structural parts.

1. pontic (**PON**-tick): artificial tooth part of the bridge that replaces the missing tooth and restores function to the bite.

2. **abutment** (ah-**BUT**-ment): natural tooth or teeth that are prepared to hold or support the retaining part of the bridgework in position.

3. **adjacent** (ah-**JAY**-cent = *nearby or adjoining*) teeth: may be included in units if they are involved in the bridge area.

▌ REMOVABLE DENTAL PROSTHESES

Prostheses that the patient can take in and out at will are called removable prostheses. These devices include full mouth dentures, as well as a replacement for single teeth. Terminology includes:

complete denture (**DENT**-chur = *removable appliance composed of artificial teeth set in an acrylic base*): full denture designed to replace the entire dentition of an upper or lower arch.

partial denture: removable appliance, usually composed of framework, artificial teeth, and acrylic material; replaces one or more teeth in an arch.

immediate denture: denture prosthesis that is placed into the mouth at the time the natural teeth are surgically removed.

overdenture: prosthetic denture that is prepared to fit and be secured upon implant posts or prepared retained roots.

Although all removable appliances are constructed to fit in a designated area and to return the mouth to a proper function, not all are fabricated in the same manner or using the same materials. The structural components of dental appliances used in removable prostheses described in this section are illustrated in Figure 12-2.

framework: metal skeleton or spine onto which a removable prosthesis is constructed.

saddle: the part of the removable prosthesis that strides or straddles the gingival crest; used to balance the prosthesis, and serves as a base for placement of artificial teeth.

rests: small extensions of removable prosthesis made to fit or sit atop the adjoining teeth; provide balance and stability for the partial denture appliance. Rests are named for the area that is in contact with the tooth surface—occlusal, lingual, incisal, etc.

clasp: extension of partial framework that grasps the adjoining teeth to provide support and retention of the prosthesis.

retainer (ree-**TAIN**-ur): in fixed prosthesis, the part of the appliance that joins with the abutting, natural tooth to support the appliance, like the pillar holding the span of a bridge over the water. Some retainers are thin bars extending from quadrant to quadrant, called lingual bars or palatial bars.

connector (kon-**ECK**-tore = *device used to unite or attach two or more parts together*): used to connect quadrants of a partial denture or connect and support an overdenture.

stress breaker: a connector applied in stress-bearing areas to provide a safe area for breakage.

artificial teeth: anatomical substitutes for natural teeth; made of porcelain or acrylic material in various shades and shapes, called molds.

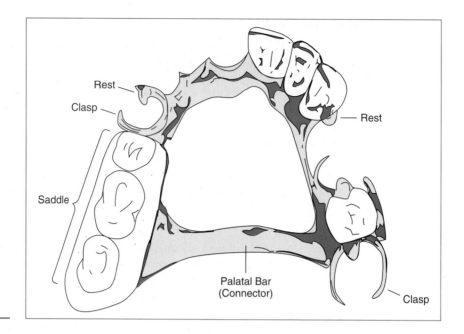

FIGURE 12-2
Removable partial denture.

denture base: acrylic part of the denture prosthesis that substitutes for the gingival tissue.

flange (flanj): projecting rim or lower edge of prosthesis.

post dam: posterior edge of the maxillary denture; helps to maintain the denture and suction.

PROCEDURES AND METHODS USED IN PROSTHODONTIC PRACTICE

Many of the operative procedures for fixed and removable prosthodontic appliances are similar in nature, with a few variations. Table 12-1 compares the operative steps for fixed and removable dental prostheses. The discussion of prosthesis fabrication is concluded in Chapter 19.

TABLE 12-1 Comparison of Operative Steps for Dental Prostheses

FIXED PROSTHODONTICS	REMOVABLE PROSTHODONTICS
Exam, shade, mold selection, impression	Same procedure
Preparation of tooth and/or site	Mouth preparation, surgical adjustment
Impression of prepared tooth/site	Multiple impressions-custom trays
Try-in, unit adjustment	Try-in, wax adjustment
Adjustment, seating, and cementation	Adjustment and delivery

Impression Procedure

Throughout the prosthodontic appointment, various impressions of the teeth and tooth preparations are taken. The choice of the material to be used and the necessary items required for the procedure depend upon the reason for the treatment and the condition or physical properties of the item to receive the impression. Impression materials must be **elastomeric** (**ee**-las-toh-**MARE**-ick = *having properties similar to rubber*), to be pliable during the impression process. Elastic impression items include hydrocolloids, rubber bases, and compounds.

Hydrocolloids. An impression material that is both reversible and irreversible is **hydrocolloid** (**high**-droh-**KOHL**-oyd, *hydro = water, colloid = suspension of material*), an agar-like material that can change from one form to another.

reversible hydrocolloid: impression material that can change from a solid or gel state to a liquid form and back again, depending upon temperature changes. This material is used in a water-cooled tray.
thermoplastic (**therm**-oh-**PLAS**-tick; *thermo = heat, plastic = moveable*): quality of a material that changes from a rigid to plastic or movable form as a result of application of heat.
irreversible hydrocolloid: quality that, once chemically set or in gel form, cannot be reversed or used again. An example of an irreversible hydrocolloid is **alginate** (**Al**-jih-nate). Humidity can affect the water balance and stability of irreversible hydrocolloid. Swelling from absorption of water is called **imbibition** (**im**-bih-**BISH**-un = *fluid absorption*), and evaporation or fluid loss causes shrinkage.

Rubber Bases. Rubber bases are common impression materials. They exhibit rubberized characteristics and are supplied in tubes, wash, and putty consistency or in a twin-cartridge (base and accelerator/activator), calibrated mixing dispenser called an **extruder** (ecks-**TRUE**-dur) **gun**. The base mixture requires an activator or **catalyst** (**CAT**-ah-list = *substance that speeds up a chemical reaction*) to instigate mixing together into a homogenous mass. The basic types of rubber bases are **silicone** (**SILL**-ih-kone), **polyether** (**pohl**-ee-**EE**-thur), **polysulfide** (**pohl**-ee-**SUL**-fide), and **polyvinylsiloxane** (**pohl**-ee-vine-uhl-sil-**ox**-ain).

Compound. Another thermoplastic impression material is **compound** (**CAHM**-pound), a non-elastic impression material that may be used in edentulous impressions. Compound is supplied in cakes or blocks and is heated to a soft, pliable mass, placed in an impression tray, and put into the mouth. After cooling in the mouth, it is removed, cooled further, and used as a customized impression tray for a future final wash or impression.

Impression Trays. Dental impressions of the mouth are accomplished by placing the desired material into a carrying device and inserting it into the patient's oral cavity. The specific device used to transport the impression material depends upon the site to be reproduced. Impressions can be of one tooth, a few teeth, or an entire **edentulous** (ee-**DENT**-you-luss = *without teeth*) arch. Some transport devices are

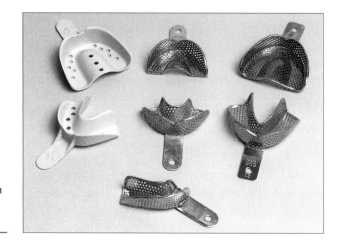

FIGURE 12-3
Impression trays.

Note: Impression trays can be rim-locked style or with holes to help hold in the material.

copper tubes. Some are trays of *stock* metal or plastic purchased through dental suppliers. Trays may be custom-constructed or purchased as full arch, quadrant, or sectional and anterior trays. Impression trays come in various sizes and shapes to accommodate specific areas of the mouth. Figure 12-3 shows a few examples.

Preparation of Teeth and Site

Site preparation must be accomplished before a prosthesis can be placed. The teeth and the area involved could receive one or a combination of a variety of preparations.

alveolectomy (al-vee-oh-**LECK**-toe-mee): surgical removal of alveolar bone crests, may be required to provide smooth alveolar ridge for denture seating.

alveoplastomy (al-vee-oh-**PLASS**-toe-me): surgical reshaping or contouring of alveolar bone.

extraction (ecks-**TRACK**-shun): surgical removal of teeth may be necessary. If completed before the insertion of an immediate denture, a clear template (**TEM**-plate = *guide or pattern*) may be used as a guide to prepare the alveolar surface.

coping (**KOH**-ping = *coverings*): metal cover placed over the remaining natural tooth surfaces to provide attachments for overdentures.

reduction (ree-**DUCT**-shun = *reducing or lessening in size*): removal of tooth decay and surfaces to receive the appliance. Various margin edges are prepared on the natural tooth to accommodate the thickness and material of the covering artificial crown, as illustrated in Figure 12-4.

  chamfer (**SHAM**-fur = *tapered margin at tooth cervix*): preparation for crown placement.

  shoulder (**SHOAL**-dur = *cut gingival margin edge*): preparation to provide junction of the crown and tooth.

  bevel (**BEV**-el = *slanted edge*): tooth preparation for seating and holding a crown.

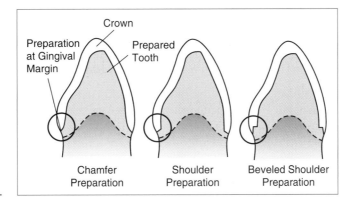

Crown

Preparation
at Gingival
Margin

Prepared
Tooth

FIGURE 12-4
Tooth margins.

| Chamfer Preparation | Shoulder Preparation | Beveled Shoulder Preparation |

core buildup: use of synthetic material to enlarge tooth core area to provide support for an artificial crown and to protect the pulpal tissues. Small brass pins may be inserted into the material to aid retention and strength.

post placement: addition of a metal retention post to teeth that have had pulp removal and root canal enlargement, to aid in stability and strength.

undercut: removal of tooth structure near the gingival edge to provide a seat or placement for the extending edge of the appliance.

retraction cord: chemically treated cord placed in the gingival sulcus to obtain chemical or physical shrinking of the gingiva. These twisted or braided cords are plain or impregnated (im-**PREG**-nay-ted = *saturated*) with chemicals and packed into the gingival area to cause temporary shrinkage of tissue and/or to control bleeding. A retraction paste may be ejected into the sulcus prep for one to two minutes and rinsed away prior to taking the impression.

bite registration: impression of the teeth while in occlusion. A bite registration is taken to assist with fabrication of the prosthesis. The impression may be obtained from biting into a wax sheet, or stock trays and prepared frames filled with impression material. Some dentists eject impression material on the surfaces of the teeth to make a bite pattern for later use. Bite registrations are classified in various ways.

open bite: patient bites into the impression material.

closed bite: the material is injected and expressed around the desired teeth while they are in occlusion.

opposing arch: impressions of the occlusal surfaces of both arches are taken in the same procedure.

work order: written directions from the dentist to the laboratory completing the case; the impressions, bite registration, and orders are sent together.

temporary or provisional coverage: temporary protection for the prepared tooth while laboratory work is being completed. Coverage may be in form of an aluminum cap, acrylic custom cover, or preformed resin crown form cemented onto the prepared teeth for protection until the final try-in and delivery.

Try-In, Adjustment, and Delivery

During the preparation, construction, and delivery of the dental prosthesis, the patient will return for various appointments. Some visits require adjustment and recordings of measurements that will be sent to the laboratory to assist in final fabrication.

seating: placement and fitting of appliance for try-in and final cementation. The patient bites on a stick or device, applying pressure for application of the crown or prosthetic item.

condylar inclination (**KHAN**-dih-lahr = *pertaining to the condyle*) (**in**-klih-**NAY**-shun = *tendency, bending, bias*): observation of bite relationship and TMJ involvement. The following articulation movements involve the condyle:

    centric (**SEN**-trick = *central, center*): occuring when the condyle rests in the temporal bone during biting, resting, and mouth movements.

    protrusion (pro-**TRUE**-zhun = *projecting or thrust forward*): measurement with the mandible thrust forward, with the lower jaw out.

    retrusion (ree-**TRUE**-zhun = *forcing backward*): measurement with the mandible drawn backward.

    lateral excursion (**LAT**-er-al = *side*, ecks-**KERR**-shun = *movement*): measurement with side-to-side movement of the mandible.

appearance indicators: notations of the smile line and the length of the cuspid point.

USE OF IMPLANTS IN PROSTHDONTICS

In cases where prosthodontic appliances do not fit properly or are difficult to retain in the mouth, the dentist may suggest implants to provide stabilization and retention. There are different types of implants and each is used in a specific area, depending upon available bone, type and amount of stabilization needed.

implant (**IM**-plant = *insertion of object*): surgical insertion of implant posts or prepared frame to provide stabilization for overdentures or appliance retention. A surgical implant may be:

    root form implant-endosseous (**en**-**DOE**-see-us = *within the alveolar bone*): screw-type device that is screwed or cemented into the mandibular bone; used for a single tooth or post implant.

    plate form implant: used for the narrow jaw bone; flat plate style.

    subperiosteal (**sub**-pear-ee-**OSS**-tee-ahl = *under the gingival and alveolar tissues*): implant plate or frame placed under the periodontium and stabilized on the mandibular bone. It is used when bone height or width is insufficient; rests on top of the bone.

    transosteal (trans-**OSS**-tee-ahl = *through the mandibular bone*): larger plate stabilized on the lower border of the mandibular bone with posts extending through the gingiva; used to anchor prostheses in difficult situations.

All implant appliances must bond with the bone tissue in order to obtain stability. This process is called **osseointegration** (*osseo = bone, integrate = bonding*).

REVIEW EXERCISES

MATCHING

Match the following word elements with their meaning:

1. _____veneer
2. _____acrylic

3. _____abutment

4. _____titanium

5. _____ductility

6. _____pontic

7. _____amalgam

8. _____alginate

9. _____tensile strength

10. _____rest

11. _____elasticity

12. _____clasp

13. _____porcelain

14. _____flange

15. _____malleability

a. implant metal
b. thin surface shell or layer applied to tooth surface
c. ability to be pressed or hammered into a shape
d. claw-like framework extension to grasp teeth
e. hard, translucent ceramic shell or cover material
f. resin material used in denture gingiva fabrication
g. natural tooth used to support bridge-work retainer
h. projecting rim or lower edge of denture or saddle
i. ability of material to stretch and return to shape
j. the part of the partial that sits on tooth to retain stability
k. ability to be drawn out into a thin line without breaking
l. part of bridgework replacing missing tooth/teeth
m. ability to be stretched
n. base metal or combination of metals
o. hydrocolloid that is irreversible

DEFINITIONS

Using the selection given for each sentence, choose the best term to complete the definition.

1. A full mouth maxillary denture is an example of what type of prosthesis?
   a. fixed
   b. removable
   c. immediate
   d. compound

2. A measurement taken with the mandible drawn back in occlusion is termed:
   a. centric
   b. protrusion
   c. retrusion
   d. lateral

3. A measurement taken with the mandible thrust forward in occlusion is termed:
   a. centric
   b. protrusion
   c. retrusion
   d. lateral

4. A solid, cast restoration fabricated to fit into a prepared tooth is a/an:
   a. inlay
   b. onlay
   c. crown
   d. composite

5. A thin layered sheath to be placed over the surface of a tooth is a/an:
   a. taper
   b. bridge
   c. veneer
   d. jacket

6. A smile line and cuspid point length are considered indicators of:
   a. appearance
   b. function
   c. condyle placement
   d. occlusion

7. Aluminum caps, preformed crowns, and custom crowns used between appointments are:
   a. permanent coverage
   b. try-in applications
   c. temporary coverage
   d. restorations

8. A natural tooth used to support and become part of a fixed bridge is a/an:
   a. restoration
   b. adjacent
   c. apperature
   d. abutment

9. Which of the following metals is not considered a noble metal?
   a. gold
   b. amalgam
   c. palladium
   d. platinum

10. A retraction cord saturated with a chemical to resorb tissue is said to be:
    a. impregnated   b. medicated
    c. resorptive   d. regulated

11. A denture prosthesis placed in the mouth at the time of tooth removal is a/an:
    a. overdenture   b. partial denture
    c. immediate denture   d. Maryland bridge

12. A hard, translucent, non-metallic block material used in milling crowns and inlays at chairside is a/an:
    a. composite   b. ceramic
    c. acrylic   d. amalgam

13. The ability of a material to withstand penetration is an example of:
    a. hardness   b. ductility
    c. tensile strength d. elasticity

14. The ability to be hammered or pressed into shape is an example of:
    a. elasticity   b. elongation
    c. ductility   d. malleability

15. The part of a partial denture that straddles the alveolar crest and gives support is a/an:
    a. saddle   b. retainer
    c. clasp   d. rest

16. The lower edge of a denture is called the:
    a. oblique ridge   b. rest
    c. post dam   d. flange

17. Alginate impression material is considered:
    a. thermoplastic   b. hydrocolloid
    c. gypsum   d. alloy

18. The term for a human dentition containing no teeth is:
    a. edentulous   b. abutting
    c. undentated   d. furnicated

19. A full gold crown with a porcelain facing is which type of prosthodontia?
    a. fixed   b. removable
    c. immediate   d. complete

20. A prosthesis constructed to fit over and attach to anchor post in the alveolar bone is a/an:
    a. immediate denture b. composite denture
    c. overdenture   d. Maryland bridge

BUILDING SKILLS

Locate and define the prefix, root/combining form, and suffix (if present) in the following words:

1. **thermoplastic**
   prefix   _____
   root/combining form   _____
   suffix   _____

2. **edentulous**
   prefix   _____
   root/combining form   _____
   suffix   _____

3. **impregnated**
   prefix   _____
   root/combining form   _____
   suffix   _____

4. **imbibition**
   prefix   _____
   root word   _____
   suffix   _____

5. **malleability**
   prefix   _____
   root/combining form   _____
   suffix   _____

FILL-INS

Write the correct word in the blank space to complete each statement.

1. The impressions and _____ that are sent to the lab are physical records of the patient's mouth form and occlusion.

2. A machine that holds two materials, unites them, and expresses one mixed material is a/an_____syringe.

3. The acrylic crown cover placed upon the prepared tooth between visits is called _____coverage.

4. _____is the taking on or absorbing of moisture by alginate material.

5. To provide support and aid retention in a large prep of a non-vital tooth, a/an _____ may be placed and

cemented into the enlarged nonfunctional root canal.

6. A/an _____ is a material or chemical that enables or quickens the chemical reaction.

7. A mouth without teeth is said to be _____.

8. The process of gross removal of tooth structure during a crown prep is called _____.

9. A/an _____ is a slanted edge prep of a tooth being prepared for a crown.

10. After gross removal of tooth structure, a/an _____ may be required to provide crown support and pulp protection.

11. A retraction core containing chemicals to decrease blood flow is said to be _____.

12. A registration of a bite while in occlusion is a/an _____ registration.

13. A prescription describing desired labor that is sent to the lab with the impressions is called a/an _____.

14. A/an _____, or removal of some tooth surface, may be placed along the gingival area of a natural tooth to assist in holding clasps from a bridge.

15. A tapered margin at the tooth cervix placed in preparation for a crown is a/an _____.

16. An extension of bridge framework that sits on the occlusal surface to support and stabilize the bridge is a/an _____.

17. A claw-like extension of a bridge that encircles a natural tooth and aids in retention of a crown is a/an _____.

18. A full cover resembling the natural shape of the tooth that is placed over a large preparation is a/an _____.

19. The metal skeleton of a partial appliance is the _____.

20. A resin material that may be used in the core build-up of a tooth is _____.

WORD USE

Read the following sentences and define the bold-faced word.

1. To control bleeding and to provide a better impression of the prep site, the dentist may request a piece of retraction cord **impregnated** with alum or another chemical.

_____

2. The dentist used the shadeguide to choose the correct shade for the **pontic**.

_____

3. Special care is given to the procedure for packing and shipping a dental **prosthesis**.

_____

4. This appointment for dental crown work is mainly for preparation of the **abutments.**

_____

5. Always replace the lid of the alginate container to prevent **imbibition** to the material.

_____

AUDIO LIST

This list contains selected new, important, or difficult terms from this chapter. You may use the list to review these terms and to practice pronouncing them correctly. When you work with the audio for this chapter, listen to the word, repeat it, and then place a checkmark in the box. Proceed to the next boxed word and repeat the process.

- ❏ abutment (ah-**BUT**-ment)
- ❏ acrylic (ah-**KRIL**-ick)
- ❏ adjacent (ah-**JAY**-sent)
- ❏ alveolectomy (al-vee-oh-**LECK**-toe-mee)
- ❏ alveoplastomy (al-vee-oh-**PLASS**-toe me)
- ❏ bevel (**BEV**-el)
- ❏ cantilever (**KAN**-tih-lee-ver)
- ❏ catalyst (**CAT**-ah-list)
- ❏ centric (**SEN**-trick)
- ❏ chamfer (**SHAM**-fur)
- ❏ condylar inclination (**KAHN**-dih-lahr in-klih-**NAY**-shun)
- ❏ connector (kon-**ECK**-tore)
- ❏ coping (**KOH**-ping)
- ❏ ductility (duck-**TILL**-ih-tee)
- ❏ edentulous (ee-**DENT**-you-luss)
- ❏ elasticity (ee-las-**tiss**-ih-tee)
- ❏ elastomeric (ee-las-toh-**MARE**-ick)
- ❏ endosseous (en-**DOE**-see-us)
- ❏ extraction (ecks-**TRACK**-shun)
- ❏ extruder (ecks-**TRUE**-dur)
- ❏ hydrocolloid (high-droh-**KOHL**-oyd)
- ❏ imbibition (im-bih-**BISH**-un)
- ❏ impregnated (im-**PREG**-nay-ted)
- ❏ malleability (mal-ee-ah-**BILL**-ih-tee)
- ❏ polyether (pohl-ee-**EE**-thur)
- ❏ polysulfide (pohl-ee-**SUL**-fide)
- ❏ polyvinylsiloxane (pohl-ee-vine-uhl-sil-**OX**-ain)
- ❏ pontic (**PON**-tick)
- ❏ porcelain (**PORE**-silh-lin)
- ❏ prosthesis (prahs-**THEE**-sis)
- ❏ protrusion (proh-**TRUE**-zhun)
- ❏ reduction (ree-**DUCT**-shun)
- ❏ retainer (ree-**TAIN**-ur)
- ❏ retrusion (ree-**TRUE**-zhun)
- ❏ shoulder (**SHOAL**-dur)
- ❏ silicone (**SILL**-ih-kone)
- ❏ subperiosteal (sub-pear-ee-**OSS**-tee-uhl)
- ❏ tensile (**TEN**-sill)
- ❏ thermoplastic (therm-oh-**PLAS**-tick)
- ❏ transosteal (trans-**OSS**-tee-ahl)

CHAPTER 13

Endodontics

OBJECTIVES   Upon completion of this chapter, the reader should be able to identify and understand terms related to:

1. **Science and practice of endodontic dentistry.** Define the practice of endodontia and discuss the need for pulp treatment.

2. **Diagnostic procedures to determine pulpal conditions.** Identify and explain the diagnostic tests used to determine pulpal conditions.

3. **Endodontic treatment procedures.** Discuss the treatment steps required in pulpal and endodontic procedures.

4. **Endodontic treatment equipment and materials.** List and identify the equipment and materials necessary for endodontic treatment.

5. **Surgical endodontic treatments.** Describe the surgical treatment plans employed in endodontic care.

6. **Endodontic treatment of traumatized teeth.** Describe and discuss the treatment involved in the care of traumatized teeth.

7. **Tooth replantation procedures.** List and identify the various methods and types of replantation procedures available in endodontic practice.

SCIENCE AND PRACTICE OF ENDODONTIC DENTISTRY

Endodontia (**en**-doh-**DAHN**-she-ah = *within the tooth*) is the branch of dentistry concerned with the diagnosis, treatment, and prevention of diseases of the dental pulp and its surrounding periradicular (pear-ee-rah-**DICK**-you-lar; peri = *around*, radi = *root*) tissues. The dental specialist who is limited to and performing this practice is the endodontist (en-doh-**DON**-tist). The endodontic treatment or procedure necessary to treat an inflamed pulpal condition, also known as pulpitis (pul-**PIE**-tis), depends upon the condition of the inner tooth tissues. The inflamed pulp tissue may be afflicted with a reversible condition and, because the fibers are vital or alive, may recover.

Diseased pulp tissue that cannot recover and repair itself is said to be **necrotic** (neh-**KRAH**-tick = *dead or non-vital*), an irreversible condition. Diagnosis and future treatment is determined by endodontic diagnostic testing of the affected tooth and its surrounding tissues.

DIAGNOSTIC PROCEDURES TO DETERMINE PULPAL CONDITIONS

Evaluation of the vitality of the pulp involves an assortment of tests. All evaluations begin with a review of the patient's dental history and a clinical examination. An exam will reveal clues that are either objective or subjective.

objective signs: conditions observed by someone other than the patient. Examples are a tooth **hyperextension** (hyper = *over*, extension = *movement*), a condition in which the tooth arises out of the socket, or a noticeable, unpleasant odor known as **putrefaction** (pyou-trih-**FACK**-shun = *decaying animal matter*).

subjective symptoms: conditions as described by the patient, who may complain of **hypersensitivity** (**high**-per-**sen**-sih-**TIV**-ih-tee; hyper = *over*; sensitivity = *abnormal reaction to stimulus*) or **pulpalgia** (pul-**PAL**-jee-ah) (pulp = *inner tooth tissue*, algia = *pain*).

Clinical Examinations

Clinical examination of the affected tooth or teeth is conducted to diagnose the dental conditions. Clinical examinations may include any of a number of tests.

palpation (pal-**PAY**-shun): application of finger pressure to body tissues, including gingiva.

percussion (per-**KUSH**-un = *tapping of body tissue, tooth*): usually done by tapping a dental mirror handle on an affected tooth and comparing the sensation to tapping on a healthy or *control* tooth.

mobility (moh-**BIL**-ih-tee = *capable of movement*): movement of a tooth in its socket during outside force or application of pressure.

transillumination (**trans**-ill-**oo**-mih-**NAY**-shun = *passage of light through object/tissue*): a light refraction test to reveal fractured tooth tissue.

thermal (**THER**-mahl = *pertaining to temperature*): pulp sensitivity test with reaction to application of heat and/or cold to tooth surface.

anesthesia: numbing the specific root or nerve ending to dissipate pain.

direct dentin stimulation: scratching the exposed dentin with an explorer; the presence of pain indicates inflamed or irritated pulp tissue.

electric pulp testing: applying an electrical current on the enamel surface of the tooth to register the tooth's pulpal sensitivity and presence of irritability. (Figure 13-1 shows two examples of testers.)

radiograph: x-ray examination and other technology such as digital radiometric analysis, radiovisiongraphy, and magnetic resonance imaging (MRI) to demonstrate early changes of bone structure and periapical involvement of suspected tooth with an inflamed pulp.

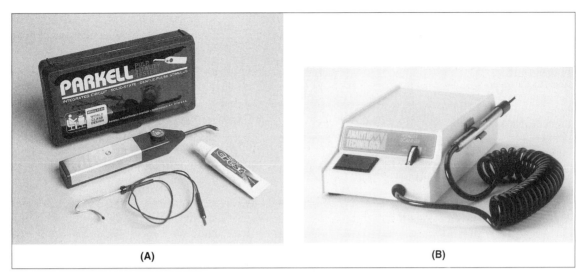

(A) **(B)**

FIGURE 13-1
Examples of pulp vitality testers. (Courtesy of Analytic Endodontics)
(A) Manual Tester
(B) Digital Scanner

Periradicular Diagnosis

Once the clinical testing has been completed, the dentist can determine the nature of the disease, or diagnosis, and develop a treatment plan. The principal diagnosis involving pulp tissues is to determine if the pulp is vital or non-vital. The periradicular tissue diagnosis may involve more pathologic conditions, such as:

periodontitis (**pear**-ee-oh-don-**TIE**-tis; peri = *around*, don = *tooth*, it is = *inflammation*): in acute apical periodontitis, a sharp, painful inflammation of tissues around an affected tooth. Pain is lessened or eliminated by removing the inflamed or necrotic pulp. A chronic apical periodontitis (CAP) requires management similar to the acute symptoms.

abscess (**AB**-cess = *local pus infection*): an infection that may be an acute or chronic apical abscess: also called **suppurative** (**SUP**-you-rah-tiv = *producing or generating pus*).

pericementitis (**pear**-ih-see-men-**TIE**-tiss (peri = *around*, cement = *cementuis*, it is = *inflammation*): inflammation and necrosis of alveoli of the tooth.

cyst (**SIST**): abnormal, closely walled fluid or exudates-filled sac in or around periapical tissues.

cellulitis (sell-you-**LIE**-tiss): inflammation of cellular or connective tissue.

osteomyelitis (oss-tee-oh-my-**LYE**-tiss): an inflammation of the bone and bone marrow, usually caused by bacterial infection.

ENDODONTIC TREATMENT PROCEDURES

After the diagnosis has been completed, a treatment plan is developed to provide dental care. An affected or irritated pulp may need one of several treatment procedures.

pulpotomy (puhl-**POT**-oh-mee): partial excision of the dental pulp.

FIGURE 13-2
Pulpectomy proce-
dure. (A) Gaining
canal access
(B) Enlarging the
canal (C) Cleansing
the canal (D) Filling
the canal
(E) Finished RCT.

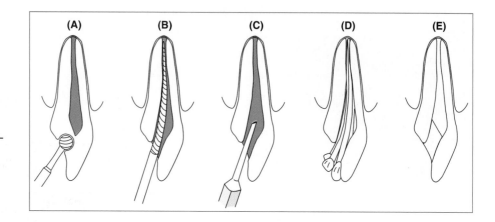

pulpectomy (puhl-**PECK**-toh-mee): surgical removal of pulp from the tooth, also known as root canal treatment (RCT) (see Figure 13-2 for steps in the procedure).

apicoectomy (ay-pih-koh-**ECK**-toh-mee): surgical amputation of a root apex.

Root Canal Treatment

The standard treatment for a root canal has the following steps.

1. **anesthesia**: local injection to relieve pain occurring during the procedure.
2. **isolation** of the operative area: accomplished to provide safety and to assure an **aseptic** (ay-**SEP**-tick = *without disease*) site.
3. **extirpation** (ecks-ter-**PAY**-shun = *to root out*): removing the pulpal tissue after the pulpal opening.
4. **debridement** (deh-**BREED**-ment = *removal of foreign or decayed matter*): removing necrotic pulpal tissue and cleaning out the area.
5. **irrigation and cleansing**: using chemicals and instruments to remove tissue dust and material matter from the pulp and pulp canals.
6. **obturation** (ahb-too-**RAY**-shun = *to close or stop up*): filling and closing the canal area. This may consist of filling from the pulp to the apex or may be complete in a **retrograde** (**REH**-troh-grade = *backward step*), process of filling the canal beginning from the apex of the tooth to the pulp, also called a retrofill endodontic restoration.
7. **restoration**: returning the tooth to normal function and purpose.

ENDODONTIC TREATMENT EQUIPMENT AND MATERIALS

Specialized equipment is needed to perform endodontic treatment and procedures. Dental dam material is used to isolate the endodontic site.

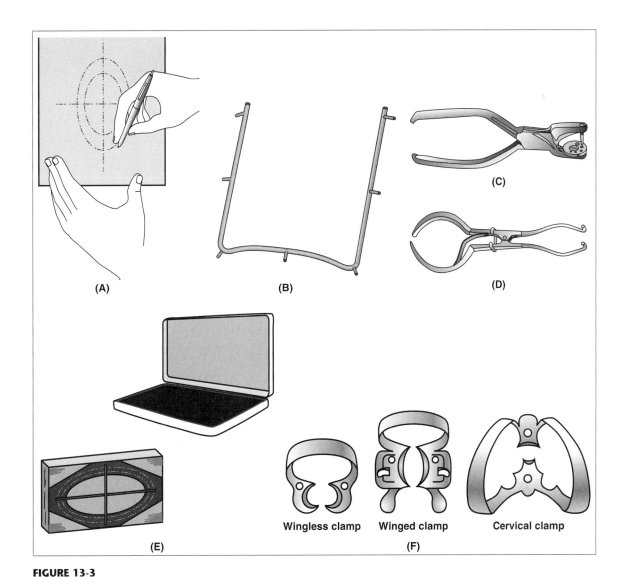

FIGURE 13-3
Dental dam equipment. (A) Dam Material (B) Dam Frame (C) Dam Punch (D) Dam Forceps (E) Dam Stamp and Pad (F) Dam Clamp Assortment

Dental Dam

The purposes and procedures of the dental dam are discussed in Chapter 10, Tooth Restorations. The components of the dental dam (sometimes called rubber dam) isolation equipment are listed below and illustrated in Figure 13-3.

dental dam material: thin sheet of latex or non-latex rubber, that varies in thickness, color and size (view A).

dental dam frame: device used to hold material in place; may be metal or plastic, rigid or adjustable (view B).

dental dam punch: device used to place selected holes in the dam material for isolating a tooth or teeth (view C).

dental dam forceps: hand device used to transport and place clamps or retainers around the selected tooth (view D).

rubber dam stamp and pad: marking stamper and pad devices used to indicate alignment spots for puncturing the material with the punch (view E).

dental dam clamp: retaining device used to hold the material around the tooth; may be metal or resin and vary in size, shape, and style. A clear plastic "hat dam" may be closely fitted and trimmed to fit a damaged tooth crown and temporarily cemented onto the tooth crown with glass ionomer cement. The rubber dam material fits under the device that is removed after treatment. Isolation also may be assisted by use of sealing materials that adhere tooth structure or gingiva to rubber dam material for a short time, approximately 1 hour (view F gives examples of clamps).

dental dam ligature: material used to hold and secure the dam material in the mouth; can be dental floss, latex stabilizing cord, or a small piece of dental dam.

RCT Instrumentation

Root canal instruments are specially designed to be used in small, cramped areas such as the tooth pulp chambers and canals. These instruments may be engine-driven but must be used in special endodontic handpieces that usually are electric and do not exceed speeds of 390 rpm. Many RCT instruments are small, held and rotated by finger control only. Others have longer shafts to accommodate the length of the canals. Each instrument completes a specific task in the RCT.

Preparation Instruments. Endodontic instruments used to debride and obturate the canal may be classified as hand-operated, engine-driven, or ultrasonic and sonic. These endodontic instruments, illustrated in Figure 13-4, are quite small and delicate.

broach: a thin, barbed, wired instrument, inserted into the root canal to ensnare and remove the pulp tissue and any natural or placed matter, such as paper points or cotton pellets. (view A).

reamer (**REE**-mer): a thin, twisted, sharp-edged instrument inserted into the canal and rotated clockwise to enlarge and taper the root canal. Reamers are available in various sizes and can be color-coded for easy identification; they also may be engine-driven at slow speeds (view B).

file: a thin, rough-edged, instrument used to plane and smooth pulpal walls. Types of files are:

K-file: has twisted edges and is used to enlarge as well as to smooth walls; color-coded to denote size.

Hedstrom file (U- and S-shaped): cone-shaped, twisted-edge instrument used for enlarging and smoothing; nickel titanium alloy files provide more flexibility.

flex file: stainless steel or nickel titanium alloy file that is stronger and provides more flexibility; used in narrow, curved canals.

pesso (**PESS**-oh) reamer: thicker, engine driven, reamer with larger and longer parallel cutting edges for use in canal openings (view C).

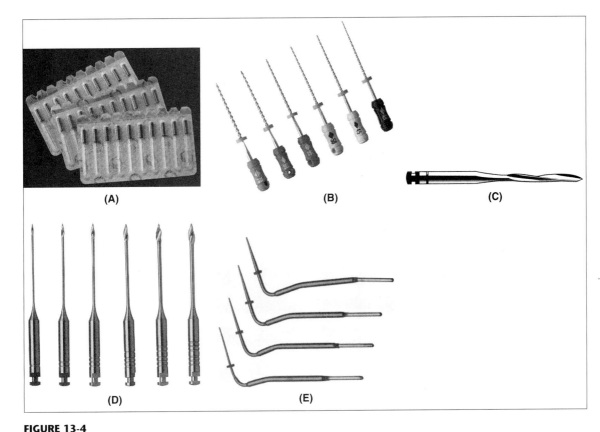

FIGURE 13-4
Endodontic instruments. (A) Barbed Broach (B) Reamers (C) Peeso Reamer (D) Gates–Glidden Drills (E) Spreaders

Note: A, B, D, and E are courtesy of Sybron Endo; C is courtesy of Premier Dental Products Company.

Gates–Glidden drills: engine-driven, latch-type burs with flame-shaped tip; used to provide an opening and access (view D).

paper points: small, narrow, absorbent, paper tips that may be inserted into the obturated canal; used to dry the prep site or to carry medication to the area; available in various gauges and lengths or may have tips cut off to accommodate needed size.

stopper: a small piece of elastic band or commercial plug that is moved up or down the shaft of the endo instrument; used to mark and indicate the length of penetration.

rotary burs and stones: friction grip burs with diamond or carbide tips used to gain access through restorations and crowns.

Filling Instruments. Some endodontic instruments used for filling canals are finger-style for more curved canals. Others are constructed with a handle, shaft, and nib for hand control and may be used with or without heat application. Figure 13-4 illustrates endodontic instruments.

root canal (endodontic) spreader: longer shank with pointed nib; used to carry and insert cement or filling material (view E).

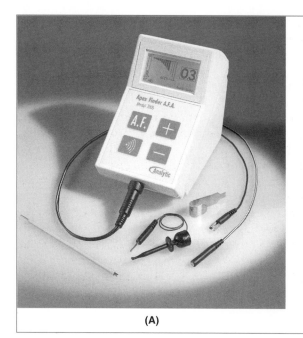
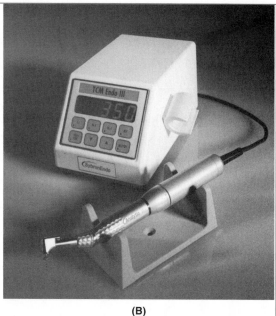

(A)　　　　　　　　(B)

FIGURE 13-5
Endodontic
machines.
(Courtesy of Sybron
Endo) (A) Apex
Locator Machine
(B) Electric
Endodontic
Handpiece

root canal plugger: longer-shanked with a flat tipped nib. It is used to condense and adapt the canal filling material.

root canal condenser: handled, long-tip instrument that may be heated and used to condense gutta-percha to the canal walls.

Lentulo spiral drill: thin, twisted wire, latch-type rotary instrument used to spread calcium hydroxide or cement into the canal.

Assorted RCT Instruments. Ultrasonic and sonic instruments used in endodontic treatment include machines that vibrate energy waves for debridement and irrigating canals and are used in conjunction with hand instrumentation. Figure 13-5 shows two of these machines. **Apex locator machines** (view A) are used to determine the proximity of the test file to the root apex and relate the information to PC board screen during preparation of the canal.

Heat carrier machines provide adjustable heat to soften, deliver, and condense gutta-percha to the canal. **Electric endodontic handpieces** (view B) permit use of instruments at slow speeds for finger instrumentation. Other assorted instruments include the explorer, spoon excavator, and paddle-ended blades. These dental hand instruments have increased nib, blade, or neck length to accommodate extra depth to the working surfaces.

Endodontic Materials

Some specialized materials are used during the treatment of pulpal tissue.

Luer-loc syringe: a barrel-type syringe with piston force plunger, used to inject fluids into the cavity.

gutta-percha points: tapered points made of a thermoplastic compound; similar in size to silver points, or endodontic instruments, and used to fill the root canal.

silver points: tapered silver points comparable in size to files and reamers; used to fill canals.

cement pastes and fillers: zinc oxide and eugenol mixes and commercial materials; used to cement points in canal.

chemicals: chemical action used in conjunction with operator treatment produce a result termed a **biomechanical** (bye-oh-meh-**KAN**-ih-kuhl) action. Endodontic chemicals may be used to clean and sterilize (sodium hypochlorite, hydrogen peroxide), lubricate the canal (soap or glycerin), and soften dentin walls. A **chelator** (**KEY**-lay-tor = *chemical ion softener*), citric acid, and EDTA (ethylenediaminetetraacetic acid) are used to soften tissue.

desiccant (**DES**-ih-kant = *dry up, remove*): methanol or ethanol alcohol, used to dry the area or clear away other chemical traces.

medicament (meh-**DICK**-ah-ment = *medicine or remedy*): used for antimicrobial action, to prevent pain, and to neutralize the pulpal area. Major medicaments are phenols, aldehydes, halines, steroids, calcium hydroxides, and antibiotics.

SURGICAL ENDODONTIC TREATMENTS

Not all treatments of inflamed or necrotic pulps require RCT. Some endodontic procedures involve surgical treatment that may or may not be included in the endodontic RCT. Figure 13-6 depicts three of these.

curettage (**CURE**-eh-tahj = *scraping of a cavity*): scraping of the apical area; may be necessary to remove necrotic tissue.

apicoectomy (ay-pih-koh-**ECK**-toh-mee): a procedure that may be necessary to remove the root apex, particularly where there is a radicular cyst involvement of the affected tooth; also called *root end resection*. (13-6A).

root amputation (**am**-pew-**TAY**-shun = *surgical removal of body part, root*): separating and removing molar roots of an affected tooth at the junction into the crown. (13-6B).

FIGURE 13-6
Endodontic surgical treatments.
(A) Apicoectomy
(B) Root Amputation
(C) Root Hemisection

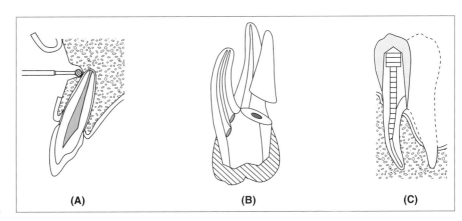

(A)   (B)   (C)

root hemisection (**HEM**-ih-seck-shun = *cutting tissue or organ in half*): surgical division of a multi-rooted tooth that may be performed in a lengthwise manner. (13-6C).

bicuspidization (bye-**cuss**-pih-dih-**ZAY**-shun): surgical division of a tooth retaining both sides.

ENDODONTIC TREATMENT OF TRAUMATIZED TEETH

Besides treating the infected pulp, the endodontist performs varied procedures for traumatized (**TRAW**-mah-tized = *wounded*) teeth, with a variety of pulp injuries.

luxation (luck-**SAY**-shun= *dislocation*): tooth movement that may be classified in one of four ways:

1. **concussion** (kun-**CUSH**-un = *shaken violently*): tooth loosened as a result of a blow; usually recovery occurs with minimal attention.
2. **subluxation** (**sub**-lucks-**AY**-shun; sub = *under*, luxation = *displacement*): tooth partially dislocated; may evidence bleeding but require only minor attention.
3. **lateral luxation**: tooth may be partially displaced with the root apex tilted forward.
4. **extruded** (ecks-**TRUE**-ded = *pushed out of normal position*) **luxation**: tooth may be forced partially out of its socket.

avulsion (ah-**VULL**-shun = *forced or torn away*): **replantation** (ree-plan-**TAY**-shun; re = *again*, plant = *place*) of teeth that have been accidentally lost; may undergo RCT at this time or at a future appointment.

fracture: breakage; may be a broken cusp, broken crown, broken root, or split tooth.

TOOTH REPLANTATION PROCEDURES

Some additional endodontic procedures, although not common, are an essential part of the pulpal therapy.

replantation: replacing an avulsed tooth in its tooth socket. In some rare cases, if RCT cannot be completed in a conventional manner, the tooth may be extracted, undergo RCT, and then be reinserted and stabilized into the same alveolus.

transplantation (**trans**-plan-**TAY**-shun; trans = *across*, planta = *plant*): transfer of a tooth from one alveolar socket to another; may be completed in one of three ways.

1. **autogenous** (awe-**toh**-**JEE**-nus; auto = *self*, geneous = *origin*): moving a tooth from one position in the oral cavity to another area in the same cavity.
2. **homogeneous** (hoh-**MAH**-jen-us; homo = *same*, geneous = *origin*): transferring and inserting a tooth from one patient to another.
3. **heterogenous** (**het**-er-oh-**JEE**-nus; heter = *other*, geneous = *origin*): transfer from one species to another, not yet a feasible practice.

implantation (**im**-plan-**TAY**-shun; in = *into*, planta = *place*): placing titanium metal extensions into the tooth root; may be performed endodontically to provide a longer crown–root ratio and stabilize the tooth.

Occasionally, traumatized teeth or other damaged and affected teeth may appear darker than adjacent teeth. Lightening of tooth color may be attempted by opening, debriding the canal, and placing an oxidizer chemical, such as sodium perborate, inside. Heating or photo-oxidizing with ultraviolet rays may help to lighten the tooth color. This **intracanal bleaching** process is not to be confused with external or cosmetic bleaching.

REVIEW EXERCISES

MATCHING
Match the following word elements with their meanings.

1. _____percussion
2. _____hemisection
3. _____mobility
4. _____gutta-percha
5. _____palpation
6. _____isolation
7. _____reamer
8. _____apicoectomy
9. _____necrotic
10. _____curettage
11. _____pulpotomy
12. _____cellulitis
13. _____thermal
14. _____endodontist
15. _____broach

a. inflammation of cellular or connective tissue
b. detachment, removal, or separation from others
c. thin, twisted sharp-edged instrument used to enlarge canal
d. dental specialist dealing with disease of pulp tissues
e. pertaining to heat
f. capable of movement
g. thin, barbed-wired instrument used to remove pulp tissue
h. cutting tissue or organ in half
i. tapping of body or tooth tissue
j. scraping of a cavity
k. finger or hand pressure on body tissue
l. synthetic material used to fill root canals
m. dead or non-vital
n. surgical removal of root apex
o. partial removal of pulp tissue

DEFINITIONS
Using the selection given for each sentence, choose the best term to complete the definition.

1. The removal of foreign or decayed matter is called:
   a. debridement   b. necrosis
   c. apicoectomy   d. isolation

2. The closing or stopping up of the root canal is a procedure called:
   a. amputation   b. obturation
   c. transillumination   d. curettage

3. A thin, wire instrument with barbed edges that is used to remove pulpal tissue is a:
   a. broach   b. reamer
   c. file   d. gutta-percha

4. A thin blade instrument with sharp edges used to widen and enlarge root canals is a:
   a. broach   b. reamer
   c. file   d. gutta-percha

5. A synthetic material point used to fill the root canal is:
   a. broach
   b. reamer
   c. file
   d. gutta-percha

6. The process of placing or separating an object from others is:
   a. amputation
   b. isolation
   c. pulpotomy
   d. pulpectomy

7. Infection of the pulp tissue is called:
   a. pulpectomy
   b. pulpotomy
   c. pulpitis
   d. pulpalgia

8. The surgical procedure of cutting an organ or tissue in half is called:
   a. amputation
   b. pulpectomy
   c. curettage
   d. hemisection

9. The surgical removal of the apex of a root is called:
   a. apicoectomy
   b. pulpotomy
   c. pulpectomy
   d. amputation

10. The diagnostic application of finger or hand pressure upon body parts is called:
    a. percussion
    b. healing hands
    c. handling
    d. palpation

11. Of the four diagnostic tests listed below, which one requires heat and cold applications?
    a. thermal
    b. mobility
    c. transillumination
    d. anesthesia

12. An objective complaint by a patient is one that is:
    a. observed by the patient
    b. observed by other than the patient
    c. described by the patient
    d. described by other than the patient

13. A subjective complaint by a patient is said to be a/an:
    a. sign
    b. symptom
    c. observation
    d. registration

14. Pulp tissue that is alive and healthy is:
    a. pulpitis
    b. necrotic
    c. regenerated
    d. vital

15. The removal of all pulpal tissue in a tooth is termed:
    a. pulpectomy
    b. pulpotomy
    c. alveolectomy
    d. amputation

16. An abnormal, closely walled fluid- or exudate-filled sac in or around periapical tissues is a/an:
    a. cyst
    b. cellulitis
    c. fistula
    d. osteomyelitis

17. Which of the following instruments does *not* have to be adapted for endodontic procedures?
    a. spreader
    b. files
    c. mirror
    d. plugger

18. The dentist who specializes in the treatment of the inner tooth tissues is a/an:
    a. periodontist
    b. denturist
    c. pedodontist
    d. endodontist

19. The type of endodontic file that is thicker and is used for larger canal openings is the:
    a. Hedstrom
    b. Endo
    c. Pesso
    d. K-file

20. A diagnostic sign is also considered to be which type of observation?
    a. objective
    b. verbal
    c. subjective
    d. related

BUILDING SKILLS

Locate and define the prefix, root/combining form, and suffix (if present) in the following words.

1. **apicoectomy**
   prefix _____
   root/combining form _____
   suffix _____

2. **endodontics**
   prefix _____
   root/combining form _____
   suffix _____

3. **transillumination**
   prefix _____
   root/combining form _____
   suffix _____

4. **pulpotomy**
   prefix _____
   root/combining form _____
   suffix _____

5. **endodontist**

prefix _____

root/combining form _____

suffix _____

FILL-INS

Write the correct word in the blank space for each question:

1. The detachment or separation of an object or person from others is termed

_____.

2. A diagnostic test using hot and cold applications to the tooth surface is a/an _____ diagnostic test.

3. _____ is the act of applying hand or finger pressure to body tissue to diagnose soreness and infection.

4. Bisecting a molar root in a lengthwise manner is a/an _____.

5. The science that deals with the pulp tissues located in the tooth is

_____.

6. The total removal of the pulp tissue from a tooth is _____.

7. _____ is the name for the procedure for stopping up and closing the root canal.

8. The _____ is a small thin, rough-edged instrument used to smooth and taper canal walls.

9. Scraping a cavity wall or enclosed area is called _____.

10. The surgical removal of a limb or organ is termed _____.

11. _____ is the act of removing foreign or decayed matter.

12. Passage of light through an object or tissue is called _____.

13. RCT is another term for

_____.

14. The partial excision of dental pulp is termed

_____.

15. The test used to determine the movement capability of a tooth in the oral cavity placement is called _____.

16. An inflammation of the bone and bone marrow usually caused by bacteria is

_____.

17. Tapping a mirror handle on the biting surface of a tooth is an example of the diagnostic testing called _____.

18. _____ is a term denoting inflamed, infected pulp.

19. A specialist who is limited to the practice of endodontia is called a/an _____.

20. _____ is a synthetic material used to fill the canal root in root canal treatment.

WORD USE

Read the following sentences and define the bold-faced word.

1. Dr. Allen's office phoned us to request an appointment for an **apicoectomy** of tooth number 8 for Mr. Jarvis.

_____

2. Most patients show the symptom of **hypersensitivity** when endodontic treatment is needed.

_____

3. The endodontist will perform several diagnostic tests to determine if the tooth pulp is vital or **necrotic.**

_____

4. Mrs. Baker brought her fourteen-year-old son to the office to receive treatment for an **avulsion** of his two central incisors.

_____

5. During a root canal treatment, the tooth chamber will be opened and the assistant will help with the **extirpation** and debridement procedures.

_____

AUDIO LIST ⊙

This list contains selected new, important, or difficult terms from this chapter. You may use the list to review these terms and to practice pronouncing them correctly. When you work with the audio for this chapter, listen to the word, repeat it, and then place a checkmark in the box. Proceed to the next boxed word and repeat the process.

❏ apicoectomy (ay-pih-koh-**ECK**-toh-mee)
❏ aseptic (ay-**SEP**-tick)
❏ autogenous (aw-toh-**JEE**-nus)
❏ bicuspidization (bye-cuss-pih-dih-**ZAY**-shun)
❏ biomechanical (bye-oh-meh-**KAN**-ih-kuhl)
❏ cellulitis (sell-you-**LIE**-tiss)
❏ chelator (**KEY**-lay-tor)
❏ concussion (kun-**CUSH**-un)
❏ curettage (**CURE**-eh-tahj)
❏ cyst (**SIST**)
❏ desiccant (**DES**-ih-kant)
❏ endodontia (**en**-doh-**DAHN**-she-ah)
❏ extirpation (ecks-ter-**PAY**-shun)
❏ extruded (ecks-**TRUE**-ded)
❏ hemisection (**HEM**-ih-seck-shun)
❏ heterogenous (het-er-oh-**JEE**-nus)
❏ homogenous (hoh-**MAH**-jeh-nuss)
❏ hyperextension (high-per-eck-**STEN**-shun)
❏ hypersensitivity (high-per-sen-sih-**TIV**-ih-tee)
❏ implanation (im-plan-**TAY**-shun)

❏ luxation (luck-**SAY**-shun)
❏ medicament (meh-**DICK**-ah-ment)
❏ mobility (moh-**BIL**-ih-tee)
❏ necrotic (neh-**KRAH**-tick)
❏ obturation (ahb-too-**RAY**-shun)
❏ osteomyelitis (oss-tee-oh-my-**LYE**-tiss)
❏ palpation (pal-**PAY**-shun)
❏ percussion (per-**KUSH**-un)
❏ pericementitis (pear-ih-seh-men-**TIE**-tiss)
❏ periradicular (pear-ee-rah-**DICK**-you-lar)
❏ pulpectomy (puhl-**PECK**-toh-mee)
❏ pulpotomy (puhl-**POT**-oh-mee)
❏ putrefaction (pyou-trih-**FACK**-shun)
❏ reamer (**REE**-mer)
❏ retrograde (**REH**-troh-grade)
❏ subluxation (sub-lucks-**AY**-shun)
❏ suppurative (**SUP**-you-rah-tiv)
❏ thermal (**THER**-mahl)
❏ transillulmination (trans-ill-oo-mih-**NAY**-shun)
❏ traumatized (**TRAW**-mah-tized)

CHAPTER 14

Oral and Maxillofacial Surgery

Oral and
Maxillofacial Surgery

OBJECTIVES   Upon completion of this chapter, the reader should be able to identify and understand terms related to:

1. **Duties and functions of an oral and maxillofacial surgeon.** Describe the functions and roles of an oral or maxillofacial surgeon.

2. **Instrumentation related to oral surgery.** List and identify the instruments commonly used in the practice of oral surgery.

3. **Surgical procedures involved in exodontia.** Discuss the various types of tooth extractions and the assorted types of tooth impactions.

4. **Procedures involved in soft tissue surgery.** List and describe the common tissue surgeries performed in the oral and maxillofacial practice.

5. **Procedures involved in minor bone surgery.** Discuss the various minor bone surgeries performed with or without tooth extraction.

6. **Surgical procedures involved in fracture fixation.** Identify and determine the differences between open and closed reduction of bone fractures.

7. **Procedures involved in maxillofacial surgery.** List and describe the various types of complicated bone surgery including arthrotomy and genioplasty alterations.

8. **Surgical procedures involved in implantology.** Identify the various types of implants and their composition materials.

DUTIES AND FUNCTIONS OF AN ORAL AND MAXILLOFACIAL SURGEON

A dentist who completes training and board certification in dentistry is able to perform extractions and dental surgery. Prescription writing and hospital privileges are afforded to members of the dental profession, but in many cases a dentist may not wish to perform some surgical procedures. Because of the complex measures, patients' health problems, or lack of specific training, a dentist may refer a patient to an oral and maxillofacial surgeon for treatment.

An **oral maxillofacial surgeon** is a dentist who has completed additional oral surgical studies of two to three years, as well as a hospital internship and residency program. This specialist performs **exodontia** (ecks-oh-**DAHN**-shah = *extraction of a tooth*), repair of a fractured maxilla and/or mandible, reconstruction of irregular facial bones, biopsies and surgical treatment of diseased gingiva and periodontal tissues, placement of implant prostheses, and other miscellaneous surgery in the oral cavity.

The oral surgeon may work as a participant on a cleft palate team, for example, or one of several specialists combining their talents on a specific case, such as an implant patient. Oral surgeons work mainly with referred patients who return to their family dentist after the surgical treatment is complete.

▌ INSTRUMENTATION RELATED TO ORAL SURGERY

Each specialization requires instruments that are designed, adapted, or modified to complete certain desired effects. In addition to regular dental implements, there are numerous specialized oral surgical instruments. See Figure 14-1 for illustrations of common surgical instruments.

forceps (**FOUR**-seps = *pincers for seizing, holding, or extracting*): instrument made for maxillary or mandibular use. Tooth forceps have a handle, a neck, and nib or beaks, which are angled and designed to grasp, hold, and provide leverage to a specific tooth for extraction. Many forceps come in right- and left-sided pairs and are numbered with an R or an L, such as 88R or 88L molar forceps. Forceps that can be used on both the right and left sides are called *universal* (view A).

scalpel: a small, surgical knife that is used to cut open or excise tissue from a surgical area. Made of metal or disposable plastic, may be a one-piece style or composed of a detachable blade and handles of varying lengths. Blades are designed to work in a certain area and are numbered according to their design and shape (view B).

bone file: heavier and thicker than the file used on tooth and restoration surfaces. Bone files may be single-ended, but most are double-ended with serrated file edges and different head sizes on opposite sides. They are used to smooth off irregular bone edges remaining from extracted teeth or bone restructure (view C).

elevators: device used to raise the tooth; of three types as used in oral surgery (view J).

periosteal (pear-ee-**OSS**-tee-al = *concerning the periosteum*): used to loosen the periosteum tissue from bone, or detach the tissue around the cervix of the tooth and retract tissue in the surgical site; also called the **periosteotome** (pear-ee-**OSS**-tee-oh-tome = *cutting tissue around bone*).

exolever (**ECKS**-oh-lee-ver = *device to raise or elevate*): used to elevate or *luxate* a tooth from its natural socket. Tips are designed to be used in the mesial or distal, and maxillary or mandibular area. Handles may be grasp-type or T-handed for extra leverage; also called root elevators.

apical (**AY**-pih-kal = *pertaining to apex or tip*): used to elevate or pick out remains of a fractured root tip. These elevators have thinner handles and longer-shanked tips than other tooth elevators; also called root tip elevators/picks.

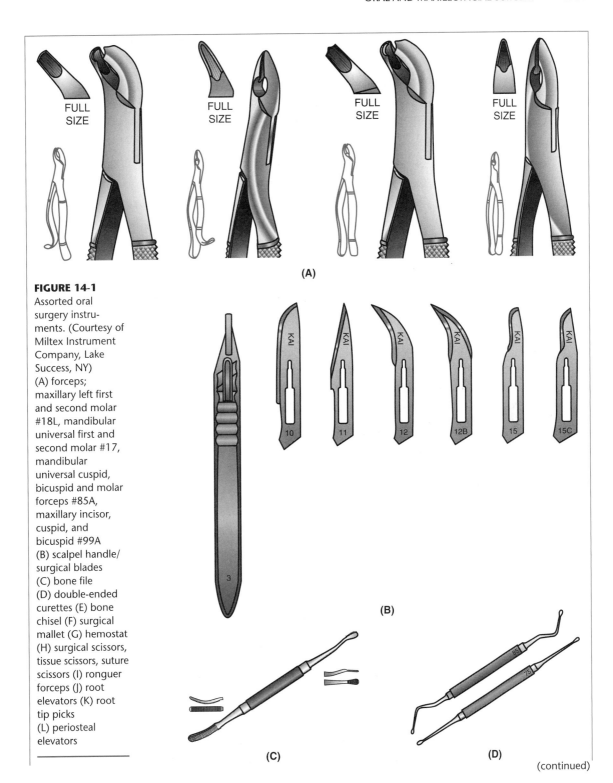

FIGURE 14-1
Assorted oral surgery instruments. (Courtesy of Miltex Instrument Company, Lake Success, NY)
(A) forceps; maxillary left first and second molar #18L, mandibular universal first and second molar #17, mandibular universal cuspid, bicuspid and molar forceps #85A, maxillary incisor, cuspid, and bicuspid #99A
(B) scalpel handle/ surgical blades
(C) bone file
(D) double-ended curettes (E) bone chisel (F) surgical mallet (G) hemostat (H) surgical scissors, tissue scissors, suture scissors (I) ronguer forceps (J) root elevators (K) root tip picks
(L) periosteal elevators

(A)

(B)

(C)

(D)

(continued)

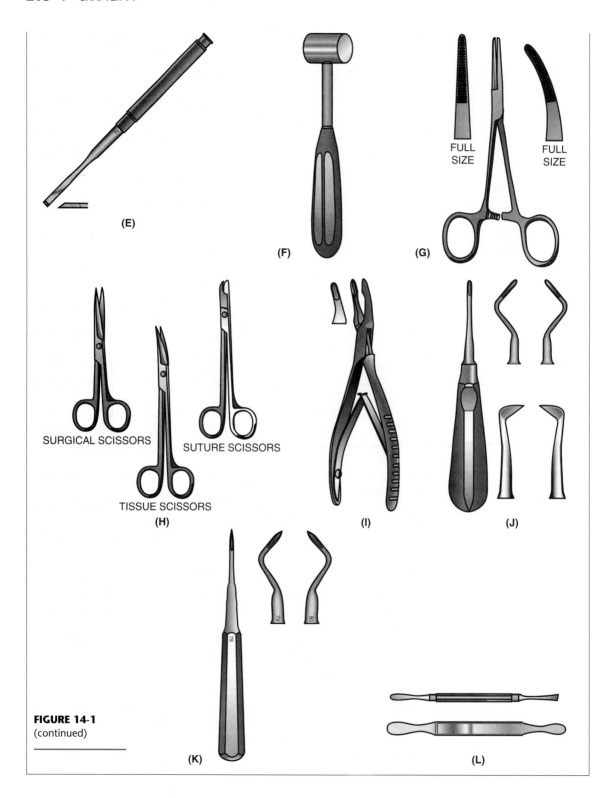

(E)

(F)

(G)

FULL SIZE   FULL SIZE

SURGICAL SCISSORS

SUTURE SCISSORS

TISSUE SCISSORS

(H)

(I)

(J)

(K)

(L)

FIGURE 14-1
(continued)

hemostat (**HE**-moh-stat = *device or drug used to arrest blood flow*): scissors-style device with a locking joint and serrated beaks; used to clamp off or hold onto and transfer. Hemostats come in various lengths and may have straight or curved beaks (view G).

needle holder: similar to a hemostat except that the nose of the instrument is rounded and blunted with serrated criss-crossed edges inside its beaks to assist with holding a needle. Suture needles are curved and triangular in shape to avoid tissue trauma during puncturing. Needles are numbered according to their sizes.

scissors: various specialized scissors used in oral surgery (view H).

> tissue: longer-handled scissors with a serrated blade edge that is used to grasp and hold the tissue during cutting.
>
> suture: smaller scissors with one curved, half-moon blade that is inserted under the suture thread during cutting.
>
> bandage: scissors used to cut materials and dressings during surgery; usually have one longer, blunted blade tip to insert under material.

rongeurs (**RON**-jeers = *bone cutting*): grasp-handled instrument similar to forceps, but with a spring in the handle to provide a "nipping" action. Beaks may be sharp cutting points (ends) or round-sided (blades); used to snip off bony edges and rough areas (view I).

aspirating tips: suction tips with longer handles and narrower tip openings. Disposable or metal, they are used to aspirate sockets, deeper throat areas, and surgical sites.

chisel: device that is longer, thicker, and heavier than tooth chisels. Available in small, medium, and large blade-width tips. Chisels are used to chip away bone and to apply force enough to break impacted molar teeth that will be removed in sections (view E).

mallet (**MAL**-ett = *surgical hammer*): device used to apply pressure to chisels. A mallet may have a plain metal face or removable nylon, padded facing (view F).

curette: hand instrument with a spoon-shaped face that is inserted in the socket or surgical site to scrape out infection and debris. A surgical curette is larger than a dental operative curette. Curettes may be single- or double-ended (view D).

retractor (ree-**TRACK**-tore = *draw back*): of three types, as used in surgery:

> tissue: may be hemostat-type device with notched tips to hold tissue or claw-like blade with holding tips; used to retract and hold tissue during surgical procedures.
>
> cheek retractor: may be bent wire-shaped device or flat, curved handles used to scoop and hold cheek tissue; may be metal or plastic.
>
> tongue retractor: scissor-type instrument with longer shaft and padded or serrated edges; used to grasp and hold the tongue.
>
> mouth prop: small, medium, or large pieces of hard rubber; also called a bite-block. Another style of prop, or gag, is a scissors-like instrument with padded ends instead of blades. The padded ends are placed into the tooth occlusion while in a "bite," and later used to spread the jaws apart while the patient is asleep during surgery.

suture (**SOO**-chur = *closure*): used to close up a wound or incision. To remove the suture, suture thread of silk or nylon material is required. Resorbable suture material of gut or collagen substances does not require removal.

surgical bur: similar to dental burs but larger in size; used to remove bone, to expose root tips, or to score and divide teeth in preparation for forced sectioning and removal.

SURGICAL PROCEDURES INVOLVED IN EXODONTIA

Tooth removal (exodontia) can be a simple or a complex procedure, depending on the tooth or teeth involved, the condition or disease of the site, and the patient's general health.

Single Extraction

A single extraction is a removal of one tooth during the procedure. The tooth may require a routine extraction, as in a single extraction of an impacted tooth. A single extraction also may entail additional surgical intervention, as when a tooth has to be sectioned or severed in half.

Impacted Teeth

A soft-tissue-impacted tooth occurs when the tooth is covered with tissues of the periodontium. Consequently, an incision is required to expose the tooth for extraction. A bone-and-tissue-impacted tooth is covered with tissue and bone. Bone-impacted teeth are typed and named for the tilt angle of the impaction. Examples of the impact classifications are given in Figure 14-2.

horizontal impaction: the tooth is horizontally tilted (14-2A); may be leaning parallel to the floor at various angles; crown may be perpendicular to an adjacent tooth crown.

vertical impaction: tooth is in upright position but in close proximity to, or under, the crown of a nearby tooth (14-2B).

distoangular impaction: crown of the tooth is slanted toward the distal surface and covered by tissue and/or bone (14-2C).

mesioangular impaction: crown of the tooth is mesially tilted and covered by tissue and/or bone (14-2D).

transverse impaction: tooth is situated sideways to the adjacent teeth and occlusal plane, and is covered by tissue and/or bone.

Multiple Extraction

A multiple extraction involves the removal of two or more teeth during one procedure. When multiple teeth are extracted, the alveolar bone crests have to be removed and smoothed to prepare the ridges for denture or appliance wear. This reduction procedure is termed an **alveolectomy** (al-vee-oh-**LECK**-toh-me).

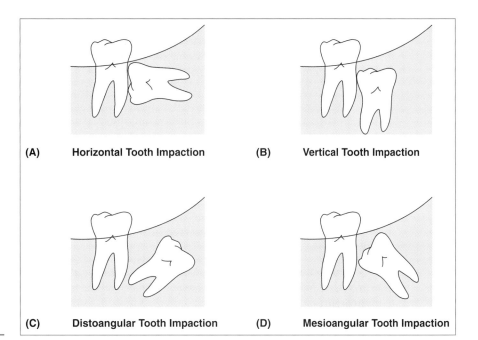

FIGURE 14-2
Examples of impaction classifications.

(A) Horizontal Tooth Impaction

(B) Vertical Tooth Impaction

(C) Distoangular Tooth Impaction

(D) Mesioangular Tooth Impaction

Full Mouth Extraction

In a full mouth extraction, all remaining teeth in the oral cavity are removed. Immediate dentures may be inserted over the sutured site at the time of surgery. A surgical template (**TEM**-plate = *pattern*) is used as a guide for the alveolectomy and resection of the area before placement of the immediate denture.

One potential complication resulting from extraction of teeth is alveolitis (al-**vee**-oh-**LIGH**-tiss = *infection or inflammation of the alveolar process*). This loss of the natural clotting is commonly called a dry socket.

PROCEDURES INVOLVED IN SOFT-TISSUE SURGERY

Many procedures performed by the oral surgeon are limited to, or involve, soft tissue of the oral cavity. Some of these soft tissue surgeries are commonly completed by the general dentist and other specialists, particularly the periodontist, as well.

gingivectomy (**jin**-jih-**VECK**-toh-me): surgical excision of unattached gingival tissue.
gingivoplastomy (**jin**-jih-voh-**PLAS**-toh-me): surgical recountour of gingival tissues.

periodontal flap surgery (*surgical excision and removal of pocket or tissue extensions*): sectioning and tissue removal that may be necessary for extensive singular pocket involvement or when, during tooth eruption, tissue flap coverage of incoming teeth, particularly third molars, obstructs or impacts food around the crown, causing gingival irritation and an infection termed **pericoronitis**.

frenectomy (freh-**NECK**-toh-me = *surgical removal or resectioning of a frenum*): surgery that may be performed on the maxillary labial frenum to correct **diastema** (die-ah-**STEE**-mah = *a space between two teeth*), or on the mandibular lingual frenum to correct **ankyloglossia** (**ang**-kill-oh-**GLOSS**-ee-ah = *shortness of tongue frenum; tongue-tied*).

incision and drainage (I & D): procedure performed for a periodontal abscess. An incision is made into the affected area and an opening is obtained to remove and drain infected matter. In some case, a small piece of rubber dam, or Iodoform gauze, is inserted into the incision to maintain the opening for drainage.

Other tissue surgery may involve removal of the salivary glands, cysts, or other **malady** (**MAL**-ah-dee = *disease or disorder*) of the mucous membranes and oral structures.

Tissue Biopsy

Another tissue surgical procedure performed by an oral surgeon is a **biopsy** (**BYE**-op-see = *small tissue incision*). The three types of biopsies are:

incision biopsy: removing a wedge-shaped section of affected tissue along with some normal adjacent tissue.

excision biopsy: removing the entire lesion of affected tissue with some underlying normal tissue.

exfoliative (ecks-**FOH**-lee-ah-tiv) **biopsy:** scraping with glass slide or tongue depressor to collect tissue cells for microscopic study.

Tissue Diseases

The term applied to cancerous tumors is **malignant** (mah-**LIG**-nant = *harmful or growing worse*). By contrast, **benign** (bee-**NINE** = *not malignant*) tumors are not considered life-threatening or deadly.

leukoplakia: formation of white patches on mucous membrane of oral cavity that cannot be scraped off and have the potential for malignancy.

fibroma: benign, fibrous, encapsulated tumor of connective tissue.

papilloma (pap-ih-**LOH**-mah): benign epithelial tumor of skin or mucous membrane.

hemangioma (he-**man**-jee-**OH**-mah): benign tumor of dilated blood vessels.

granuloma (gran-you-**LOH**-mah): grandular tumor usually occurring with other diseases.

melanoma (mel-ah-**NO**-mah): malignant, pigmented mole or tumor
basal or squamous cell carcinoma: malignant growth of epithelial cells.

▌ PROCEDURES INVOLVED IN MINOR BONE SURGERY

Some tissue surgeries involve treatment of the alveolar bone (osteoplasty = **OSS**-tee-oh-**plas**-tee = *forming bones*).

alveolectomy (al-vee-oh-LECK-toh-me): usually performed to remove alveolar bone crests remaining after tooth extraction in preparation for a smooth bone ridge for denture wear (A).

apicoectomy (ay-pih-koh-**ECK**-toh-me): usually requires opening of the periodontium, including some alveolar bone, and exposure with removal of the root apex (B). Many times this surgery is followed with a retrofill root canal treatment.

Figure 14-3 illustrates these two procedures. Related terminology is:

exostosis (ecks-ahs-TOH-sis = *bony outgrowth*): removing overgrowths and smoothing in preparation for dentures.

torus (TORE-us = *rounded elevation*): an excessive bone growth; a torus on the lingual side of the mandible is termed torus **mandibularis** (man-dib-you-**LAIR**-iss = *concerning the mandible*). In the roof of the mouth, it is termed torus **palatinus** (**pal**-ah-**TEEN**-us = *in the palate*).

Cysts (**SISTs =** *abnormal, closed walled sac present in or around tissue*) found and removed in the oral cavity are described as:

dentigerous (den-**TIJ**-er-us): cystic sac containing teeth.

radicular (rah-**DICK**-you-lar): cyst located alongside or at the apex of a tooth root.

ranula (RAN-you-lah): cystic tumor found on underside of the tongue or in the sublingual or submaxillary ducts.

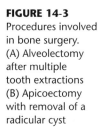
FIGURE 14-3
Procedures involved in bone surgery. (A) Alveolectomy after multiple tooth extractions (B) Apicoectomy with removal of a radicular cyst

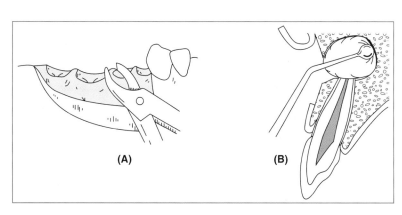

(A)   (B)

SURGICAL PROCEDURES INVOLVED IN FRACTURE FIXATION

Repair of fractured maxillae and mandible bones are reserved for treatment by an oral maxillofacial specialist. Fracture reduction can be completed in two ways—closed or open reduction.

1. **Closed fracture reduction**: repair with interoral fixation, tooth wiring, or ligation methods in which the teeth are "wired together" in proper alignment awaiting bone healing.
2. **Open fracture reduction**: a more complicated procedure involving osteotomy and rigid fixation, perhaps bone plate, mesh, pins, grafts and other fixation devices. Open reduction requires not only alignment by fixation of the teeth but also repositioning and correction of fractures after surgical access through the periosteum.

PROCEDURES INVOLVED IN MAXILLOFACIAL SURGERY

More complicated or involved surgical intervention with tissue and bone elements is termed maxillofacial reconstruction. Such adjustments usually are completed in conjunction with orthodontic involvement and may involve a team of specialists.

genioplasty (**JEE**-nee-oh-**plas**-tee): plastic surgery of the chin or cheek. Chin size is classified in six ways.

1. **macrogenia** (mack-roh-**JEE**-nee-ah): large or excessive chin.
2. **microgenia** (my-kroh-**JEE**-nee-ah): undersized chin.
3. **lateral excessive/deficient**: excessive bone in one direction and deficient bone in another.
4. **asymmetrical** (ay-sim-**EH**-trih-kal): lack of balance of size and shape on opposite sides.
5. **pseudomacrogenia** (soo-doh-mack-roh-**JEE**-nee-ah): excess of soft tissue presenting a chin with the look of abnormal size.
6. **"witch's chin"**: soft tissue ptosis (**TOH**-sis = *drooping or sagging of an organ*).

Chin size may be altered by chin augmentation, which involves implanting bone cartilage, grafts, or alloplastic materials. **Osteotomy** (oss-tee-**OT**-oh-me = *bone incision*), surgical movement of bone, or **osteoplasty** (**OSS**-tee-oh-**plas**-tee = *to form bones*) removal of bone, usually is completed with surgical burs.

orthognathic surgery: surgical manipulation of the facial skeleton to restore facial esthetics and proper function to a congenital, developmental, or trauma-affected patient.
ridge augmentation: use of bone grafts to build or correct an underdeveloped or missing ridge.
arthrotomy (ar-**THRAH**-toh-me = *cutting into a joint*): reconstruction and alignment of the mandible for TMJ (temperomandibular joint) disorders. The mandible may be altered to obtain one of these three movements.

1. **retrusive** (ree-**TRUE**-sive): position with mandible backward.

TABLE 14-1   Wilkes Classification of TMJ Internal Derangement

STAGES	SYMPTOMS	MOTION FUNCTION
Stage I Early	Painless clicking	No restrictive motion
Stage II Early/Intermediate	Occasional painful clicking, headaches	Intermittent locking
Stage III Intermediate	Frequent pain, joint tenderness, headaches	Painful chewing, locking, restricted motion
Stage IV Intermediate/Late	Chronic pain, headache	Restricted motion <35 mm
Stage V Late	Variable pain, joint crepitus (**KREP**-ih-tus): *grinding*	Painful function

2. protrusive (proh-**TRUE**-sive): position with mandible forward.
3. lateral (**LAT**-er-al): position to the side: mesiolateral is toward center of face, distolateral is toward outside of face.

The temporomandibular joint, composed of condyle of the mandible and the fossa eminence of the temporal bone, is responsible for vertical and lateral movement of the lower jaw. Any misposition or derangement of these parts of the TMJ may cause pain and dysfunction. Repair of a dysfunctional TMJ depends upon the severity of the malady. One classification of internal derangement is listed in Table 14-1.

Medical tests used to determine malpositioning of the TMJ are:

Computerized mandibular scan (CMS): 3-D tracking device to record functional movement of the jaw during opening, closing, chewing, and swallowing,

Electyromyograph (EMG): surface electrodes instrument to determine muscle activity during function; healthy muscles have low levels of electrical activity, and disarranged muscles register high activity.

Electrosonograph (ESG): recording of sounds during opening and closing of the jaw; also observed by use of a stethoscope.

CT (computed tomography, also known as CAT scan): uses x-ray images taken at different angles and computerized into a cross section of anatomical features. It is used for diagnosis as well as for the preparation of Co-Cr-Mo (Cobalt–Chromium–Molybdenum) prostheses.

Treatment of TMJ Dysfunction

Although some minor cases of TMJ dysfunction can be treated by selective grinding and aligning of tooth surfaces, night sleep guards, or temporary stabilization of the bite process, more severe cases of TMJ dysfunction require oral surgical services. Surgical intervention in TMJ treatment includes a variety of techniques.

hemiarthroplasty: surgical repair of a joint with a partial joint implant reconstruction. This may be completed in two ways:
1. **alloplastic reconstruction:** rebuilding of the joint using manmade materials.
2. **autogenous reconstruction:** rebuilding of the joint using organic material, such as toe and rib bone grafts.

total joint reconstruction: surgical intervention and use of artificial prostheses for the condyle, disc, and fossa of the temporal bone.

revision surgery: surgical correction of an area that has been operated upon previously, occurring when further degeneration happens, when previous implants have failed, or when going from a partial joint implant to a total implant.

Team Oral Surgery

The practice of oral surgery sometimes is performed in conjunction with other professionals as part of a combined project. For example, team members consisting of maxillofacial surgeons, prosthodontists, orthodontists, dentists, speech therapists, and others alter and repair cleft lips, palates, and tongues.

cleft lip: tissue fissure or incomplete juncture of maxillary lip tissues.
cleft palate: congenital fissure in roof of mouth with an opening into the nasal cavity; may be unilateral (one-sided) or bilateral (two-sided); also may be complete or incomplete.
cleft tongue: bifid or split tongue; usually split at the tip.

In conjunction with the orthodontist and/or the prosthodontist, the oral surgeon may expose and band or peg erupting teeth to prepare the mouth for orthodontic treatment or may remove hidden or retained root tips, cysts, or foreign bodies before taking denture impressions.

SURGICAL PROCEDURES INVOLVED IN IMPLANTOLOGY

The oral maxillofacial surgeon may work in association with a prosthodontist or dentist in the construction and completion of a dental appliance involving a single or multiple dental bone implants. The surgeon may perform one of the following types of dental implants shown in Figure 14-4.

endosteal (en-**DOSS**-tee-ahl = *placement within the bone*): also known as **osseointegrated** implants (14-4A).
subperiosteal (sub-pear-ee-**OSS**-tee-ahl = *beneath the periosteum and placed onto the bone*): usually a cast framework implant with protruding pegs that is placed over the bone and under the periosteum (14-4B).
transosteal (trans-**OSS**-tee-ahl = *through the mandibular bone*): anchor implants that are placed all the way through the mandible. These are also called staple implants (14-4C).

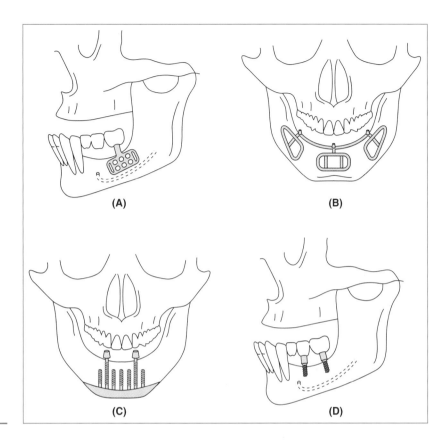

FIGURE 14-4
Dental Implants
(A) Endosteal
Implant
(B) Subperiosteal
Implant
(C) Transosteal
Implant
(D) Endodontic
Implant

endodontic (**en**-doh-**DAHN**-tick = *within the tooth*): titanium post placed in the apex of an endodontically treated tooth to improve the crown-root length ratio (14-4D).

Implant Material

Implant pins or frameworks may be fabricated using any of several materials.

titanium: has high strength; oxidizes readily on contact with tissue fluid and has a minimum amount of corrosion.

ceramic: is biocompatible but is not used in stressful areas.

polymers and composites: in the research stage, may be used as abutments in partially edentulous mouth.

stainless steel and cobalt–chromium alloys: older but less used metal materials.

cobalt–chromium–molybdenum: implant material used in prosthesis construction for TMJ replacement.

REVIEW EXERCISES

MATCHING
Match the following word elements with their meaning:

1. _____fibroma
2. _____malady
3. _____diastema
4. _____implant
5. _____exodontia
6. _____gingivec-tomy
7. _____alveolitis
8. _____crepitus
9. _____template
10. _____periosteal
11. _____biopsy
12. _____torus
13. _____suture
14. _____leukoplakia
15. _____pericornitis

a. extraction of a tooth
b. inflammation of the alveolar process
c. surgically placed device for denture retention
d. surgical removal of unattached gingival tissue
e. infection of tissue surrounding crown of tooth
f. white, precancerous patch on mucous membrane
g. concerning or about the periosteum
h. open space between two teeth
i. disease or disorder
j. bony overgrowth or rounded elevation
k. surgical incision for microscopic study
l. fibrous, encapsulated connective tissue tumor
m. surgical stitch or union
n. pattern for surgical adaptation
o. grinding

DEFINITIONS
Using the selection given for each sentence, choose the best term to complete the definition.

1. Another word for a bony elevation or overgrowth in the palate or mandible is:
   a. fibroma
   b. biopsy
   c. osteograndus
   d. torus

2. Anklyloglossia is an immobility or fixation of which tissue?
   a. uvula
   b. tongue
   c. tooth
   d. cheek

3. Which instrument is used to nip or cut off bony tissue ridges?
   a. rongeurs
   b. scissors
   c. forceps
   d. hemostats

4. A biopsy technique taking some normal tissue and the entire removal of the lesion is:
   a. excision
   b. general
   c. incision
   d. exfoliative

5. A biopsy technique taking tissue samples by a tissue scraping method is:
   a. excision
   b. general
   c. incision
   d. exfoliative

6. A biopsy technique taking some normal tissue and a partial sample of the lesion is:
   a. excision
   b. general
   c. incision
   d. exfoliative

7. A surgical hammer is a:
   a. retractor
   b. mallet
   c. chisel
   d. periosteal

8. The surgical contouring of the gingival tissue is termed:
   a. gingiveoplastomy
   b. osteoplastomy
   c. gingivectomy
   d. osteoectomy

9. A surgical instrument used to scrape and remove matter from tooth socket areas is a/an:
   a. curette
   b. chisel
   c. exolever
   d. bone file

10. An impaction of a tilted third molar in which the crown surface is parallel to the floor is termed:
    a. mesioangular
    b. distoangular
    c. vertical
    d. horizontal

11. The loss of natural clotting of a tooth socket following an extraction may result in a condition called:
    a. alveolectomy
    b. alveolitis
    c. apicoectomy
    d. apicalgia

12. A noncancerous tumor is termed:
    a. onocologious   b. benign
    c. malignant   d. biopsy

13. A torus of the mandibular bone is termed:
    a. palatinus   b. lingualis
    c. mandibularis   d. subosteolaris

14. In the Wilkes classification of TMJ internal derangement, which stage is characterized by variable pain, crepitus, and limited motion?
    a. Stage II   b. State III
    c. Stage IV   d. StageV

15. When the mandible is situated in a drawn-backward position, it is said to be:
    a. anterior   b. prognastic
    c. retrusive   d. posterior

16. A cystic sac containing a tooth or tooth bud is termed:
    a. radicular   b. cystic
    c. fibromic   d. dentigerous

17. A cystic tumor found under the tongue or in sublingual ducts is called a:
    a. ranula   b. radicular
    c. fibroma   d. lingualitis

18. An implant appliance that is placed within the bone is termed:
    a. osseous   b. exosteal
    c. subperiosteal   d. endosteal

19. The surgical removal of alveolar bone crests is:
    a. periosteumectomy   b. gingivectomy
    c. alveolectomy   d. apicoectomy

20. A type of surgical forceps designed to remove a maxillary or mandibular tooth is called:
    a. multipurpose   b. universal
    c. omnipotent   d. general

BUILDING SKILLS

Locate and define prefix, root/combining form, and suffix (if present) in the following words.

1. **arthrotomy**
   prefix   _____
   root/combining form   _____
   suffix   _____

2. **anklyloglossia**
   prefix   _____
   root/combining form   _____
   suffix   _____

3. **subperiosteal**
   prefix   _____
   root/combining form   _____
   suffix   _____

4. **alveolectomy**
   prefix   _____
   root/combining form   _____
   suffix   _____

5. **exostosis**
   prefix   _____
   root/combining form   _____
   suffix   _____

FILL-INS

Write the correct word in the blank space to complete each statement.

1. Another word for a bifid tongue that is usually split at the tip is a/an _____ tongue.

2. A surgical implant appliance that is placed beneath the periosteum and onto the bone is a/an _____ implant.

3. _____ is the term given to a tooth extraction.

4. A/an _____ is a cystic tumor found on the underside of the tongue or in a sublingual or submaxillary gland.

5. A person with a malfunctioning temporomandibular joint is said to have a/an _____ problem.

6. A mandible in a forward position during a bite registration is said to be _____.

7. Another term given to the condition alveolitis is a/an _____.

8. The surgical removal of bony alveolar crests that remains after tooth extractions is called _____.

9. _____ is the term for surgical contouring of gingival tissue.

10. The rebuilding of a joint with manmade materials is termed _____ reconstruction.

11. A/an _____ is a fibrous, encapsulated tumor of connective tissue.

12. The removal of the entire lesion during a biopsy is termed a/an _____biopsy.

13. The surgical removal or resectioning of a frenum is a/an _____.

14. A/an _____ is a tumor of dilated blood vessels.

15. A rounded bone elevation in the palate area is termed a torus _____.

16. A cyst that contains a tooth or tooth bud is called a/an _____ cyst.

17. A malignant, pigmented mole or tumor is termed a/an _____.

18. An implant device that is placed within the mandible bone is a/an _____ implant.

19. A/an _____ is a pattern that is used during the procedure for immediate dentures.

20. An open gap or space area between two teeth is a/an _____.

WORD USE

Read the following sentences and define the bold-faced word.

1. To avoid **pericornitis,** the dental hygienist instructed the teenager to carefully maintain a clean area round the erupting third molar.

   _____

2. The dental assistant is preparing a surgical tray for the removal of a lower third molar situated in a **distoangular** impacted position.

   _____

3. The **biopsy** specimen must be preserved and sent to the laboratory for evaluation.

   _____

4. The **radicular** cyst is to be removed during the apicoectomy.

   _____

5. The surgeon advised Mr. Towers that there must be a long waiting period between the implant appointments to allow for **osseointegration.**

   _____

AUDIO LIST

This list contains selected new, important, or difficult terms from this chapter. You may use the list to review these terms and to practice pronouncing them correctly. When you work with the audio for this chapter, listen to the word, repeat it, and then place a checkmark in the box. Proceed to the next boxed word and repeat the process.

❑ **alveolectomy** (al-vee-oh-**LECK**-toh-me)
❑ **alveolitis** (al-vee-oh-**LIGH**-tiss)
❑ **ankyloglossia** (ang-kill-loh-**GLOSS**-ee-ah)
❑ **apicoectomy** (ay-pih-koh-**ECK**-toe-me)
❑ **arthrotomy** (ar-**THRAH**-toh-me)
❑ **asymmetrical** (ay-sim-**EH**-trih-kal)
❑ **benign** (bee-**NINE**)

❑ **crepitus** (**KREP**-ih-tus)
❑ **cyst** (**SIST**)
❑ **dentigerous** (den-**TIJ**-er-us)
❑ **diastema** (die-ah-**STEE**-mah)
❑ **endodontic** (en-doh-**DAHN**-tick)
❑ **endosteal** (en-**DOSS**-tee-ahl)
❑ **exfoliative** (ecks-**FOH**-lee-ah-tiv)

- ❏ exodontia (ecks-oh-**DAHN**-shah)
- ❏ exolever (**ECKS**-oh-lee-ver)
- ❏ exostosis (ecks-ahs-**TOH**-sis)
- ❏ forceps (**FOUR**-seps)
- ❏ frenectomy (freh-**NECK**-toh-me)
- ❏ genioplasty (**JEE**-nee-oh-plas-tee)
- ❏ gingivectomy (**jin**-jih-**VECK**-toh-me)
- ❏ ginvivoplastomy (**jin**-jih-voh-**PLAS**-toh-me)
- ❏ hemangioma (heh-man-jee-**OH**-mah)
- ❏ hemostat (**HE**-moh-stat)
- ❏ macrogenia (mack-roh-**JEE**-nee-ah)
- ❏ malady (**MAL**-ah-dee)
- ❏ malignant (mah-**LIG**-nant)
- ❏ mallet (**MAL**-ett)
- ❏ melanoma (mel-ah-**NO**-mah)
- ❏ microgenia (my-kroh-**JEE**-nee-ah)
- ❏ osteoplasty (**OSS**-tee-oh-plas-tee)
- ❏ osteotomy (oss-tee-**OT**-oh-me)
- ❏ papilloma (pap-ih-**LOH**-mah)
- ❏ periosteal (pear-ee-**OSS**-tee-al)
- ❏ periosteotome (pear-ee-**OSS**-tee-oh-tome)
- ❏ pseudomacrogenia (soo-doh-mack-roh-**JEE**-nee-ah)
- ❏ ptosis (**TOH**-sis)
- ❏ radicular (rah-**DICK**-you-lar)
- ❏ ranula (**RAN**-you-lah)
- ❏ retractor (ree-**TRACK**-tore)
- ❏ rongeurs (**RON**-jeers)
- ❏ subperiosteal (sub-pear-ee-**OSS**-tee-ahl)
- ❏ suture (**SOO**-chur)
- ❏ torus (**TORE**-us)
- ❏ transosteal (trans-**OSS**-tee-ahl)

CHAPTER 15

Orthodontics

Orthodontics

OBJECTIVES   Upon completion of this chapter, the reader should be able to identify and understand terms related to:

1.   **Orthodontic practice and malocclusion.** Discuss the orthodontic practice, and describe the classifications and causes of malocclusion.

2.   **Types and methods of orthodontic treatment.** Describe the primary methods of treatment for malocclusion and the different approaches that may be taken.

3.   **Requirements for diagnosis and treatment planning for malocclusion.** Identify the various diagnostic tests and records for planning orthodontic care.

4.   **Types and purposes of headgear and traction devices.** Discuss the need, purposes, and uses of headgear and traction devices used in orthodontics.

5.   **Assorted and specialized appliances and retainers.** Identify the assortment of special appliances and retainers necessary for orthodontic treatment.

6.   **Instrumentation for the orthodontic practice.** List and identify the specialized instruments used in the orthodontic practice.

ORTHODONTIC PRACTICE AND MALOCCLUSION

Orthodontia (ore-thoh-**DAHN**-shah; ortho = *straight*, dont = *tooth*) is the study dealing with the prevention and correction of abnormally positioned or misaligned teeth. The dentist specializing in this practice, the orthodontist, is concerned with the causes and treatment of malocclusion.

Classifications of Malocclusion

Dr. Edward Angle divided malocclusion into three classifications with the teeth set in centric relation, the most retruded position of the mandibular condyle into the

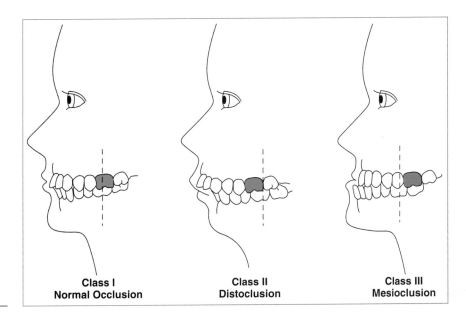

FIGURE 15-1
Classifications of malocclusion.

Class I	Class II	Class III
Normal Occlusion	**Distoclusion**	**Mesioclusion**

glenoid fossa (biting on the back teeth), also known as the *terminal hinge position*. The three classifications are illustrated in Figure 15-1.

1. neutroclusion (**new**-troh-**KLOO**-zhun): Class I condition, in which the antero-posterior occlusal positions of the teeth or the mesiodistal positions are normal but other malocclusion or positioning of the individual teeth occurs.
2. distoclusion (**dis**-toh-**KLOO**-zhun): Class II condition, in which the mesiobuccal cusp of the maxillary first molar is anterior to the buccal groove of the mandibular first molar, resulting in an appearance of a retruded mandible. Class II is further separated into two divisions, according to the individual placement of the anterior teeth.
   a. Division 1: maxillary incisors protruding, with a V-shaped arch instead of a U-shaped arch.
   b. Division 2: maxillary incisors having a lingual incline with an excessive over-bite and a wider than normal arch.
3. mesioclusion (**me**-zee-oh-**KLOO**-zhun): Class III condition, in which the mesiobuccal cusp of the maxillary first molar occludes in the interdental space of the mandibular permanent first molar's distal cusp and the mesial cusp of the mandibular permanent second molar, resulting in an appearance of a protruded mandible.

Causes of Malocclusion

Malocclusion occurs from diverse causes and in various forms. Causes include trauma, habits, poor mouth conditions, or congenital (kahn-**JEN**-ih-tahl = *present at birth*)

FIGURE 15-2
Assorted malocclusion conditions.
(A) Open Bite: anterior teeth failing to meet and posterior teeth occluding
(B) Overjet: increased horizontal distance between incisal edges of central incisors
(C) Vertical Overbite: vertical overlap that is not on incisal third of central incisor
(D) Crossbite: midsagittal balance between maxillary and mandibular central incisors not in alignment; posteriors in improper occlusion
(E) Underjet: maxillary incisors lingual to mandibular incisors.
(F) End-to-End: edges of maxillary and mandibular incisors meeting each other.

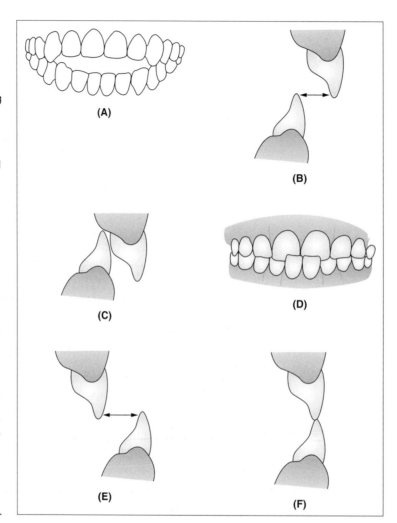

factors, such as **supernumerary** teeth, or **ectopic** (eck-**TOP**-ic = *out of place*) eruption of teeth. Some occlusion problems, as illustrated in Figure 15-2, are:

open bite: anterior teeth do not contact with each other (A).
overjet: also know as horizontal overbite, increased horizontal distance between the incisal edges of maxillary and mandibular central incisors (B).
vertical overbite: excessive amount of overlap of maxillary and mandibular central incisors when they are in occlusion (C).
crossbite: midsagittal alignment between central incisors not in agreement (D).
underjet: maxillary incisors lingual to mandibular incisors (E).
end to end: edges of maxillary and mandibular incisors meeting each other (F).

TYPES AND METHODS OF ORTHODONTIC TREATMENT

Malocclusion is treated with a variety of methods or treatment plans.

preventive orthodontics: action taken to preserve the integrity of a normal developing occlusion by protecting current conditions or preventing situations that would interfere with growth, such as correction of caries, poor nutrition, elimination of habits through **myotherapeutic** (my-oh-thare-ah-**PYOU**-tick = *muscle healing treatment*) exercises, or by placing space maintainers in areas of missing teeth.

interceptive orthodontics: procedures taken to lessen the severity of any existing malfunctions or problems from genetic or environmental factors, such as placement or use of appliances to correct improper growth patterns. Examples of these appliances are a tongue retrainer or incline biteplane to move a crossbite.

corrective orthodontics: procedures taken to reduce or eliminate malocclusion; treatment plans include the application of intraoral and extraoral appliances and auxiliary forces for tooth direction.

> rotation (**ROH**-tay-shun = *turn around on an axis*): altering the position of a tooth around its long axis.
>
> translation: bodily tooth movement; a change of teeth to alternate positions.
>
> tipping: change of tooth position to a more upright direction.
>
> intrusion (in-**TROO**-zhun): movement of the tooth into the alveolus.
>
> extrusion (ecks-**TROO**-zhun): movement of the tooth out of the alveolus.
>
> torque (**tork**): movement of the root without movement of the crown.

Corrective orthodontic treatment is determined by many factors, including age, degree of malocclusion, cause of malocclusion, the patient's general health and attitude, and economics, as well as the orthodontist's expertise and training. Today's patient has many choices or methods of correction, including:

banding: placing metal band around entire selective tooth or teeth. Brackets, tubes, hooks, springs, and other devices are placed on these bands and are used to attach push/pull pressure to the teeth movements and archwire shaping.

direct bonding: cementing stainless steel or golden metal brackets, composite brackets, or *Inspire* (monocrystalline sapphire) brackets on the surface of the tooth to attach needed pressures and archwire forms. Two independently designed metal braces developed by dentists are the **Viazis**, a triangular bracket using a low-force square or rectangular bracket; and the **Damon** self-ligating system bracket, which does away with elastics and requires fewer appointments and adjustments.

Invisalign braces: strong plastic custom trays used in mild malocclusion cases. The specially trained orthodontist takes impressions for fabrication of trays at the Align laboratory. These trays are changed every few weeks, making adjustment in the bite until the desired occlusion is obtained, and then maintained until stabilized.

lingual braces: braces that are placed on the tongue side of the teeth. Some orthodontists use 3-D CAM/CAD technology by *iBraces* to prepare custom braces that fit the lingual tooth surfaces, and precision bent wires that are delivered in a *itray* for indirect bonding to the tooth's lingual surfaces.

accelerated osteogenic orthodontic treatment: surgical orthodontic team approach that involves incising the gingiva to expose the alveolar bone, where a surgical drill is used to place holes to weaken and demineralize the bone. An antibiotic bone graft mixture is placed in the site and the area is closed. While the bone is in a weakened condition, the teeth are banded and moved quickly into position and retained there while the bone remineralizes and strengthens. This procedure is also termed *Wilckodontics* (see Chapter 11, Cosmetic Dentistry).

adjunctive orthodontics: procedures taken to facilitate other dental procedures that are necessary to correct or restore function, such as cleft palate surgery, TMJ dysfunction, periodontal damage, pulp changes, closing of diastemas, or jaw reduction. Usually completed along with services of oral surgery and/or prosthodontic dental care for adult patients.

REQUIREMENTS FOR DIAGNOSIS AND TREATMENT PLANNING FOR MALOCCLUSION

Diagnosing the type of malocclusion to enable the identification of subsequent treatment depends upon a thorough exam that includes a clinical exam, patient history, intraoral and extraoral photos, impressions for diagnostic casts, and periapical, occlusal, panoramic, and cephalometric radiographs.

Cephalometric Measurements

Cephalometric (**sef**-ah-low-**MEH**-trik = *measurement of the head*) **radiographs** are used for evaluation of dentofacial development in tracings for future growth patterns and directions. Geometric images may be determined from an analysis of markings made from various anatomical points and planes. Different methods, such as the Downs, Steiner, Ricketts, Moyers, Johnson, and even a computer-generated analysis, have been developed to estimate the degree of malocclusion and projected growth, and to prepare a treatment plan.

Intraoral Appliances and Auxiliaries Used in Orthodontics

Treatment of malocclusion is accomplished by applying forces through an intraoral or an extraoral source, or a combination of both. They may be fixed or removable. The most common orthodontic appliances, known as "braces," are fixed bands or brackets to which auxiliary devices are applied. Figure 15-3 shows a variety of fixed orthodontic appliances.

bands: stainless steel circles or rings that are sized and cemented around a tooth. Bands are supplied as maxillary or mandibular in varying sizes, and may be supplied with or without brackets or tubes attached.

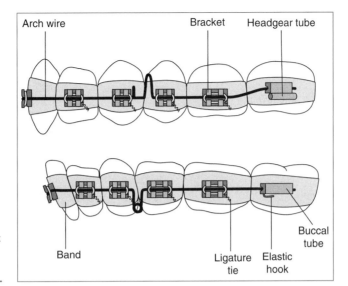

FIGURE 15-3
Popular orthodontic appliances with parts identified.

bracket (**BRACK**-et = *support*): a metal or clear resin holding device used to support and stabilize the archwire in the mouth. A bracket may be either gas-**soldered** (**SOD**-erd =,*joining of two metals*) or spot-welded onto an orthodontic band. Other brackets may be cemented directly onto the facial surface of tooth and are called **DBs** (direct-bonded) brackets when cemented onto pre-etched tooth surface.

archwire: horseshoe-shaped stainless steel or nickel titanium wire that may be round, rectangular, or square and removable or fixed. For the first year, round wires normally are used to move the tooth crown, and during the second year, square or rectangular wires are used to move the root of the tooth. The archwire is attached and held by ligatures to the brackets and tubes and maintains a pattern for development.

buccal tubes: support devices soldered on bands into which headgear and archwires are inserted. They also may serve as stabilization for elastics or power devices.

button, cleats, hooks, eyelets: devices used for support and holding power devices, elastics, and wires.

ligature (**LIG**-ah-chur = *binder or tie off*): thin, stainless steel wires used to tie on or attach archwires and any necessary attachments.

elastics: sized latex circles providing various pull forces, or elastomeric ties for holding.

auxiliary springs: noble metal or stainless steel attachment to apply directional force.

separators (**SEP**-ah-ray-tors = *device to set aside*): brass wire, steel springs, or elastomeric materials placed between the teeth to obtain space before placing the bands.

TYPES AND PURPOSES OF HEADGEAR AND TRACTION DEVICES

Many cases of corrective orthodontics require the application of external forces to obtain proper movement and alignment. The application of force stimulates the osteoclast cells to resorb the alveolar bone. After the misaligned tooth has moved into the proper place and are retained in that position, the osteoblast cells deposit mineral salts necessary to strengthen the alveolar bone, making the movement permanent. A combination of fixed, intraoral appliances and removable extraoral devices are used to apply the proper amount of force.

headgear: device composed of facebow and traction. It is used to apply external force.

facebow: stainless steel external archbow device that is inserted into the fixed molar tubes on the maxillary first molars; the open wing ends extending from the oral cavity are connected with the prepared elastic traction strap devices. The facebow is used to move the molars distal for more anterior space.

traction device: fitted, expandable device to be hooked onto a facebow after placement on the head. The traction device is custom-made and placed to achieve desired movement of teeth. Figure 15-4 gives examples of three of these orthodontic traction devices.

cervical device: circles the patient's neck and attaches to facebow to pull in a parallel position to retract teeth (A).

high-pull device: fits on top of the patient's head and hooks in a downward position, perpendicular to occlusion, to retract anterior teeth and control maxillary growth (B).

combination high-pull and cervical device: traction combining both forces (C).

chin device: placed on the chin, incorporates high-pull and cervical forces and is used to control mandible growth.

FIGURE 15-4
Examples of orthodontic traction devices. (A) Cervical Traction Device (B) High-Pull Traction Device (C) Combination High-Pull and Cervical Traction Device

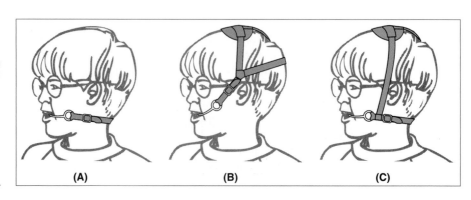

(A)   **(B)**   **(C)**

ASSORTED AND SPECIALIZED APPLIANCES AND RETAINERS

Each orthodontic treatment case is individualized for the patient. Devices and appliances are developed to accomplish a specific goal.

aligner: an *Invisalign* system of computer-imaged and computer-generated clear plastic overlay trays used with milder cases of misaligned teeth. The patient wears this removable, personal aligner tray for a designated period of weeks and then progresses to the next tray until movement has been completed and the teeth are in position.

activator: appliance designed to guide, change, or alter facial and jaw functions for a more favorable occlusion position. Most popular is the Anderson activator, constructed to conform to the inside of the mouth with the teeth occluding and holding against it.

Hawley appliance: removable, customized, acrylic and wire appliance designed to maintain newly acquired tooth positions

Stev plate: maxillary bite plane covering incisal edges of maxillary incisors; may be used in conjunction with headgear or for retention of the bite.

Crozat appliance: removable appliance made of precious alloy with body wires, lingual arms, and a high labial archwire (maxillary); molar clasps hold the appliance in place.

lingual retainer: mandibular lingual bar with cuspid-to-cuspid cemented unions, to maintain lower incisors in position. When extended and attached to the mandibular molar to molar areas, it is known as a lingual arch retainer.

orthodontic tooth positioner: customized mouth device constructed of soft acrylic or rubberized material surrounding the crowns of all the teeth in both jaws; worn by the patient to maintain the newly acquired tooth placement until calcification and positioning are assured.

palatal expanders: known as RPE (rapid palatal expanders), a fixed appliance cemented to the maxillary molar teeth with a spring insert in the palate area. The spring is activated by a key rotation to expand the appliance. This expansion applies force that rapidly expands the midpalatal suture and increases the size of the maxilla (see Figure 15-5).

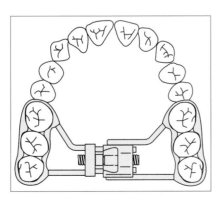

FIGURE 15-5
Rapid palate
expander.

fixed space maintainer: custom-constructed appliance attached to the remaining teeth to hold a tooth pattern or to maintain space from premature loss of tooth.

oral shield: device that fits into the vestibule space between the teeth and the lips; helps to train and maintain lip function by correcting habits, strengthening lip action, or correcting mouth breathing faults.

mouthguard: though not considered a treatment appliance, protects the tooth position while the patient is involved in sport activities.

dental appliances: specialized mouth appliances for health disorders such as sleep apnea, thumb sucking, nail biters, and tongue thrusters.

▌INSTRUMENTATION FOR THE ORTHODONTIC PRACTICE

Each practice requires specialized instruments to complete assigned tasks. Among orthodontic instruments are:

band-remover pliers: used to remove bands from teeth.

bird-beak pliers: used to bend and shape appliance wires.

loop-forming pliers: used to form and shape loops in wires.

Howe pliers: used to make archwire adjustment; sometimes called How pliers.

three-prong pliers: used to close or adjust clasps.

contouring pliers: used to contour bands for concave or convex tilt.

ligature-tying pliers: used to tie or bind off ligature wires and to place elastics.

arch-forming pliers: used for bending or holding dimensional wires.

stress and tension gauge: narrow, hand-held instrument with interior 1-oz. and 4-oz. marked sliding scale; used to measure intraoral forces.

band seater: rounded, serrated end used to "seat" band onto tooth.

ligature tucker: straight-handled instrument with claw-like end that is used to guide ligatures and assist with the bending of cut wire edges.

bracket tweezers: reverse-action, small-ended tweezers used to place direct-bond brackets.

ligature cutter: used to cut ligature wire, intraorally or extraorally.

pin and fine wire cutter: used to cut or snip off ends of tied ligature wires.

Weingart utility plier: used for placing archwires.

anterior band slitter: used to shear upper and lower bands.

distal end cutter: used to cut and hold arch wire that was inserted into the buccal tube.

band pusher: used to push and seat bands onto the teeth.

ligature director: used to direct and place ligature wires.

scaler: hand instrument used to remove excess cement from bands, and to direct wires, bands, and elastics into place.

direct-bonding bracket holder: used to hold DBs in position during placement.

edgewise pliers: used to hold or adjust archwires.

hemostat: scissor-like clamps, straight and curved; used to carry or hold small objects.

Boone gauge: measuring device used to establish the height of the orthodontic bands.

bitestick: plastic- or metal-handled instrument with projecting serrated steel area that is used to help "seat" posterior bands.

protractor (orthodontic): triangular premarked form used to make cephalometric tracing.

REVIEW EXERCISES

MATCHING
Match the following word elements with their meaning:

1. _____retainer
2. _____cephalogram
3. _____band plugger
4. _____neutroclusion
5. _____congenital
6. _____open bite
7. _____ligature
8. _____crossbite
9. _____mesioclusion
10. _____separator
11. _____archwire
12. _____orthodontia
13. _____super- numerary
14. _____orthodontic band
15. _____distoclusion

a. Class II mal- occlusion
b. concerned with pre- venting and correct- ing malocclusion
c. midsagittal alignment not in agreement
d. customized device used to maintain new tooth osition
e. exceeding normal amount
f. stainless steel circle or ring placed on tooth
g. horseshoe-shaped wire used as pattern for position
h. Class I malocclusion
i. present at birth
j. device placed between teeth to prepare for banding
k. hand instrument used to seat poste- rior bands
l. thin, stainless steel wire used to tie off or bind
m. anterior teeth not in contact with each other
n. Class III malocclusion
o. radiograph for mea- surement of head

DEFINITIONS
Using the selection given for each sentence, choose the best term to complete the definition.

1. A device used to widen maxilla suture area is a:
   a. palate retainer
   b. Boone gage
   c. How plier
   d. palatal expander

2. The type of malocclusion that displays a projected mandible is:
   a. Class I
   b. Class II
   c. Class III
   d. Class IV

3. Bird-beak pliers are used to:
   a. secure brackets
   b. tie off ligatures
   c. bend and shape wires
   d. hold bands

4. Which type of traction device is placed around the patient's neck?
   a. cervical
   b. high-pull
   c. combination
   d. facebow

5. Placement of a tongue retainer to correct improper growth patterns is a form of which kind of treatment?
   a. interceptive
   b. preventive
   c. corrective
   d. orthodontic

6. The radiograph that best exposes head markings for measurement is:
   a. periapical
   b. cephalometric
   c. occlusal
   d. panoramic

7. To change a tooth position to a more "upright" direction is an example of:
   a. moving   b. expanding
   c. rotating   d. tipping

8. Correction of bad habits or carious conditions is an example of which type of orthodontics?
   a. preventive   b. interceptive
   c. corrective   d. constructive

9. An increase of horizontal distance between incisal edges of central incisors is called:
   a. crossbite   b. overjet
   c. overbite   d. open bite

10. Teeth affected by ectopic eruption are:
    a. missing
    b. malpositioned
    c. macrosized
    d. microsized

11. The class of malocclusion that is signified by a protrusive maxillary jaw is:
    a. Class I   b. Class II
    c. Class III   d. Class IV

12. Congenital factors for malocclusion are:
    a. present at puberty
    b. a result of trauma
    c. present at birth
    d. a result of habit

13. A corrective treatment device cemented upon the tooth surface is a/an:
    a. retainer   b. archwire
    c. band   d. bracket

14. Which of the following is not considered a "force" or power device:
    a. springs   b. headgear
    c. elastics   d. tubes

15. Which devices are placed between teeth to prepare for placement of bands?
    a. separators   b. pins
    c. buttons   d. ligatures

16. Support devices placed on molar bands to hold facebow inserts are called:
    a. bars   b. tubes
    c. brackets   d. bands

17. Application of appliances and auxiliaries to improve occlusion is which form of orthodontics?
    a. interceptive   b. preventive
    c. corrective   d. activated

18. A bracket or a band is considered which type of orthodontic appliance?
    a. intraoral   b. extraoral
    c. combination   d. neutral

19. The process of moving a tooth on its axis is termed:
    a. expanding   b. moving
    c. rotating   d. tipping

20. A condition of normal jaw position but malpositioned teeth is:
    a. Class I   b. Class II
    c. Class III   d. Class IV

BUILDING SKILLS

Locate and define the prefix, root/combining form, and the suffix (if present) in the following words.

1. **mesioclusion**
   prefix   _____
   root/combining form   _____
   suffix   _____

2. **orthodontia**
   prefix   _____
   root/combining form   _____
   suffix   _____

3. **cephalometric**
   prefix   _____
   root/combining form   _____
   suffix   _____

4. **cervical**
   prefix   _____
   root/combining form   _____
   suffix   _____

5. **supernumerary**
   prefix   _____
   root/combining form   _____
   suffix   _____

FILL-INS

Write the correct word in the blank space to complete each statement.

1. A Boone gauge is used to measure the _____ of the bands.

2. A Howe pliers is used to make _____ or _____ in archwires.

3. Another name for the Crozat appliance is a/an _____ appliance.

4. _____ are placed between teeth to establish space prior to banding.

5. _____ orthodontics consists of procedures taken to reduce or eliminate malocclusion.

6. When anterior teeth do not contact with each other, the condition is termed _____.

7. Class II malocclusion may be indicated by a/an _____ mandible.

8. _____ is the science that deals with the prevention and correction of abnormally positioned teeth and oral structures.

9. Classification of types of malocclusion is credited to Dr. _____.

10. The term for extra teeth present in the mouth is _____.

11. The amount of overlapping of maxillary and mandibular central incisors while set in occlusion is called vertical _____.

12. Teeth that have erupted in a malposition are said to result from _____ eruption.

13. Cephalometric radiographs are used to determine measurements of the _____.

14. Stainless steel rings or circles that are cemented onto teeth are orthodontic _____.

15. _____ are thin, stainless steel wires used to tie or bind off.

16. _____ may be soldered to molar bands to serve as a place to insert headgear and provide support.

17. A high-pull traction device applies pressure _____ to the occlusal surfaces so the forces may retract maxillary incisors.

18. A Hawley appliance is constructed to be used to retain _____ of the newly aligned teeth.

19. A triangular measurement device used for completing cephalometric tracings is an orthodontic _____.

20. A/an _____ is a hand instrument used to remove excess cement from bands and may assist with placement of elastics.

WORD USE

Read the following sentences and define the bold-faced words.

1. The patient was advised to notify the office if any of the **separators** were to become loose or were lost.

   _____.

2. A diagnosis of Class III, **distoclusion**, has been determined, and a treatment plan for the correction of the problem has been prepared.

   _____.

3. The presence of supernumerary teeth in a patient's dentition may be the result of a **congenital** factor.

   _____.

4. The child received instructions for wearing a **headgear** apparatus that is part of the treatment plan.

   _____.

5. The assistant measures and prepares the **ligatures** prior to the archwire replacement appointment.

   _____.

AUDIO LIST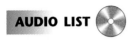

This list contains selected new, important, or difficult terms from this chapter. You may use the list to review these terms and to practice pronouncing them correctly. When you work with the audio for this chapter, listen to the word, repeat it, and then place a checkmark in the box. Proceed to the next boxed word and repeat the process.

❑ bracket (**BRACK**-et)
❑ cephalometric (sef-ah-low-**MEH**-trik)
❑ cervical (**SIR**-vih-cull)
❑ congenital (kahn-**JEN**-ih-tahl)
❑ distoclusion (dis-toh-**KLOO**-zhun)
❑ ectopic (eck-**TOP**-ic)
❑ extrusion (ecks-**TROO**-zhun)
❑ intrusion (in-**TROO**-zhun)

❑ ligature (**LIG**-ah-chur)
❑ mesioclusion (me-zee-oh-**KLOO**-zhun)
❑ myotherapeutic (**my**-oh-thare-ah-**PYOU**-tick)
❑ neutroclusion (**new**-troh-**KLOO**-zhun)
❑ orthodontia (ore-thoh-**DAHN**-shah)
❑ rotation (roh-**TAY**-shun)
❑ torque (**TORK**)

CHAPTER 16

Periodontics

Upon completion of this chapter, the reader should be able to identify and understand terms related to:

1. **Anatomy of the periodontium.** Identify and describe the major tissues comprising the periodontium.

2. **Etiology and symptoms of periodontal diseases.** Describe the cause of periodontal diseases and the symptoms involved.

3. **Classification of periodontal diseases.** List the various classes and types of gingivitis and periodontitis.

4. **Periodontal examination and evaluation.** Describe the examination measures required to evaluate periodontal diseases.

5. **Measurement and recording of periodontal conditions.** Describe the methods used to measure and record various periodontal conditions, and identify and explain the index ratings for tooth and periodontal conditions.

6. **Periodontal treatment methods.** Identify the nonsurgical and surgical methods used to care for periodontal problems.

7. **Periodontal involvement with dental implants.** Identify the various types of bone implants and describe the methods for care of periodontal implants.

8. **Instrumentation for periodontics.** Explain the use of instruments commonly used in periodontal treatment and care.

ANATOMY OF THE PERIODONTIUM

Periodontology (pear-ee-oh-dahn-**TAH**-loh-jee) is the field of dentistry that deals with the treatment of diseases of the tissues around the teeth, commonly called the periodontium. The periodontium serves as an attachment apparatus and is composed of four major tissues.

1. **gingiva:** fibrous, epithelial tissue surrounding a tooth; may be divided into three types:
   a. **attached:** the portion that is firm, dense, stippled, and bound to the underlying periosteum, tooth, and bone. The **keratinized** (**KARE**-ah-tin-ized = *hard or horny*) tissue, also called *masticatory mucosa*, where the gingiva and mucous membrane unite, is indicated by the color change from pink gingiva to red mucosa, and is called the **mucogingival** border.
   b. **marginal:** the portion that is unattached to underlying tissues and helps to form the sides of the gingival crevice; also called the *free margin gingiva* and forms the gingival **sulcus** (**SUL**-kus = *groove*), approximately 1 to 3 mm in depth.
   c. **papillary:** the part of the marginal gingiva that occupies the interproximal spaces. Normally this tissue is triangular and fills the tooth embrasure area, and also is called the **interdental papilla**.
2. **periodontal ligaments:** bundles of fibers that support and retain the tooth in the socket (see Figure 16-1).
3. **cementum:** outer, hard surface covering of the root section of the tooth.
4. **alveolar bone process:** compact bone that forms the tooth socket; supported by stronger bone tissue of the mandible and maxilla and accepts periodontal fiber attachment. The alveolar process makes up the **cribriform** (**KRIB**-rih-form = *sieve-like*) plate to form and line the tooth socket. This outline is called **lamina dura** (**LAM**-ih-nah= *lining, thin layer*) and is easily viewed on radiographs.

The five principal types of periodontal membrane are:

1. **alveolar crest fibers:** found at the cementoenamel junction; help to retain the tooth in its socket and protect the deeper fibers.
2. **horizontal fibers:** connect the alveolar bone to the upper part of the root and assist with control of lateral movement.

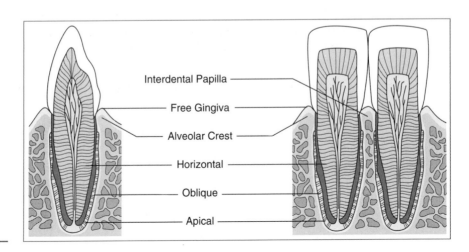

FIGURE 16-1
Principal fibers of periodontal membrane.

Interdental Papilla

Free Gingiva

Alveolar Crest

Horizontal

Oblique

Apical

3. **oblique fibers:** attach the alveolar socket to the majority of the root cementum and assist in resisting the axial forces.
4. **apical fiber bundles:** running from the apex of the tooth to the alveolar bone, fibers that help to prevent tipping and dislocation, as well as protect nerve and blood supply to the tooth.
5. **interradicular fiber bundles:** are present in multirooted teeth, extending apically from the tooth furcation; help the tooth resist tipping, turning, and dislocation.

ETIOLOGY AND SYMPTOMS OF PERIODONTAL DISEASES

In the **etiology** of problems affecting the periodontium, the major contributing factors are **plaque** (**PLACK** = *plate or buildup*) and **calculus** (**KAL**-kyou-lus). Teeth acquire an adhering film, or **pellicle** (**PELL**-ih-kul), which harbors an assortment of bacterial pathogens and enables plaque to build up. With the addition of calcium and phosphorus salts found in saliva and mouth fluids, a hard substance called calculus (also known as tartar) forms. These gingival irritants are classified as either supragingival (found on the tooth crowns) or subgingival (found on root surfaces below the gingival margin). When this collection of calculus and plaque with pathogens extends into periodontal pockets, it causes irritation and disease.

Indications of periodontal disease are:

▶ **erythema.** The gingiva is red and appears inflamed.
▶ **edema.** The tissue is overgrown from **hyperplasia** (high-per-**PLAY**-zee-ah = *excessive number of tissue cells*) and **hypertrophy** (high-per-**TROE**-fee = *excessive cellular growth*). The gingiva looks swollen and irritated. Hyperplastic gum tissue may be caused by drug reactions, allergies, and hormonal changes, as well as response to local irritants and disease.
▶ loss of **stippling** (**STIP**-ling = *spotting*). Tone or tissue attachment loosens and puffy gums become smooth and shiny.
▶ pocket formation. Gingiva is unattached, recession occurs, and the root surface may be observed.
▶ alveolar bone loss with **exudate** (**EX**-you-dayt = *passing out of pus*). A foul odor is present as supporting bone resorbs; retention is lessening.
▶ mobility. The tooth seems loose and moves under pressure because of loss of attachment.

The tooth eventually is lost from lack of support or from extraction.

CLASSIFICATION OF PERIODONTAL DISEASES

Periodontal diseases can be divided into two main divisions:

1. gingivitis, an inflammation of gingival tissue with no supporting tissue loss and periodontitis,
2. inflammation of gingival tissue with involvement of other tissues of the periodontium.

Destruction of these tissues varies in degree, intensity, and overall action. To identify each stage and type of periodontal involvement, the American Academy of Periodontology (AAP) devised a classification system for periodontal diseases, which is examined and revised periodically. Following is an outline of this classification.

A. Gingival disease:

1. **dental plaque involvement** (most common). Tissues react to irritants.
2. **dental plaque with systemic factors included.** Pregnancy, hormone, medication, or malnutrition may modify and intensify the disease course of action; sometimes called **induced gingivitis.**
3. **non-dental plaque lesions.** These are of specific bacterial, viral, fungal, or genetic origin, such as gonorrhea, herpes, and candida infections.
4. **allergies.** The patient may be allergic to dental restorative materials, reactions to foods, additives, and so forth.
5. **traumatic lesions, injury.** The patient may have been subjected to an external force or have been injured in some way.

B. Periodontal disease

1. **chronic periodontitis.** Previously termed *adult periodontitis*, this is the most common type of slowly progressive periodontal disease. May be subdivided according to extent and severity into localized with <30% involvement and generalized with >30% involvement. Severity is measured based on the amount of clinical attachment loss (CAL) as slight, moderate, or severe.
2. **aggressive periodontitis.** Previously termed early-onset periodontitis, this is a rapidly progressive disease. Subclassifications are:
   a. localized aggressive periodontitis, formerly termed localized juvenile periodontitis (LPJ) affecting young adults; and
   b. generalized aggressive periodontitis, formerly termed prepubertal or rapid-progressing periodontitis (RPP).
3. **refractory periodontitis.** The periodontitis progresses in spite of excellent patient compliance and provision of periodontal therapy; may be applied to all types of periodontitis. Tissues that are painful, red, and sloughing are said to be **desquamative** (des-**KWAM**-ah-tiv = *shedding or scaling off*).
4. **periodontitis as manifestation of systemic disease.** Periodontal inflammatory reactions occur as a result of diseases and genetic disorders, such as leukemia, HIV, malnutrition, and hormones.
5. **necrotizing periodontal diseases:** Rapid gingival tissue destruction with bacterial invasion of connective tissue may be a manifestation of systemic disease, such as HIV infection. This category is subdivided in two divisions:
   a. **necrotizing ulcerative gingivitis** (NUG) with a foul odor and a loss of interdental papilla, sometimes called "trench mouth."
   b. **necrotizing ulcerative periodontitis** (NUP) with bone pain and rapid bone loss.

C. **Abscesses of the periodontium.** Abscesses are classified according to location, such as gingival, periodontal, and pericoronal.

D. **Periodontitis associated with endodontic lesions.** This simple classification was added to distinguish between periodontitis and periodontitis with endodontic inflammation involvement.

E. **Developmental or acquired deformities and conditions.** Deformities appear around teeth, edentulous ridges, and from trauma.

PERIODONTAL EXAMINATION AND EVALUATION

The patient must receive a thorough exam and evaluation before treatment can be established. This procedure involves:

medical history: questions regarding diabetes, pregnancy, smoking, hypertension, dedication, substance abuse, and so forth.
dental history: chief complaint, past dental records, and radiographs; complete assessment of restoration condition, tooth position, mobility.
extraoral structure assessment: exam of oral mucosa, muscles of mastication, lips, floor of mouth, tongue, palate, salivary glands, and the oropharynx area.
periodontal probing depths: charting and recording findings of probe depths, assessing plaque and calculus presence, soft tissue, and implant conditions.
assessing intraoral findings: exam for tories, abnormal frenum placement and size, furcation involvement.

MEASUREMENT AND RECORDING OF PERIODONTAL CONDITIONS

The periodontal examination involves charting and recording tooth conditions and the status of the oral mucosa, particularly the periodontium. Clinical examination requires obtaining and recording an **index** (**IN**-decks = *measurement of conditions to a standard*), which rates the status of a particular patient and provides a method to measure the progress of the tested item, such as bleeding or plaque.

To be effective, the index procedure must be followed for each patient and the same method must be used from one dental source to another. Different indices apply to different conditions. The common indices used in periodontics cover plaque, oral hygiene, calculus, debris, periodontal conditions, bleeding, mobility, periodontal disease and involvement, among others. Some examples of periodontal indices follow, and Figure 16-2 provides an example of indexing.

FIGURE 16-2
Guideline for indexing. 0 = none present 1 = coverage of one-third or less of tooth surface 2 = coverage of more than one-third but less than two-thirds of tooth surface 3 = coverage of more than two-thirds of tooth surface

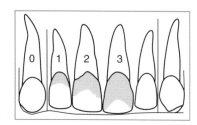

(PI I) Plaque Index (Silness and Loe)

Selected teeth: All teeth or any selected tooth or teeth

Method: Examine distofacial, facial, mesiofacial, and lingual tooth surfaces. Total the score for measured surfaces and divide by the number of surfaces; or obtain total "mouth score" by adding the total tooth scores and divide by the number of involved teeth.

0 = Gingival area of tooth is plaque-free.

1 = No visible plaque, but evidence of plaque on probe or explorer point is observed.

2 = Gingival area is covered by thin to moderate layer of visible plaque.

3 = Heavy accumulation of soft matter, filling gingival margin and covering tooth surface.

(DI-S) Simplified Oral Debris Index (Greene and Vermillion)

Selected teeth: #3, 8, 14, 24 facial view, and #19, 30 lingual view.

Method: Draw explorer from incisal third toward gingival third. Total the score per tooth and divide by number of surfaces examined. (See Figure 16-2 for an example of scoring areas.)

0 = No debris or stain present.

1 = Soft debris covering no more than one-third of the tooth surface; or the presence of extrinsic stains without other debris on any surface area.

2 = Soft debris covering more than one-third but not more than two-thirds of exposed surface.

3 = Soft debris covering more than two-thirds of exposed tooth surface.

(CI-S) Simplified Calculus Index (Greene and Vermillion)

Selected teeth: #3, 8, 14, 24 facial view, and #19 and 30 lingual view.

Method: Draw explorer subgingivally from the distal contact to the mesial contact. Total calculus score per tooth surfaces and divide by total examined tooth surfaces.

0 = No calculus present.

1 = Supragingival calculus covering no more than one-third of the exposed tooth surface.

2 = Supragingival calculus covering more than one-third but not more than two-thirds of the exposed tooth surface, or the presence of some subgingival calculus around cervical portion of the tooth, or both.

3 = Subgingival calculus covering more than two-thirds of the exposed tooth surface, or a continuous band of heavy calculus around the cervical area of the tooth, or both.

Note: Combining the simplified calculus (CI-S) and the simplified oral debris (DI-S) indices produces the simplified oral hygiene index (OHI-S).

(PI) Periodontal Index (Russell)

Selected teeth: All
Method: The score for each tooth is added for a total that is divided by the number of teeth examined.

0 = Negative finding; no bone loss or inflammation.
1 = Mild gingivitis with free gingiva inflammation but lacking entire tooth involvement.
2 = Gingivitis, normal probing depth but total circumscribing inflammation.
6 = Gingivitis, pocket formation, deepened gingival sulcus but no mobility or drifting present.
8 = Advanced destruction with loss of function, mobility present, may have socket. depression, may sound dull on percussion.

(SBI) Sulcus Bleeding Index .

Selected teeth: All or any chosen tooth
Method: Insert probe into sulcus of tooth at medial, buccal, distal, and lingual surfaces. Withdraw probe. Wait 30 seconds. Observe conditions.

0 = Healthy gingiva with no bleeding upon probing.
1 = Healthy gingival with some bleeding upon probing.
2 = Gingival color change with no swelling. Bleeding present upon probing.
3 = Bleeding upon probing, color change, and some swelling of gingiva.
4 = Bleeding upon probing, with obvious swelling and color change.
5 = Spontaneous bleeding or bleeding upon probing, color change, significant swelling, possible ulceration.

Tooth Mobility Index (Miller)

Selected teeth: Suspected tooth or teeth
Method: Place one metal instrument handle on each opposing sides of tooth to be tested. Apply pressure to observe mobility.

0 = No movement when force is applied.
1 = Barely observable tooth movement.
2 = 1 mm tooth movement in any direction.
3 = 1 mm tooth movement in any direction, or the ability of tooth rotatation or depression while in the socket.

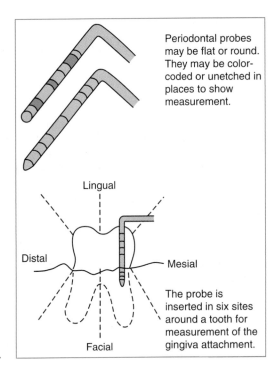

Periodontal probes may be flat or round. They may be color-coded or unetched in places to show measurement.

Lingual

Distal

Mesial

The probe is inserted in six sites around a tooth for measurement of the gingiva attachment.

Facial

FIGURE 16-3
Periodontal probe.

The Periodontal Probe

The most common instrument used in measuring the gingival pocket index records is the **periodontal probe**, a round or a flat-bladed hand instrument marked in millimeter increments (see Figure 16-3). The probe normally is inserted into six specific areas with the deepest pocket marking measurement recorded for that spot. The six areas are: facial (F), mesiofacial (MF), distofacial (DF), lingual (L), mesiolingual (ML), and distolingual (DL).

When connected by a continuous line, measurement marks placed on a dental chart give a visual indication of the gingival crest, indicating the heights of the interdental papilla and the depths of gingival pockets, including furcation involvement. Dental radiographs are examined to determine bone resorption and loss. The tooth is palpated and tested for mobility, and the patient's health history is elicited.

▌ PERIODONTAL TREATMENT METHODS

Treatments for periodontal conditions vary with the severity of the disease. Treatment may be of a non-surgical nature, conducted in the dental office with a program of home care, or it may involve extensive surgical care.

Non-Surgical Treatment of the Periodontium

The non-surgical treatment of periodontal irregularities and diseases involves a variety of procedures and therapies.

periodontal debridement: removing supragingival and subgingival plaque, calculus, stain, and irritants through tooth-crown and root-surface scaling and root planing.

tooth and surface polishing: polishing surfaces to remove accumulated extrinsic (ex-**TRIN**-sick = *outer*) stains on the tooth surfaces and endotoxins (en-doh-TOCKS-inz = *absorbed pathogens*) on the accessible surfaces.

selective polishing: term applied to the polishing of chosen tooth sites or areas.

prophylaxis: term applied to the combination of debridement and tooth polishing; used for purposes of insurance and scheduling.

patient education: customized instruction in oral hygiene, the care of teeth and gingival tissue; may include antimicrobal (an-**tie**-my-**KROH**-bee-al = *against small life*) therapy and antiplaque agents, diet and habit control, stress reduction, and fabrication of occlusal guards to prevent tooth grinding.

correction of plaque retention factors: dental intervention in existing conditions of open contacts, overcrowding, open or overhanging restoration margins, narrow embrasures, and ill-fitting appliances.

monitoring of patient: determination of progress and reevaluation of patient condition and efforts.

Periodontal Surgery Techniques

Various specialized surgical treatments are applied in cases of extensive disease of the periodontium.

mucogingival excision: used to correct defects in shape, position, or amount of gingiva around the tooth; eliminates the pocket formation and pericoronitis typically found on erupting third molars.

gingivectomy: excision of gum tissue area. (See Figure 16-4 for an example of tissue marking for the gingivectomy procedure.)

gingivoplasty: surgical contour of gingival tissue.

periodontal flap surgery: separating a loosened section of tissue from the adjacent tissues to enable elimination of deposits and contouring of alveolar bone. The several types of flap surgery include:

> envelope flap: no vertical incision with the mucoperiosteal flap retracted from a horizontal incision line.
>
> mucoperiosteal: mucosal tissue flap including the periosteum, reflected from the bone; also called full thickness flap.
>
> partial-thickness flap: surgical flap including mucosa and connective tissue but no periosteum.
>
> pedicle flap: tissue flap with lateral incisions.
>
> positioned flap: flap that is moved to a new position, apically, laterally, or coronally.

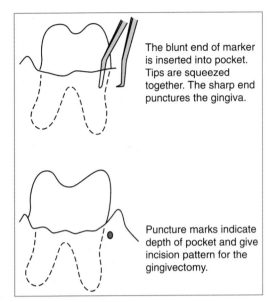

The blunt end of marker is inserted into pocket. Tips are squeezed together. The sharp end punctures the gingiva.

Puncture marks indicate depth of pocket and give incision pattern for the gingivectomy.

FIGURE 16-4
Pocket marking for tissue removal.

repositioned flap: surgical flap replaced in its original position.

sliding flap: pedicle flap re-situated in a new position.

osseous surgery: tissue surgery with alteration in bony support of the teeth.

re-entry: second-stage surgical procedure to enhance or improve conditions from a previous surgical procedure.

vestibuloplasty (ves-**TIB**-you-loh-**plas**-tee): surgical alteration of gingival mucous membrane in vestibule of the mouth, including frenum reposition and change in muscle attachment.

ENAP (excisional new attachment procedure): removal of chronically inflamed soft tissue to permit formation of new tissue attachment.

guided tissue regeneration: placement of a semipermeable membrane (Gore-Tex) beneath the flap to prevent ingrowth of epithelium between the flap and the defect; encourages the growth of new periodontal attachment.

Periodontal dressing packs are placed over the surgical site to assist with protection and healing. These packs are mixed, prepared, and expressed on the surgical site. They are supplied in four ways:

1. Zinc oxide and eugenol powder and liquid that is mixed to a paste, rolled, and pressed over the site.
2. Zinc oxide paste and a non-eugenol base paste that are mixed together and applied to the area.
3. Syringe-dispensed periodontal paste that is expressed upon the site and light cured.
4. Gelatin packs that dissolve and do not have to be removed.

Bone Grafting

Some periodontal surgical techniques will require bone tissues. Bone grafts involve transplants to restore bone loss from periodontal disease.

allograft (**AL**-oh-graft) : human bone graft from someone other than the patient.
autograft (**AW**-toh-graft): bone graft from another site in the same patient.
xenograft (**ZEE**-no-graft): graft taken from another species, such as cow or pig bone (experimental).
allogenic (al-loh-**JEN**-ick): addition of synthetic material to repair or build up bone.

▌ PERIODONTAL INVOLVEMENT WITH DENTAL IMPLANTS

Dental implants are titanium or ceramic devices that are surgically placed into the alveolar bone to provide firm, fixed anchors for dental appliances or dentures. The bone and the implant complete a process of uniting called osseointegration (**oss**-ee-oh-in-teh-**GRAY**-shun = *union of bone and device*). Implants are explained and illustrated in Chapter 14, Oral and Maxillofacial Surgery, and terminology relevant to periodontics is defined below.

endosteal: implants of various designs placed within the bone.
subperiosteal: implant placement beneath the periosteum and onto the bone.
transosteal: implant placement through the bone.
endodontic: implant set within the apex of the root.

Periodontal cleaning and scaling procedures performed on implants must be completed with plastic or sonic instruments to protect the implants.

▌ INSTRUMENTATION FOR PERIODONTICS

Periodontal treatment requires specialized instruments, most of which are hand instruments, although ultrasonic, sonic, laser, and power-driven tools also are part of the necessary setup.

Periodontal Hand Instruments

Hand instruments employed in periodontal treatment, illustrated in Figure 16-5, are used in a push or pull method to accomplish a desired outcome. Push instruments use a push stroke direction with a blade-to-tooth angle of less than 45 degrees perpendicular to the instrument's shaft. An example is the chisel. Pull instruments use a pull stroke direction with a blade-to-tooth angle of between 45 and 90 degrees perpendicular to the instrument's shaft. The most effective pull angle is approximately 75 degrees. Examples include scalers, curettes, hoes, and files.

periodontal probe: used to measure the depth of the periodontal pocket by determining the amount of gingival tissue attachment. A probe may be flat- or

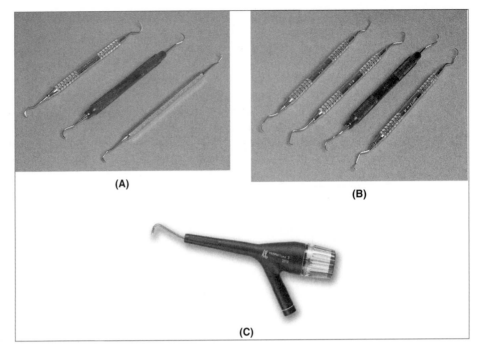

FIGURE 16-5
Examples of periodontal instruments. (A) Scalers (B) Curettes (Courtesy of Hu-Friedy) (C) Power Polishing Unit (Courtesy of Kavo Dental Corporation)

(A)

(B)

(C)

round-bladed and is marked in measured increments. Automatic periodontal probes are available and are used by inserting the probe wire into the sulcus area to determine and record the measurement on a computer.

explorer: instrument with a longer, tapered, thin wire tip to determine calculus formation, restoration overhangs, and any root **furcation** involvement.

scaler: instrument with a sharpened blade to remove supragingival calculus deposits and stains. Scalers (Figure 16-5A) are available in various shapes such as sickle for universal use, straight for anterior areas, and contra-angled for posterior areas.

hoe: instrument with long shank and hoe-like tip, used to remove heavy or thick supragingival calculus in posterior areas.

chisel: instrument with longer shaft and chisel-bladed tip, used to break off and remove heavy calculus in the anterior region.

curette: instrument with longer shank and working end with a rounded toe and back to access and remove subgingival deposits. A **universal curette** has a cutting edge on each side of the blade to enable use in all areas. Other curettes are designed for specific areas, such as the Gracey curettes with a cutting edge on one side of blade, shown in Figure 16-5 B.

file: hand instrument with multiple cutting edges, used to smooth rough and uneven tissues and remove stubborn calculus deposits.

ultrasonic and sonic instrument tip: inserted into the ultrasonic handle; sonic forces move the tip in rapid, short (0.001 inch) waves at speed frequencies of 20,000 to 35,000 vibrations per second to break apart and dislodge deposits from the tooth surface. The tips or inserts are designed for specific areas and designated use. Machine tips are cooled with a water spray to lessen friction heat. Some handpieces have light sources for better viewing.

Polishing Instruments

Instruments used to polish the tooth surfaces include straight handpieces, prophylaxis contra-angles, and rubber cups, as well as polishing agents such as pumice, cleaners, and chemically impregnated rubber points. Polishing and stain removal is completed by using an air power-driven calcium carbonate powder spray unit (Figure 16-5C) or a slow handpiece rotary rubber cup with pumice.

Surgical Periodontal Instruments

The following are instruments used in surgery.

periodontal pocket marker: set of instruments similar to tweezers with a sharp point on one tip for insertion into the depth of the pocket and then compressed to make puncture marks indicating pocket depth. There is one marker for each side of pocket.

periodontal knives: used to make incisions to remove tissue or to obtain flap design. Blade shape may be round or pointed and long-edged.

electrosurgery tips/unit: apparatus using electrical current to incise tissue and coagulate blood at the same time; useful in periodontal flap, tissue grafting, crown lengthening, and other tissue surgeries.

laser tip/unit: apparatus delivering energy in light form at different wavelengths; can be used in soft or hard tissue curettage surgery when regulated to the specific bacterial target.

REVIEW EXERCISES

MATCHING

Match the following word elements with their meaning:

1. _____ papillary gingiva
2. _____ gingivectomy
3. _____ file
4. _____ allograft
5. _____ curette
6. _____ transosteal implant
7. _____ sulcus
8. _____ endodontic implant

a. free marginal gingiva
b. used to measure depth of attached gingiva
c. tissue redness
d. used to access attached gingiva in subgingival areas
e. implant placed within apex of tooth root
f. hard gingival tissue, called masticatory mucosa
g. hand instrument with multiple cutting, rasping edges
h. bone graft from another site on the same patient

9. _____ furcation

i. used to mark depth of tissue pocket for excision

10. _____ periodontal probe

j. marginal gingiva occupying inter-proximal space

11. _____ periodontal pocket marker

k. branching or forking of tooth roots

12. _____ erythema

l. implant placed through the mandibular bone

13. _____ etiology

m. excision and removal of gingival tissue

14. _____ autograft

n. bone graft from someone other than patient

15. _____ keratinized gingiva

o. study of the cause of a disease

DEFINITIONS

Using the selection given for each sentence, choose the best term to complete the definition.

1. Transplanting bone to restore bone lost from periodontal disease is termed:
   a. osteoplasty
   b. bone graft
   c. bone therapy
   d. osseotectomy

2. Splinting, wire ligating, or bonding teeth together are forms of tooth:
   a. stabilization
   b. mobility
   c. transplantation
   d. adjustment

3. An increase in the size of affected gingiva is termed:
   a. hypertrophy
   b. hypotrophy
   c. hypoextension
   d. hyperextension

4. Gingivitis that may be modified by a systemic factor such as pregnancy, puberty, or hormone is called:
   a. ulcerated gingivitis
   b. induced gingivitis
   c. irritant gingivitis
   d. severe gingivitis

5. Debridement and shining of tooth surfaces and exposed tooth tissue is termed:
   a. prophylaxis
   b. scaling
   c. root planning
   d. tooth polishing.

6. Which is not considered a periodontal pull hand instrument?
   a. periodontal probe
   b. scaler
   c. currette
   d. hoe

7. Ultrasonic periodontal tips vibrate at _____ per second.
   a. 10–20
   b. 100–250
   c. 9,000–15,1000
   d. 20,000–35,000

8. Which is not considered a tooth polishing agent?
   a. pumice
   b. impregnated points
   c. hoes
   d. rubber cups

9. Which is not considered an indexing record-ing of conditions?
   a. calculus
   b. bleeding
   c. radiograph
   d. stain

10. The term for "trench mouth" is:
    a. halitosis
    b. gingivitis
    c. NUG
    d. periodontia

11. The hard substances formed from calcium and phosphorous salts deposits on teeth is called:
    a. stains
    b. calculus
    c. plaque
    d. pellicle

12. Interradicular periodontal fibers may be found around which teeth?
    a. incisors
    b. cuspids (canines)
    c. bicuspids (premolars)
    d. molars

13. Which is not considered a tissue of the periodontium?
    a. gingiva
    b. alveolar bone
    c. dentin
    d. cementum

14. An oral hygiene index (OHI) of 3 indicates which degree of oral tooth debris?
    a. none
    b. slight
    c. moderate
    d. heavy

15. What is considered the proper number of probe sites per tooth for pocket data?
    a. 1   b. 2
    c. 4   d. 6

16. Painful, red, sloughing gingival epithelium is called:
    a. irritated   b. desquamative
    c. gingivitis   d. refractory

17. Which of the following is not a symptom of gingivitis?
    a. redness   b. mobility
    c. foul odor   d. coral stippling

18. Calculus deposits found on the exposed coronal surfaces of the teeth are termed:
    a. coronal   b. subgingival
    c. sublingual   d. supragingival

19. Which periodontal instrument is used to incise and remove diseased tissue?
    a. periodontal probe
    b. periodontal hoe
    c. periodontal file
    d. periodontal knife

20. The periodontium tissue that makes up the tooth socket is/are:
    a. alveolar bone   b. gingiva
    c. periodontal fibers   d. gums

BUILDING SKILLS

Locate and define the prefix, root/combining form, and suffix (if present) in the following words.

1. **periodontology**
   prefix   _____
   root/combining form   _____
   suffix   _____

2. **antimicrobal**
   prefix   _____
   root/combining form   _____
   suffix   _____

3. **desquamative**
   prefix   _____
   root/combining form   _____
   suffix   _____

4. **hypertrophy**
   prefix   _____
   root/combining form   _____
   suffix   _____

5. **endosseous**
   prefix   _____
   root/combining form   _____
   suffix   _____

FILL-INS

Write the correct word in the blank space to complete each statement.

1. The _____ is a periodontal hand instrument with a longer shank and working end with a rounded toe and back that is used to access subgingival areas.

2. The chisel is used to break off and remove heavy calculus deposits in the _____ region.

3. The major contributing factor to diseases of the periodontium is _____ formation.

4. Pus formation in pocket area is called pocket _____.

5. An adhering tooth film that assists with the sticking ability of plaque is called _____ film.

6. Hard tissue gingiva, also known as masticatory mucosa, is _____ gingiva.

7. The _____ is composed of the tissue surrounding the teeth.

8. _____ gingiva is unattached to the underlying tissues and forms the gingival crevice.

9. Scalpels and _____ are used to incise gingival tissue.

10. Periodontal instruments that vibrate rapidly, using little strokes to break away deposits are called _____ instruments.

11. Uniting of the implant and the bone tissue is a process called _____.

12. Using a bone graft taken from another species is term a/an _____.

13. A/An _____ implant is placed under the periosteum and onto the bone.

14. A periodontal instrument used in a pushing motion should have less than a _____ degree angle on the blade.

15. The use of prescription mouthwashes and treated fibers to destroy microbes is termed _____ therapy.

16. The selective grinding of occlusal cusps to prevent premature contacts is _____.

17. Acrylic night guards worn to protect from tooth grinding are called _____.

18. Polishing selected teeth during a prophylaxis is termed _____.

19. _____ is procedure of contouring gingival tissue.

20. The measure of a condition to determine standards is called a/an _____.

WORD USE

Read the following sentences and define the bold-faced words.

1. The dentist explained to Mrs. Bailey that her **induced gingivitis** is only temporary and will cease after the delivery of her baby.

   _____

2. Dr. Goldenberg's office called to arrange an appointment for a **gingivoplasty** procedure for her patient.

   _____

3. One of the treatment plan procedures for the NUG patient involves **antimicrobial therapy.**

   _____

4. The dental hygienist uses a periodontal probe to establish the extent of the **marginal gingiva.**

   _____

5. The laboratory returned the study cast and the **occlusal guard** prepared for Mr. Mason.

   _____

AUDIO LIST

This list contains selected new, important, or difficult terms from this chapter. You may use the list to review these terms and to practice pronouncing them correctly. When you work with the audio for this chapter, listen to the word, repeat it, and then place a checkmark in the box. Proceed to the next boxed word and repeat the process.

- ❏ allograft (**AL**-oh graft)
- ❏ antimicrobial (an-tie-my-**KROH**-bee-al)
- ❏ autograft (**AW**-toh-graft)
- ❏ cribriform (**KRIB**-rih-form)
- ❏ desquamative (des-**KWAM**-ah-tiv)
- ❏ endotoxins (en-doh-**TOCKS**-inz)
- ❏ exudate (**EX**-you-dayt)
- ❏ hyperplasia (high-per-**PLAY**-zee-ah)
- ❏ hypertrophy (high-per-**TROH**-fee)
- ❏ keratinized (**KARE**-ah-tin-ized)
- ❏ mucogingival (myou-koh-**JIN**-jih-vahl)
- ❏ osseointegration (**oss**-ee-oh-in-teh-**GRAY** shun)
- ❏ pellicle (**PELL**-ih-kul)
- ❏ periodontology (**pear**-ee-oh-dahn-**TAH**-loh-jee)
- ❏ refractory (ree-**FRACK**-tore-ee)
- ❏ somatic (soh-**MAT**-ick)
- ❏ stippling (**STIP**-ling)
- ❏ vestibuloplasty (ves-**TIB**-you-loh-**plas**-tee)

Pediatric Dentistry

OBJECTIVES   Upon completion of this chapter, the reader should be able to identify and understand terms related to:

1. **Scope of pediatric dentistry.** Discuss the practice and duties of a pedodontist and the types of teeth involved with children's dentistry.

2. **Development and growth concerns of pediatric dentition.** List and identify the common concerns related to children's dental care.

3. **Maintenance and preservation of pediatric dentition.** Describe the preventive, operative, and home care procedures provided to the deciduous teeth.

4. **Restorative dental care for the primary dentition.** Discuss the restorative care given the primary dentition and explain the various pulp treatment procedures available.

5. **Control and sedation of the child patient.** Explain the need for control and/or sedation of the child patient and the methods employed to accomplish this state.

6. **Treatment for trauma and abuse.** List and explain the classifications and treatment methods for fractured and traumatized teeth.

7. **Use of dental records for patient identification.** Discuss the various methods used to establish patient identification from the use of dental and personal records.

8. **Miscellaneous child health conditions.** Identify common childhood diseases that may affect the development and condition of the human dentition.

SCOPE OF PEDIATRIC DENTISTRY

Pediatric dentistry is concerned with the care of teeth and oral tissues of the child patient. The dentist who specializes in this practice, called a pedodontist, generally treats the child patient until the premolars erupt or the beginning of the teen years. The first dentition to erupt is called the primary dentition. This set of teeth consists of twenty deciduous teeth, which will be replaced by secondary or permanent teeth.

The treatment and care provided in pediatric dentistry is essentially the same as for adults, although the instruments and some techniques may be modified.

DEVELOPMENT AND GROWTH CONCERNS OF PEDIATRIC DENTITION

Many of the dental problems of the child patient are the result of improper or irregular development of newly erupting teeth. Some problems arise during the growth period, when environment and habits can affect the teeth.

caries: dental decay.

epulis: fibrous, sarcomatous tumor, also called *gumboil*.

abscess: local collection of pus.

cellulites: inflammation in cellular or connective tissue.

anodontia: absence of teeth, usually of genetic origin.

macrodontia (**mack**-roh-**DAHN**-she-ah): abnormally large teeth.

hyperdontia (high-per-**DAHN**-she-ah): excess number of supernumerary teeth.

hypodontia (high-poh-**DAHN**-she-ah): congenital absence of teeth.

enamel hypoplasia: underdevelopment of enamel tissue.

dentinogenesis imperfecta: genetic defect resulting in incomplete or improper development of dentin tissue.

amelogenesis imperfecta (ah-**meal**-oh-**JEN**-ih-sis im-purr-**FECK**-tah): incomplete or improper development of enamel tissue.

aplasia (ah-**PLAY**-zee-ah): failure of an organ or body part to develop.

dens in dente: tooth within a tooth.

germinate (**JER**-mih-nay-ted = *sprout*): attempted division of a single tooth.

fusion of teeth: union of two, independently developing primary or secondary teeth.

early tooth exfoliation (ecks-**foh**-lee-**AY**-shun = *shedding or falling off*): tooth loss resulting in the shifting of teeth and loss of tooth position.

ankylosis (ang-key-**LOH**-sis): stiff joint; retention of deciduous tooth.

intrinsic (in-**TRIN**-sick = *on the inside*): internal discoloration of teeth resulting from diet, medication, or excessive fluoride intake during tooth development.

Some growth irregularities present future problems requiring interceptive or orthodontic care. These maladies include open bite, diastema, cross-bites, tooth protrusions, oral habits such as thumb sucking, and tooth crowding.

Developmental Tissue and Bone Problems

Not only are the developing teeth subject to growth problems, but sometimes the oral tissues and the child's bones develop problems associated with dental care.

odontoma (oh-dahn-**TOH**-mah = *tumor of a tooth or dental tissue*): abnormal cell proliferation of cells.

macroglossia (**mack**-roh-**GLOSS**-ee-ah; macro = *large*, glossia = *tongue*): enlarged tongue.

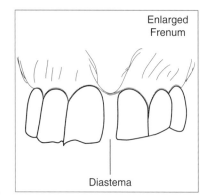

FIGURE 17-1
Diastema, correctable by a frenectomy.

Enlarged Frenum

Diastema

ankyloglossia (ang-key-loh-**GLOSS**-ee-ah): abnormally short lingual frenum, causing limited tongue movement (tongue-tied).

fissured (**FISH**-erd) tongue: grooved division, cleft, or split of tongue.

abnormal labial frenum: enlarged or thick labial frenum that may cause **diastema**, an open area between the central incisors (see Figure 17-1).

micrognathia (my-kroh-**NAY**-thee-ah): abnormally small jaw; undersized mandible.

cherubism (**CHAIR**-you-bizm): a genetic disorder resulting in enlargement of cheek tissue and other facial structures.

Tumor and Cyst Growth

Some children develop neoplasms of the oral soft tissue and bones.

papilloma: neoplasm arising from epithelial cells; benign tumor.

verruca vulgaris (ver-**OO**-kah-, vul-**GAIR**-iss = *oral warts*): viral cause, possibly from finger sucking.

fibroma: fibrous tumor, benign in nature.

granuloma: granular tumor, usually of epithelioid or lymphoid cells.

neurofibromatosis (**new**-roh-fie-**broh**-mah-**TOH**-sis): tumor on peripheral nerves.

hemangioma: vascular tumor, usually located in the neck / head area.

lymphangioma (lim-**fan**-jee-**OH**-mah): tumor made up of lymphatic vessels.

lymphoma (lim-**FOH**-mah): new tissue growth within the lymphatic system.

mucocele (**MYOU**-koh-seal): mucous cyst.

ranula: mucocele in the floor of the mouth in the sublingual duct.

MAINTENANCE AND PRESERVATION OF PEDIATRIC DENTITION

Maintenance and preservation of the primary dentition involves the same care and attention as that given to adult teeth. Visits to the dentist should begin early (at age two) and consist of the health and dental history, clinical and dental exam, prophylaxis, and radiographs that have been modified in size for the smaller mouth. Parents may benefit from receiving instruction in nutrition and home care, including toothbrushing, and other preventive measures.

Prophylaxis treatment may include gingival care for simple, eruption, **scorbutic** (skor-**BYOU**-tick = *lacking vitamin C*), or acute gingivitis, as well as periodontitis and periodontosis, herpes simplex virus, aphthous ulcer, ANUG, or **candidiasis** (**kan**-dih-**DYE**-ah-sis = *fungus infection, thrush*). Appliances may be constructed to correct bad habits, such as finger sucking or nail biting. Other professional preventive care includes the following.

Fluoride Application.   The dentist may indicate a need for professional application of fluoride to the child's teeth. Fluoride care may be provided in the form of ingestion by drinking water with fluoride or taking prescribed fluoride supplements, by topical application, placing on the teeth, or a combination of both techniques. Topical application is supplied in the form of gel, varnish, liquid, spray, or other methods. The various types of dental fluoride, as recommended by the Division of Oral Health, National Center for Chronic Disease Prevention and Health Promotion, are given in Table 17-1.

Enamoplasty.   Enamoplasty (ee-**NAM**-oh-**plas**-tee) is the selective reduction of fissures and occlusal irregularities caused by grinding. Rather than filling deep pits or fissures with sealant material, the dentist may choose to perform some selective reducing or leveling of deep crevices to permit easier cleansing and home care of the teeth.

Pit and Fissure Sealant Application.   Sealants are clear or tinted acrylic coatings that are either **self-cured** (when mixed, base and catalyst are chemically polymerized) or **light-cured** (polymerizes with the use of a curing light). Application to the enamel surface requires **etching** of the tooth before placing the topical sealant. When in place and hardened, the sealant will form an even, hard acrylic coating on the chewing surfaces, eliminating any deep pits or fissures.

Oral Surgery.   Surgical intervention may be used to prevent future problems for developing teeth. Examples include extraction to remove **ankylosed** (**ANG**-kih-lowzd = *fixed, stiff*) teeth or a large labial frenum that requires a **frenectomy** (freh-**NECK**-toh-me = *incision and suturing of frenum to the pertosteum*) to avoid a diastema (dye-ah-**STEE**-mah) of the anterior central incisors.

Space Maintenance.   Professional care may involve placement of fixed or removable appliances to maintain or reclaim premature spacing in the arch until eruption of the secondary teeth. Some common space maintainers are the **band and loop** and the **distal shoe** appliances (see Figure 17-2). An acrylic **bite plane** appliance may be constructed to correct a simple crossbite.

TABLE 17-1   Fluoride Supplementation

FLUORIDE ITEM	FORM	USE	AVAILABILITY	RECOMMENDATIONS
Fluoride Toothpaste	Paste 1,000–1,500 ppm	Brush teeth 2× daily. Fl taken up by plaque and demineralized enamel, increases Fl in saliva.	OTC (over-the-counter)	Brush 2× daily, supervise children <6 small amounts, no swallowing; tots <2 by dentist advice.
Fl Mouthrinse	0.05% sodium fluoride OTC for daily use; 0.20% sodium fluoride (NaFl) for weekly school rinse program.	Used daily or weekly for pre-scribed time. Fl retained in saliva and plaque to help prevent tooth decay.	OTC for normal use; higher con-centrations by RX.	Not for use by children <6 unless RX by DDS; danger of swallowing and causing fluorosis.
Fl Supplements	Tablets, liquid, lozenges with (NaFl) sodium fluoride bases of 1.0, 0.5, or 0.25 mg Fl.	Useful for children without fluoride in water supply. Prefer sucking or chewing tablets for 1–2 minutes to maximize effects.	RX by dentists.	Dentist to determine if child is high-risk without fluoride in water. Use proper dosage to avoid fluorosis.
Fl Gel and Foam	Gel = acidulated phosphate fluoride, gel, or foam of NaFl, or stannous fluoride.	Applied in dental office for 1–4 minutes; home use as prescribed.	Dental office = acidulated phosphate with 1.23% Fl concentration, 0.9% NaFl in office use, or 0.5% home use, or 0.15 stannous fluoride home use.	Applications at 3–12 month intervals; little risk of enamel fluorosis.
Fl Varnish	Varnishes of 2.26% NaFl, or difluor-silane 0.1% fluoride amount.	Painted on teeth by dental professional; not intended to adhere perma-nently but holds Fl to teeth for hours.	Applied by dental professional in dental office.	Reapply at regular intervals, 2× year. No fluorosis risk from application.

Source: Division of Oral Health, National Center for Chronic Disease Prevention and Health Promotion.

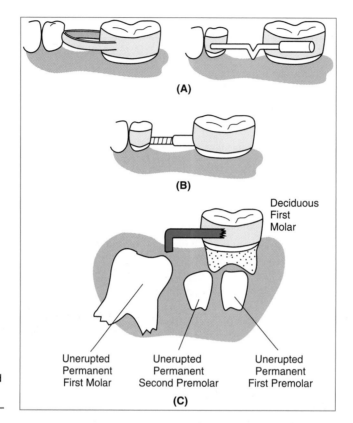

FIGURE 17-2
Examples of space maintainers.
(A) Band and Loop
(B) Spring-activated
(C) Distal Shoe Bar

Deciduous
First
Molar

(A)

(B)

Unerupted
Permanent
First Molar

Unerupted
Permanent
Second Premolar

Unerupted
Permanent
First Premolar

(C)

RESTORATIVE DENTAL CARE FOR THE PRIMARY DENTITION

Restorative care of the deciduous teeth is basically the same as for the permanent dentition. Although restorations are completed in the same manner, some instruments can be modified in size, such as a T-band matrix (see Figure 17-3) in place of a matrix and retainer. A T-band matrix may be curved or straight. These bands are bent into a circle, and the T edges are folded over to hold the shape. The strips require no retainer and take less space in a smaller mouth.

The child patient may receive straight-edge or contoured stainless steel crowns for badly decayed or broken-down teeth. The crowns are fitted or **festooned** (fes-**TUNED**= *trimmed*), and cemented onto the tooth. Children may receive composite resin bonding for tooth surfaces, ceramic and metal crowns, cores, fixed or removable partial or full dentures, implants, retainers, and protective mouthguards.

Pulpal Treatment

Because of the large opening in the **apex** of the erupting and developing tooth, pulpal treatment may be more aggressive in a child than an adult. The two types of

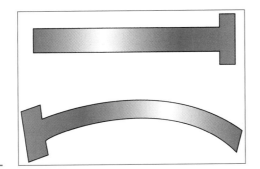

FIGURE 17-3
A curved and a straight T-band matrix.

pulpal treatment are:

1. **apexogenesis** (ay-pecks-oh-**JEN**-ih-sis): treatment of a vital pulp to allow continued natural development.
2. **apexification** (ay-pecks-ih-fih-**KAY**-shun): treatment of a nonvital tooth to stimulate closure and the development of cementum.

The affected vital pulp of a primary tooth or a permanent tooth that is not fully calcified may receive any of a number of treatment procedures, as illustrated in Figure 17-4.

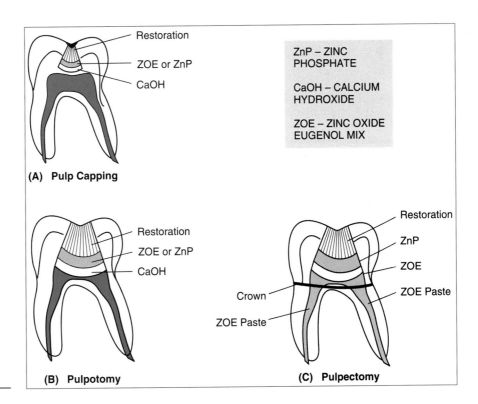

FIGURE 17-4
Pulp treatment.

pulp capping: placement of medication to sedate and treat inflamed pulp (17-4A). **Indirect capping** is needed when the pulp has not yet been exposed. In **direct capping**, the medicament is placed directly upon the exposed, affected pulp (17-4A).

pulpotomy: partial or full removal of pulpal tissue located in the crown (17-4B).

pulpectomy: removal of pulpal tissue from the crown and root sections; may be endodontically filled immediately or followed later with endodontic treatment after apexification and closure of the apex of a young, secondary tooth (17-4C).

CONTROL AND SEDATION OF THE CHILD PATIENT

Pediatric dental care requires precise techniques completed rapidly and calmly. Control and sedation of the child patient is completed in various ways.

dental (rubber) dam: provides control of tongue and saliva and maintains a sterile and open area.

papoose board: wrapping device used to restrain the patient for a difficult or precise treatment.

topical anesthesia: liquid, gel, or ointment that provides temporary numbing of the tissue surface.

Injection Anesthesia

Injection anesthesia refers to the placement of an anesthetic solution by means of an aspirating syringe to produce a loss of sensation. The various application methods are explained in Chapter 8, Pain Management/Pharmacology.

Conscious Sedation

Calming nervous anxiety without loss of consciousness is called conscious sedation. This condition may be achieved in a number of ways.

inhalation sedation: administration of nitrous oxide with at least 30 percent oxygen.

oral sedation: completed by having the patient ingest the drug.

intramuscular (in-tra-**MUSS**-kyou-lahr = *within the muscle*) sedation: parenterally administrated sedation.

rectal sedation: placement of sedation drug in the rectum.

submucosal (sub-mew-**COH**-sul = *under the mucous membrane*): deposit of the drug beneath the mucous membrane.

subcutaneous (sub-kyou-**TAY**-nee-us = *under the skin*): injection of the drug under the tissues.

intravenous (in-trah-**VEE**-nus = *into the vein, vessel*): injection of the drug into the vein.

TREATMENT FOR TRAUMA AND ABUSE

Injury to the teeth and mouth tissues can result from trauma or abuse to the head and face. The most common complaint is a tooth fracture. The four classifications of tooth fractures are

Class I: fractured enamel showing rough edges with no dentin involved.
Class II: fractured enamel with dentin involved and no pulp tissue included.
Class III: full fracture of tooth, exposing the pulp.
Class IV: tooth crown is fractured off.

Traumatized Tooth Difficulties

Traumatized primary and permanent teeth exhibit a variety of difficulties and effects.

pulpal hyperemia: congestion of blood within the pulp chamber.
internal hemorrhage: rupture of pulpal capillaries.
internal or external resorption: destructive, dissolving process caused by odonto-
    clastic action.
pulpal necrosis: pulpal death.
ankylosis: fusion of cementum of the root with the cribriform plate of the alveolar
    bone, with no intervening periodontal ligament
intrusion: tooth thrusting into the alveolus with partial crown exposure.
extrusion: tooth thrust away from the alveolus.
luxation: tooth moved out of place.
avulsion: tooth forced out of its socket.

Treatment of Traumatized Teeth

Treatment for injured primary teeth may include:

▶ smoothing of rough edge
▶ pulp capping
▶ pulpotomy
▶ pulpectomy with or without endodontic treatment
▶ stainless steel banding, metal or resin crowns, placement of posts
▶ replantation and stabilization (splinting) of replantation.

USE OF DENTAL RECORDS FOR PATIENT IDENTIFICATION

Dental records are being used extensively for identification in forensic and legal matters. The dental office offers many methods for recording and maintaining positive identification items for future reference. With particular attention to missing children, the pedodontist may supply information collected during routine visits.

personal information data: including name, address, nicknames, ethnicity, hobbies,
    eyeglasses, tattoos, scars, birthmarks, and so forth.
dental charting record: current tooth development, dentition characteristics, and
    treatment data.

radiographs: current tooth placement and expected tooth development.

photographs: frontal and side views with profile and tooth growth. Digital photos have the advantage of providing immediate images that can be transmitted in missing child cases.

toothprint: a thermoplastic wafer impression record of the child's unique occlusion.

saliva: fluid collection containing the child's DNA and scent for use with tracking dogs in missing child cases.

▌MISCELLANEOUS CHILD HEALTH CONDITIONS

Dental care delivery is dependent upon the child's total health condition. Children affected with systemic or genetic diseases may exhibit more dental distress and/or require more and specialized dental treatment. Some childhood diseases that may have additional dental concerns are:

AIDS	cystic fibrosis	learning difficulties
autism	deafness	leukemia
blindness	juvenile diabetes	rheumatic fever
asthma	Down syndrome	viral hepatitis
cerebral palsy	fragile X syndrome	
congenital heart disease	hemophilia	

▌REVIEW EXERCISES

MATCHING

Match the following word elements with their meanings.

1. _____caries
2. _____macrodontia
3. _____ankyloglossia
4. _____cellulitis
5. _____Class I fracture
6. _____epulis
7. _____toothprint

8. _____ranula
9. _____Class III fracture
10. _____deciduous
11. _____macroglossia
12. _____submucosal
13. _____avulsion
14. _____pulpotomy
15. _____hemangioma

a. primary teeth
b. abnormally large tongue
c. removal of pulp tissue in crown of tooth
d. mucocele in sublingual gland
e. full tooth fracture, exposing pulp tissue
f. inflammation in cellular tissue
g. under the mucous membrane
h. vascular tumor
i. tooth fracture of enamel; no other tissue included
j. torn or pulled away or out of
k. dental decay
l. fibrous tumor, gumboil
m. thermoplastic ID wafer
n. stiff or rigid tongue condition
o. abnormally large teeth

DEFINITIONS

Using the selection given for each sentence, choose the best term to complete the definition.

1. Another term for a common gumboil is a/an:
   a. oral wart   b. gingival abscess
   c. inflamed uvula   d. epulis

2. An abnormally short lingual frenum may cause a tongue-tied condition called:
   a. macroglossia   b. microglossia
   c. papilloma   d. ankyloglossia

3. A mucocele is a cyst present in which tissue?
   a. mucous   b. bone
   c. lymph   d. epithelial

4. Which of the following is not an accepted topical fluoride?
   a. stannous fluoride b. carbon fluoride
   c. sodium fluoride   d. acidulated phosphate

5. Selective grinding away or removal of enamel tissue and flaws is called:
   a. amelogenesis   b. enamel hypoplasia
   c. enamelation   d. enamoplasty

6. Candidiasis is a fungus infection commonly referred to as:
   a. thrush   b. ANUG
   c. gingivitis   d. periodontitits

7. Scorbutic gingivitis is a result of a deficiency of which vitamin?
   a. vitamin A   b. vitamin B
   c. vitamin C   d. vitamin D

8. Sedation by swallowing medication involves which avenue of entrance?
   a. ingestion
   b. inhalation
   c. rectal placement
   d. intravenous

9. Trimming the gingival area of a stainless steel crown is called:
   a. festooning   b. obturation
   c. crowning   d. alteration

10. Amelogenesis imperfecta is the improper development of which tissue?
    a. enamel   b. dentin
    c. pulp   d. cementum

11. Which condition involves an excessive number of teeth, supernumerary teeth?
    a. hypodontia   b. hyperdontia
    c. macrodontia   d. microdontia

12. Intrinsic pigmentation is a coloring of which tooth surface?
    a. apical   b. external
    c. gingival   d. internal

13. The full or partial removal of pulp tissue from the crown portion of a tooth is a/an:
    a. apicoectomy   b. pulpectomy
    c. pulpotomy   d. pulp capping

14. A liquid, gel, or ointment medicine placed on the mucous membrane to obtain surface anesthesia is which type of anesthesia?
    a. conduction   b. block
    c. infiltration   d. topical

15. Cellulitis denotes inflammation of which tissue?
    a. enamel   b. connective
    c. bone   d. mucous

16. Which pit and fissure sealant polymerizes without the use of the curing light?
    a. self-cure   b. etched-cure
    c. light-cure   d. polymer-cure

17. The forced removal or knocking out of a tooth is known as:
    a. avulsion   b. luxation
    c. intrusion   d. extrusion

18. A fractured tooth showing evidence of dentin and enamel involvement is which class?
    a. Class I   b. Class II
    c. Class III   d. Class IV

19. Acid conditioning of a cavity preparation prior to placement of a restorative material is called:
    a. etching
    b. sealant application
    c. composite auto-curing
    d. composite self-curing

20. Which of the following is not a name for the teeth in a child's dentition?
    a. primary   b. succedeaneous
    c. baby teeth   d. deciduous

BUILDING SKILLS

Locate and define the prefix, root/combining form, and suffix (if present) in the following words.

1. **apexogenesis**

   prefix _____

   root/combining form _____

   suffix _____

2. **infraorbital**

   prefix _____

   root/combining form _____

   suffix _____

3. **exfoliation**

   prefix _____

   root/combining form _____

   suffix _____

4. **lymphangioma**

   prefix _____

   root/combining form _____

   suffix _____

5. **anodontia**

   prefix _____

   root/combining form _____

   suffix _____

FILL-INS

Write the correct word in the blank space to complete each statement.

1. The dental specialist who treats the child patient is called a/an _____.

2. Enamel _____ is an under-development of enamel tissue.

3. A/an _____ is a mucocele in the sublingual gland in the floor of the mouth.

4. _____ is the condition of having congenital missing teeth or a lack of teeth.

5. Enlargement of the cheek tissue is called _____.

6. A/an _____ is a tumor of the tooth or dental tissue.

7. An enlarged labial frenum may cause a space between teeth called a/an _____.

8. A/an _____ is an excision of the frenum and its periosteum.

9. A/n _____ is a collection of pus and infection.

10. Failure of the development of an organ or body part is called _____.

11. _____ is the treatment of the vital pulp to permit continued natural development.

12. The death of a tissue is termed _____.

13. A/an _____ is a growth in the lymphatic system.

14. A/an _____ matrix may be used in the child patient to isolate the tooth during restoration.

15. A band and loop or a distal shoe are types or methods for _____.

16. _____ is the congestion of blood within the pulp chamber.

17. A tooth that is forced away from the alveolus is said to be _____.

18. A full fracture of the crown involving all tissues is a Class _____ fracture.

19. A toothprint is an ID dental record made of the child's _____.

20. _____ anesthesia is a gel, ointment, or liquid used to obtain anesthesia prior to injection.

WORD USE

Read the following sentences and define the bold-faced words.

1. Upon clinical examination of the child patient, the doctor observed several unattended caries and a small **epulis** in the right maxillary anterior region.

   _____

2. The dental receptionist made an emergency appointment to provide treatment for the **avulsed** primary left maxillary central incisor.

3. The dental assistant noted that the next patient was scheduled for a partial **pulpotomy**.

4. The mother of the child who has just received an extraction of his primary molar was informed that a **space maintainer** would be necessary for the child's dental health.

5. Although the child was very young, some signs of **gingivitis** were present and home care instruction was given to the child and parent.

AUDIO LIST

This list contains selected new, important, or difficult terms from this chapter. You may use the list to review these terms and to practice pronouncing them correctly. When you work with the audio for this chapter, listen to the word, repeat it, and then place a checkmark in the box. Proceed to the next boxed word and repeat the process.

❑ amelogenesis imperfecta (ah-meal-oh-**JEN**-ih-sis im-purr-**FECK**-tah)
❑ ankylosed (**ANG**-kihl-lowzd)
❑ apexification (ay-pecks-ih-fih-**KAY**-shun)
❑ aplasia (ah-**PLAY**-zee-ah)
❑ candidiasis (kan-dih-**DYE**-ah-sis)
❑ cherubism (**CHAIR**-you-bizm)
❑ diastema (dye-ah-**STEE**-mah)
❑ enamoplasty (ee-**NAM**-oh-plas-tee)
❑ exfoliation (ecks-foh-lee-**AY**-shun)
❑ fissure (**FISH**-er)
❑ frenectomy (freh-**NECK**-toh-me)
❑ hyperdontia (high-per-**DAHN**-she-ah)
❑ hypodontia (high-poh-**DAHN**-she-ah)
❑ infraorbital (in-frah-**OR**-bih-tal)
❑ intraligamentary (in-trah-ligg-ah-**MEN**-tah-ree)

❑ intramuscular (in-tra-**MUSS**-kyou-lahr)
❑ intravenous (in-trah-**VEE**-nus)
❑ lymphangioma (lim-fan-jee-**OH**-mah)
❑ lymphoma (lim-**FOH**-mah)
❑ macrodontia (mack-roh-**DAHN**-she-ah)
❑ macroglossia (mack-roh-**GLOSS**-ee-ah)
❑ micrognathia (my-kroh-**NAY**-thee-ah)
❑ mucocele (**MYOU**-koh-seal)
❑ neurofibromatosis (new-roh-fie-broh-mah-**TOH**-sis)
❑ scorbutic (skor-**BYOU**-tick)
❑ subcutaneous (sub-kyou-**TAY**-nee-us)
❑ submucosal (sub-mew-**COH**-sul)
❑ supraperiosteal (soo-prah-pear-ee-**OSS**-tee-ahl)
❑ verruca vulgaris (ver-**OO**-kah vul-**GAIR**-iss)

Dental Laboratory Materials

Upon completion of this chapter, the reader should be able to identify and understand terms related to:

1. **Impression materials.** Identify the various kinds of rigid and elastic impression materials and give examples of each.

2. **Gypsum materials.** Discuss the various types of gypsum products used in dentistry and give examples of their uses.

3. **Wax materials.** Identify the various kinds of dental waxes and discuss a use for each type of wax.

4. **Dental polymer materials.** Explain the process of polymerization and the factors that alter or modify the chemical reaction, as well as the uses for the polymer materials.

5. **Precious and base metals.** Describe the difference between precious and other metals and state uses for the assorted types of gold.

6. **Abrasive and polishing materials.** Identify the common abrasives and polishing materials used in dentistry and the desired effect of each.

7. **Cement materials.** List the various types of dental cements and state the uses for each type.

8. **Characteristics of dental laboratory materials.** Discuss the descriptive or manipulative characteristics of various dental materials.

IMPRESSION MATERIALS

Dental laboratory procedures involve a variety of procedural steps and techniques and the use of many materials. These materials may be grouped into families according to composition or use. Each material exhibits its own particular characteristic, and one substance may differ from another even within its own grouping or family.

Knowledge of the general and specific use of a dental material is essential to successfully complete many laboratory procedures.

The assortment of materials needed to complete the various dental lab procedures is not limited to the lab area. Materials may be used alone, or they may be used in conjunction with the dental operatory.

Types of Impression Materials

Impression materials are substances that are used to take and record the shape, size, or position of teeth, appliances, and oral anatomy. These materials may be rigid, plastic, or elastic.

Rigid Impression Material. **Rigid impression material** is used where no teeth are present and flexibility is not needed or of concern. The two types of rigid impression material are:

1. **impression plaster** = gypsum product, 60 cc of water to 100 grams of plaster.
2. **metallic oxide paste** = two-paste system: zinc oxide eugenol (ZOE) base with resin accelerator. This paste hardens through chemical reaction.

Plastic Impression Material. **Plastic impression material** is used with or without the presence of teeth. This material is employed where some material flexibility is needed for the impression. The three types of plastic impression material are:

1. **thermoplastic** = material that softens when heated and hardens when cooled.
2. **compound** = supplied in sheets or stick form. The material is composed of thermoplastic resin base with filers and plasticizers. It softens when heated and returns to a solid when cool.
3. **wax** = used for registration of bites or for impression of single tooth area.

Elastic Impression Materials. **Elastic impression materials** are used where teeth are present and material must be flexible for removal from the oral cavity or teeth. Elastic impression materials are either reversible or irreversible hydrocolloids.

reversible hydrocolloid: impression material that can change repeatedly from gel to solid states depending upon the thermal condition of the substance.

> **gel state** = the material is soft and pliable.
> **solid state** = the material has "set" or is rigid enough to hold the form.

irreversible hydrocolloid: agar impression material that can be changed from gel to solid state as a result of a chemical reaction, and remain in that condition after mixing and using, such as alginate powder or premixed packages that are supplied in regular or fast-set, tinted, and flavored.

Elastomeric Impression Materials. **Elastomeric impression materials** are used to make impressions of preparations and for demanding or accurate reproductions.

These substances are composed of a base and an accelerator, or a **catalyst** (**CAT**-ah-list = *substance that speeds up the chemical reaction*).

polysulfide: impression substance available in light, regular, or heavy-bodied **viscosity** (thickness or tendency to flow). Also known as mercaptan, this material will harden or set by means of chemical action.

polyether: supplied in regular viscosity, with a thinner **modifier** (**MAH**-dih-fye-er = *material to change conditions*) for reduced thickness.

vinyl polysiloxane: impression material supplied in tubes, putty, paste-to-paste system and cartridge styles. The material may be heavy, medium, or wash viscosity

silicone: supplied as a base putty with liquid accelerator drops (condensation silicone type) or as a two-paste system (addition silicone type).

Uses of Impression Materials

Impression material can be measured, mixed, and placed in a tray or syringe for use in the mouth, or it can be delivered to the preparation site by the use of an **extruder gun**, a device that contains two independent materials to be forced into a common tip, mixed, and dispensed as one material. This device eliminates measuring, mixing, and cleanup time, see Figure 18-1.

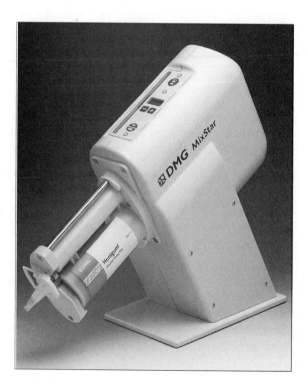

FIGURE 18-1
Example of a hands-free mix and dispense machine for impression materials. (Courtesy of Zenith DMG)

GYPSUM MATERIALS

Gypsum products generally are obtained from the same rock or ore source—calcium sulfate. The **calcination** process of preparing and handling of the gypsum material is what determines the final classification and purpose of a gypsum product.

Types of Gypsum

The five types of gypsum are:

Type I plaster—impression: used to take impression but not popular because of its weakness and replacement by better impression materials.

Type II plaster—model: also known as *plaster of Paris*, used mostly for impression and study models. Prepared by dehydrating calcium sulfate at atmospheric pressure to beta-hemihydrate form.

Type III—dental stone: white or buff-colored, Class I stone, used for orthodontic, diagnostic, and working casts. Prepared by dehydrating gypsum under pressure for alpha-hemihydrate form.

Type IV—improved or die stone: stronger Class II stone used for dental dies and casts. It is dehydrated in a solution of calcium chloride to obtain a modified alpha-hemi-hydrate form, also known as densite.

Type V—casting investment: gypsum-bonded material that can withstand extreme heat; used for casts of a prosthesis.

Other casting substances include phosphate and silica bonded investment materials.

Use of Gypsum Materials

Gypsum products have a variety of uses in the dental office and the laboratory setting in the construction and fabrication of dental prostheses.

model and cast: used for a positive reproduction of the mouth and oral conditions. The gypsum model, called a diagnostic cast or study model, consists of an art portion (base) and an anatomical (tooth) portion (see Figure 18-2). Study

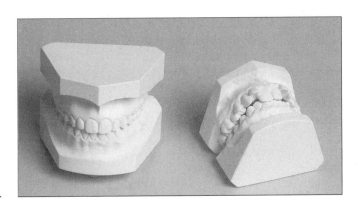

FIGURE 18-2
Study models.

models can be used as patterns for construction, legal records, and examples of before-and-after treatment, as well as planning and preparation.

die: reproduction of prepared tooth; usually Class II stone poured into an impression of the preparation. Dies can be **electroplated** (ee-**LECK**-troh-play-ted = *thin metal covering thru electrolysis*) with copper, silver, amalgam, or low-fusing metals for a stronger surface and working area.

WAX MATERIALS

Wax is supplied in sheet, stick, rope, shaped, and block forms for use in various dental procedures. Figure 18-3 gives examples of dental waxes. They include both synthetic and natural products from animal, mineral, and vegetable sources. The combination of material and the manufacturing process determines the ability of the wax to complete its designed purposes.

inlay wax: hard wax; blue, purple, green, or ivory colors; available in 3- to 4-inch sticks. Type I is for direct oral use; Type II is for laboratory or indirect use for inlay, crown, and casting patterns.

baseplate wax: supplied in 3″ × 6″ inch sheets, pink in color and soft, medium, or hard; used for denture construction, bite registration, and prosthesis construction.

casting wax: available in square sheets of various thicknesses; colors denote its softening point; used for construction of patterns for cast partial dentures.

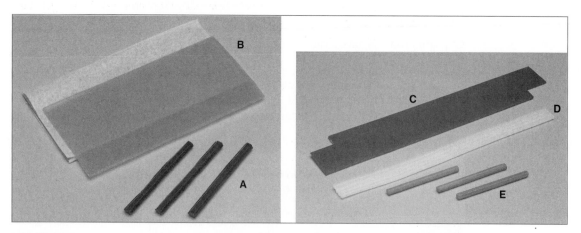

FIGURE 18-3
Examples of dental waxes. (A) Inlay Wax; (B) Base Plate Wax; (C) Boxing Wax; (D) Utility Wax; (E) Sticky Wax.

boxing wax: supplied in 1½″ width × 12″ length × 1/8″ thick strips; used to box or wrap around an impression prior to pouring. The strips hold the plaster or stone in place to form the art base of a study model.

utility wax: soft, adhesive wax, supplied in stick or sheet; used to mount casts and to adapt or modify impression tray edges; also called rope wax.

sticky wax: hard, brittle wax stick that is melted to hold dental units together.

disclosing wax: also known as pressure indicator paste; painted on an appliance, inserted into the mouth, and pressure applied to indicate high, sore, or tender areas.

DENTAL POLYMER MATERIALS

Dental polymers, known as a synthetic resin or **acrylic**, are the result of a chemical union of **monomer** and **polymer** substances. The chemical union of these chains is called **polymerization**, also know as *curing*. Among the substances included in the polymerization process are the following.

filler: inert substance added to the polymer to alter or modify the polymer properties.

initiator (ih-**NISH**-ee-ay-tore = *agent capable of starting polymerization process*): may be light, heat, radiation, or chemicals.

activator: reacts with initiator to start polymerization.

inhibitor (in-**HIB**-bih-tore = *substance that prevents polymerization*): maintains storage life.

plasticizer (**PLAS**-tih-sigh-zer = *substance that causes a softening effect*): changes hard, brittle resin into a flexible, tough material.

composite: polymer matrix bonded to glass particles, used for dental restorations.

self-curing resins: autopolymerization materials that perform the uniting process by means of a chemical union; the activator is present in the polymer powder or base and does not have to be added.

Some of the more common polymers used in dentistry are for denture bases, denture liners and repairs, denture teeth, custom impression trays, orthodontic and dental appliances, mouthguards, tooth-bleaching trays, metal-casting veneers, pit and fissure sealants, and tooth restorations. Artificial teeth used in dentures and appliances may be acrylic (resin) or may be porcelain (ceramic).

PRECIOUS AND BASE METALS

Many different metals are used in dental procedures. Some are used in their pure state, and others in combinations with other metals. A combination of metals is called an **alloy** (**AL**-oy). Combinations of two metals are **binary** (**BYE**-nar-ee); three metals are **ternary** (**TURN**-ah-ree); four metals are **quaternary** (**KWAH**-ter-nare-ee); and five different metals make up a **quinary** (**KWIN**-ar-ee) alloy.

TABLE 18-1   Types of Gold Casting Alloy

TYPE	CONSISTENCY	USE
Type I (A)	Soft	Used for simple, one surface inlays
Type II (B)	Medium	Preferred for inlay and onlay use
Type III (C)	Hard	Used for crowns and bridgework
Type IV (D)	Extra-hard	Preferred for partial denture frames, saddles, and clasps

Metals are classified as precious metals or base metals. The precious or "noble" metals—gold, platinum, palladium, and silver—are used for crowns, bridges, and dental appliances.

Gold Alloy

Pure gold (24 carat) may be used for gold foil restorations, and gold alloys formed with other precious metals, copper, or zinc may be supplied in sheet, wrought, or solder forms. Gold alloys can be **tempered** (hardened) or **annealed** (softened). They can also be whitened by adding silver, platinum, or palladium. Gold alloy solder is used to join parts of dental appliances or for repairs. Gold castings are classified into the four types shown in Table 18-1.

Base Alloy

Base metal alloys consist of chromium, nickel, and cobalt. They are used in partial denture framework or as substitutes for gold alloy. Other metals include stainless steel for crowns, orthodontic materials, nickel chromium and cobalt-chromium for orthodontic wires.

▌ABRASIVE AND POLISHING MATERIALS

Finishing a dental prosthesis is a matter of smoothing and polishing. An abrasive material reduces or removes bumps, overhangs, and excesses but leaves behind scratches and surface cuts. A polishing agent reduces these scratches to an unnoticeable flat surface that reflects light.

The technician begins the procedure with an abrasive material and then changes to a polishing agent to produce a shining surface. Abrasive and polishing materials may be supplied as powder to form a paste or **slurry** (**SLUR**-ee = *thin, watery mixture*), or luted to paper or cloth into sheets. Abrasives can be impregnated into wheels and points, or supplied in solid bricks that may be rubbed on rag or brush wheels for use with the

TABLE 18-2 Common Abrasive and Polishing Agents

MATERIAL	SUPPLIED AS	AGENT	USE
aluminum oxide	mounted stone, slurry	abrasive/polish	acrylic resin
carborundum	stones, points, disc	abrasive	metal, resin, tooth
chalk	soft powder	polishing	gold, resins
chromium oxide	powder	polishing	stainless steel
cuttle	powder of fish shell	abrasive	gold alloys
diamond	particles of various sizes	abrasive	tooth structure
emery	particle or luted to cloth	abrasive	trim acrylic
garnet	stone, points	abrasive	resin, composite
pumice	powder, slurry	abrasive	metal, enamel, resin
quartz	grits, luted to paper, discs	abrasive	general use
rouge	powder, brick	polishing	gold, denture resin
tin oxide	powder, slurry	polishing	metals
tripoli	stone, brick	polishing	gold alloy
zirconium silicate	powder	polishing	enamel

dental lathe machine. Some common abrasive and polishing materials, supplied in various grits on strips, discs, wheels, bricks, and powders are listed in Table 18-2.

CEMENT MATERIALS

Dental cements are used to temporarily or permanently lute dental castings, crowns, and bridges in place. These same cements, in thicker viscosities, can be used as bases or as restoratives in operative dentistry. The most common luting cements used with the dental laboratory products are zinc phosphate, zinc-oxide eugenol, **polycarboxylate** (**pahl**-ee-kar-**BOX**-ih-late) and resin. The common cements used in dentistry are listed in Table 18-3.

CHARACTERISTICS OF DENTAL LABORATORY MATERIALS

When working with the various dental laboratory materials, one must be aware of and understand the descriptive or manipulative characteristics of strengths of each material.

bonding: force of the union of one substance with another substance.
coefficient of thermal expansion: amount of form change that takes place in a dental material and tooth during heat exposure in the oral cavity.

TABLE 18-3 Dental Cements or Luting Agents

MATERIAL	USE
zinc phosphate	Permanent luting of casting, orthodontic appliances. Type II is used as a base.
zinc-oxide eugenol (ZOE)	Temporary luting for castings, pulp capping, cavity liner, periodontal dressing, temporary restoration, insulating base, and wash.
ZOE and EBA (orthoethoxybenzoic acid)	Type II—permanent cement for inlays, onlays, crowns, and bridges.
polycarboxylate	Luting for castings, stainless steel crowns, orthodontic cement.
silicophosphate	Luting for orthodontic appliances.
resin (light and self-cure)	Luting for castings, porcelain restorations, Maryland bridge.
glass ionomer	Type I—cementation of metal castings, direct-bond ortho bands, and core buildup.
	Type II—for anterior restorative.

color: has three components:

> *hue* = color of object, red, green blue, etc.
> *chroma* = strength of specified hue.
> *value* = darkness or brightness of specified hue.

creep: tendency of amalgam to deform under constant applied pressure.

cure process: hardening of the material through auto- (chemical) or light-activated response.

ductility: ability of the material to withstand permanent deformation without fracturing under elongation stress.

elasticity: ability of a material to return to its original form when stress is removed.

exothermic (**ecks**-oh-**THER**-mick): chemical release of heat, as in zinc phosphate cement.

flow: slow bending or movement of material under its own weight.

galvanization: tendency of certain metals to produce an electrical charge when in contact with each other.

hardness: maximum amount of resistance before penetration or scratching can occur.

hydrophilic (high-droh-**FIL**-ick = *ability to attract and hold water*): absorption of water.

hydrophobia (high-droh-**FOH**-bee-ah = *fear of water*): giving off or shedding water.

hygroscopic (high-groh-**SKAH**-pick) **expansion:** submersion into, or the addition of, water to a material prior to initial set.

initial set: period of time when material assumes shape but remains pliable.

imbibition (**im**-bih-**BISH**-un = *absorption of fluid*): taking on of water.

malleability: ability to withstand deformation without fracture while undergoing maximum compression stress.

setting time: amount of time required for the material to become
will be.

tensile strength: maximum amount of pulling stress required to rupture the

thermal conductivity: capability of the material to transmit heat.

toughness: ability of the material to resist fracture.

trituration: mixing of mercury with other alloy material to form an amalgam.

working time: period during which a material can be molded, shaped, or manipulated
without any adverse effect on the material.

yield strength: maximum amount of stress a material can withstand without
deformation.

REVIEW EXERCISES

MATCHING

Match the following word elements with their meaning:

1. _____catalyst
2. _____plasticizer
3. _____Type IV metal
4. _____filler
5. _____noble metal
6. _____boxing wax
7. _____Type IV gypsum
8. _____bonding
9. _____ternary alloy
10. _____slurry
11. _____reversible hydrocolloid
12. _____acrylic
13. _____inhibitor
14. _____modifier
15. _____die

a. inert substance added to alter properties
b. gypsum reproduction of a prepared tooth
c. substance that changes material's action
d. strip to encircle impression tray prior to pour-up
e. synthetic resin
f. mixture of three metals
g. extra-hard gold alloy
h. substance to prevent polymerization, helps storage
i. watery mix
j. elastic impression material
k. platinum
l. union of one substance with another substance
m. improved stone
n. substance that causes softening effect
o. substance to speed up chemical reaction

DEFINITIONS

Using the selection given in each sentence, choose the best term to complete the definition.

1. Which of the following is not considered a precious or noble metal?
   a. amalgam   b. gold
   c. platinum   d. silver

2. A dark blue wax used to make wax patterns for cast restorations is:
   a. baseplate wax b. boxing wax
   c. inlay wax   d. sticky wax

3. A hard, brittle stick wax that is melted to hold together dental items is:
   a. baseplate wax b. boxing wax
   c. inlay wax   d. sticky wax

4. A pink sheet wax that is used for denture construction of the gingival area is:
   a. baseplate wax b. boxing wax
   c. inlay wax   d. sticky wax

5. An inert substance added to the polymer to alter or modify the polymer's properties is a/an:
   a. composite   b. filler
   c. plasticizer   d. inhibitor

). Which type of gold alloy is preferred for use in crown and bridgework?
   a. Type I   b. Type II
   c. Type III   d. Type IV

7. Which of the following is not considered a rigid impression material?
   a. gypsum   b. amalgam
   c. compound   d. metallic oxide

8. Gypsum products may be used for all of the following uses except:
   a. restorations   b. impressions
   c. study models   d. investment

9. Which wax is supplied in strips and placed around the impression tray prior to pouring?
   a. boxing   b. casting
   c. inlay   d. sticky

10. Which class of stone is classified as improved stone and used to make dies?
   a. Class I   b. Class II
   c. Class III   d. Class IV

11. The period of time when material assumes shape but remains pliable is called:
   a. working time   b. initial set
   c. setting time   d. form time

12. A material that softens when heated and hardens when cooled is said to be:
   a. exothermic   b. intrusive
   c. rigid   d. thermoplastic

13. A substance composed of two or more different substances is called a/an:
   a. union   b. compound
   c. hydrogrosic   d. elastic

14. Which of these impression materials should be used intraorally when teeth are present?
   a. compound
   b. hydrocolloid
   c. metallic oxide
   d. gypsum

15. In a comparison of two materials, the one with a heavier viscosity would be:
   a. thicker
   b. less stable
   c. same thickness
   d. thinner

16. A substance used to take and record the shape, size, or position of items is an:
   a. implant
   b. investment
   c. inlay
   d. impression

17. How many carats are in the precious metal pure gold?
   a. 10   b. 12
   c. 20   d. 24

18. Chromium, nickel, and cobalt are considered which type of metal:
   a. base
   b. noble
   c. thermoplastic
   d. elastic

19. Which of the following finishing agents is considered an abrasive agent?
   a. chromium oxide
   b. chalk
   c. carborundum
   d. tin oxide

20. Trituration is another term for which process?
   a. heating   b. polymerization
   c. amalgamation   d. curing

BUILDING SKILLS

Locate and define the prefix, root/combining form, and suffix (if present) in the following words.

1. **thermoplastic**
   prefix   _____
   root/combining form _____
   suffix   _____

2. **exothermic**
   prefix   _____
   root/combining form _____
   suffix   _____

3. **imbibition**
   prefix   _____
   root/combining form _____
   suffix   _____

4. **malleability**

   prefix _____

   root/combining form _____

   suffix _____

5. **hydrophobia**

   prefix _____

   root/combining form _____

   suffix _____

FILL-INS

Write the correct word in the blank space to complete each statement.

1. The mixing of mercury with other metal alloys is a/an _____.

2. A thin, watery mixture of an abrasive material is a/an _____.

3. A mixture of five different metals is a/an _____alloy.

4. A/An _____is added to resin material to cause a softening effect.

5. A/An _____is a reproduction of a prepared tooth for crown or bridgework.

6. The time period when it is possible to mold, shape, or manipulate a material without an adverse effect upon the material is called _____time.

7. A/An _____is a substance that speeds up chemical reactions.

8. Model plaster is also known as _____of _____.

9. A die with a thin metal covering obtained through electrolysis has been completed in a/an _____process.

10. A polymer matrix bonded to glass particles is a/an _____.

11. A/An _____is a substance that reacts with an initiator to start polymerization.

12. A combination of two metal powders is a/an _____alloy.

13. _____ is the maximum amount of stress a material can withstand without deformation.

14. The forced union of one substance with another substance is _____.

15. Tin oxide, chalk, rouge, and tripoli are examples of a/an _____agent.

16. _____ is the maximum amount of pulling stress required to rupture a material.

17. _____is a fear of water or shedding of water.

18. The polishing agent, rouge, is used to obtain a shine on denture resin or _____.

19. _____wax may be used for constructing patterns for partial dentures.

20. The maximum amount of stress after which metal will return to the original form when stress is removed is termed _____ _____.

WORD USE

Read the following sentences and define the bold-faced words.

1. The dental technician warned the trainee to be careful of the **exothermic** chemical reaction that occurs with the cement material.

   _____

2. When discussing the crown procedure with the patient, the dentist advised Mrs. Jones of the advantages and disadvantages of base metals versus **precious metals**.

   _____

3. The dental assistant noted that the **setting time** of the new cement was different from the former brand of cement used in the office.

   _____

4. The dentist requested the assistant to pour up the **die** impression with Class II improved stone.

   _____

5. The technician noted that using some plaster **slurry** in the mix will hasten the setting time.

   _____

AUDIO LIST

This list contains selected new, important, or difficult terms from this chapter. You may use the list to review these terms and to practice pronouncing them correctly. When you work with the audio for this chapter, listen to the word, repeat it, and then place a checkmark in the box. Proceed to the next boxed word and repeat the process.

❑ alloy (**AL**-loy)
❑ binary (**BYE**-nar-ee)
❑ catalyst (**CAT**-ah-list)
❑ electroplated (ee-**LECK**-troh-play-ted)
❑ exothermic (ecks-oh-**THER**-mick)
❑ hydrophilic (high-droh-**FIL**-ick)
❑ hydrophobia (high-droh-**FOH**-bee-ah)
❑ hygroscopic (high-groh-**SKAH**-pick)
❑ inhibitor (in-**HIB**-ih-tore)

❑ initiater (ih-**NISH**-ee-ay-tore)
❑ modifier (**MAH**-dih-fye-er)
❑ plasticizer (**PLAS**-tih-sigh-zer)
❑ polycarboxylate (pahl-ee-kar-**BOX**-ih-late)
❑ quaternary (**KWAH**-ter-nare-ee)
❑ quinary (**KWIN**-ar-ee)
❑ slurry (**SLUR**-ee)
❑ ternary (**TURN**-ah-ree)

CHAPTER 19

Dental Laboratory Procedures

Upon completion of this chapter, the reader should be able to identify and understand terms related to:

1. **Range and scope of the dental laboratory.** Identify the professional personnel related to the construction of dental prostheses or appliances made in the lab setting.

2. **Dental laboratory equipment.** List and identify the assorted machinery and equipment necessary for laboratory procedures.

3. **Denture construction laboratory procedures.** Describe the divisions of prostodontia into fixed or removable sections and the major differences between these areas.

4. **Removable partial denture construction laboratory procedures.** List and describe the assorted appliances that may be included in the partial reconstruction of the oral cavity and dental care.

5. **Fixed prosthodontic dental laboratory procedures.** List and describe the major fixed prosthodontic items and the variety of crowns and bridgework available.

6. **Miscellaneous dental laboratory procedures.** Discuss the miscellaneous assortment of dental appliances and items used to protect, maintain, or correct dental care.

RANGE AND SCOPE OF THE DENTAL LABORATORY

A dental laboratory is the area where laboratory procedures necessary to complete dental health care are accomplished. The laboratory can be located in an independent building or in a specified area of a dental office facility. The dentist or prosthodontist may perform the dental laboratory work or it may be assigned to others. A dental laboratory technician is trained in this type of work through formal schooling or on-the-job experience. A denturist fabricates dentures and is legalized by the state dental boards in some states. A ceramist (sir-**AM**-ist = *an expert in ceramics*) specializes in porcelain crowns and restorations.

All dental laboratory work, when not completed specifically by the dentist, must follow prescription orders from the practicing dentist. This **work order** is attached to each case sent to the lab. The amount of time required by the laboratory to complete the prescription, termed the **working days**, is included in the appointment setup.

DENTAL LABORATORY EQUIPMENT

Various items and equipment are necessary in the dental laboratory to complete the required construction and fabrication procedures.

articulator (ar-**TICK**-you-lay-tore = *device to imitate joint action*): a machine that imitates the movement of the mandible and TMJ on mounted models. Constructed models of the patient's mouth are arranged in the patient's "bite pattern" or articulation. Figure 19-1 shows gypsum models with a denture setup, which is placed on an articulator that imitates the opening and closing of the patient's jaws.

model trimmer: grinding device used to trim or remove excess gypsum on diagnostic casts for placement on articulators or for models that may be used as visual records of mouth conditions for patient education and treatment planning.

gypsum mixing machine: device used for mixing gypsum products; the machine also has a vacuum process to eliminate air bubbles in the mixture.

vibrator: small table model appliance with a platform to hold bowls of freshly mixed gypsum to gently shake or vibrate air bubbles to the top of the mixture.

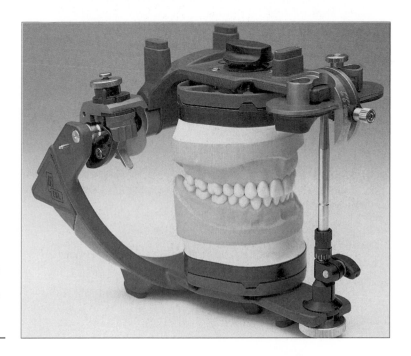

FIGURE 19-1
Gypsum models with denture setup mounted on an articular. (Courtesy of Kavo Dental Corporation)

furnace: heating device with high temperature range (up to 2,000 degrees); used to melt out the wax patterns from the investment materials.

waxing unit: heater unit to melt and hold lab wax (140–210 degrees) in a liquid state for use in procedures.

oven: hot air heat devices to prepare materials 200 to 900 degrees F (100 to 480 C).

bath: hot oil, or water–heat device to prepare materials to 350 degrees F (200 degrees C) temperature.

hydrocolloid conditioning machine: heating device that uses water to condition and prepare reversible hydrocolloid material for impressions. The machine has three compartments for graduated heated water baths.

burner: heating device to externally heat object not contained within it; e.g., Bunsen burner or micro torch used to heat wax for carving or sheets of baseplate wax for models.

vacuum former (press): device used to heat acrylic sheets and vacuum pressure them to a prepared form for construction of a custom impression tray, mouthguard, surgical template, or tooth-bleaching trays. The vacuum press in Figure 19-2 contours the acrylic sheet to the model form.

electroplating unit: electrical device used to apply alloy materials to surface objects, such as dies.

blowtorch: heating device using compressed gas or chemical fuel to melt alloys for casting.

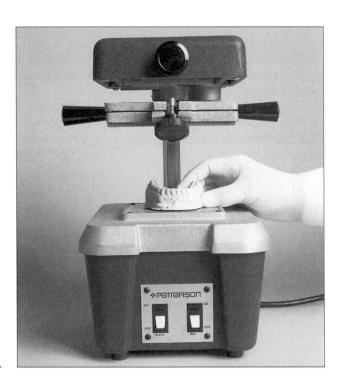

FIGURE 19-2
Vacuum press.

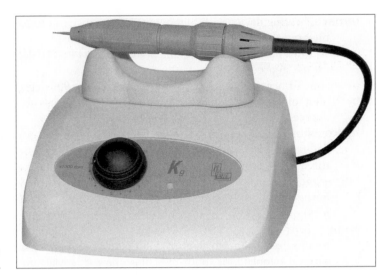

FIGURE 19-3
Example of a tabletop lab handpiece. (Courtesy of Kavo Dental Corporation)

casting machine: centrifugal spin device used to force melted alloy into an investment ring.

curing unit: device used to cure or complete the polymerization process of acrylics; may use pressurized heat or a light-curing unit for bonding materials and substances.

sandblasting machine: air abrasion machine that forces abrasive material (sand) to polish and clean items.

lathe: electrical motor that rotates attached appliances for sanding, smoothing, and shaping of materials.

splash pan: receptacle with high back that is inserted under lathe wheel ends; the pan captures and contains the splash from the attachments and helps to maintain a clean area.

dust collector: suction-powered unit to remove gypsum and acrylic dust from the lab area.

plating unit: machine to electroplate gold veneers, precious and semi-precious metals.

electric motors and **handpieces:** benchtop units providing selective handpiece power for lab operations. Figure 19-3 shows a tabletop lab handpiece used for laboratory grinding and adjusting procedures.

welder/solder machine: electric unit used to weld orthodontic bands or general soldering.

DENTURE CONSTRUCTION LABORATORY PROCEDURES

Each dental laboratory procedure, whether performed in the dental office or in a commercial lab, has terminology related to the fabrication of specific items. Some terms are more general, and others are specific to a procedure. Common terms related to denture construction procedures are *denture* and *prosthesis*. A **denture** set is a replacement for a body part, also known as a prosthesis.

Types of Dentures

An assortment of denture types accommodates all the reconstructive reasons for tooth replacement.

full-mouth denture set: a complete replacement for the maxillary and mandibular arches; composed of two trays—the maxiallary denture plate and the mandibular plate.

single denture: a denture replacement for one arch, maxillary or mandibular.

immediate denture: a denture that is placed in the mouth at the time the natural teeth are surgically removed. After removal of the teeth and an alveolectomy to prepare the bone, the tissues are sutured and the denture is inserted into place.

overdenture: acrylic denture prepared to fit on the bony ridge and gingiva while attached to the remaining teeth or implants.

Denture Construction

Specialized terms are used to describe the materials and process of fabricating a set of dentures.

denture base: pink acrylic part of the denture that fits over and covers the alveolar ridge (gum).

denture teeth: artificial teeth used in denture construction; may be porcelain or acrylic material and supplied on anterior or posterior "cards," differing in shape, color, and material (see Figure 19-4).

denture flange: extension of denture over the posterior anatomy present; it is used for stabilization.

denture post dam: suction seal of denture that extends side to side from the rear of the denture.

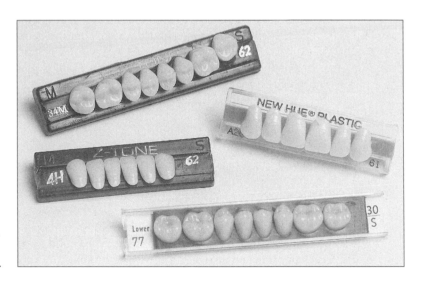

FIGURE 19-4
Denture teeth on anterior or posterior "cards."

impression tray: may be custom-made or purchased commercially as plain or perforated full arch (upper and lower), quadrant (right and left), or anterior (universal) in metal or plastic material. The trays are used to hold material for the impression procedure.

spacer: material, usually baseplate wax, that is placed on the model or cast surface to allow a space for the impression material.

stop: indents or holes cut out of the spacer in the tray to prevent the tray from being placed too deeply.

adhesive: sticky liquid that is painted or sprayed on the surface of the impression tray to help retain the impression material in the tray.

molding: finger shaping of the impression material over the edge of the tray for better adaptation; also called **muscle trimming**.

wax setup: sample prosthesis used to fit, adjust, and test jaw relationship of the wax denture. Made of baseplate wax, shellac, or thermoplastic material formed and constructed on a model of the patient's mouth. The baseplate will become a pattern for the denture base.

occlusal rims: wax block placed upon baseplate over the residual ridge of plate; the rims are used for placement of denture teeth while mounted upon the articulator.

festooning: melting, shaping, and forming of the wax rims to simulate functional and esthetic gingival tissue.

Wax Try-In Procedures

After construction of the wax denture with the positioned denture teeth, the patient returns to the dentist for a try-in appointment. This visit is to determine the proper seating and articulation of the dentures, and the correct alignment of the denture teeth. The dentist will observe and examine a number of things during this visit.

centric relationship: the most retruded, unstrained position in the mandibular condyle in the glenoid fossa, commonly stated as "biting on the posterior teeth."

retrusion (ree-**TRUE**-zhun): position of the mandible as far posterior as possible while in occlusion.

protrusion (pro-**TRUE**-shun): position of the mandible as far anterior as possible while in occlusion.

lateral excursion: sliding position of the mandible from side to side while in occlusion.

vertical dimension: space height of the denture teeth while in occlusion.

smile line: amount of denture tooth space that is viewed while the patient is smiling.

cuspid eminence: vertical length or height of the denture cuspid placement.

Laboratory Construction

Following the wax try-in, the technician invests the setup in a flask and removes the wax by boiling. A separating medium such as tinfoil solution is applied to the mold, the original denture teeth are replaced, and an acrylic is mixed, placed into the flask, and cured. When cured, the acrylic denture with the teeth is removed, cleaned, polished, and returned to the dentist.

REMOVABLE PARTIAL DENTURE CONSTRUCTION LABORATORY PROCEDURES

A dental prosthesis that replaces one or more teeth is a **partial appliance**. When it is fixed or cemented in the mouth it usually is called **crown and bridgework**. When the patient is able to remove the prosthesis at will, it is known as a **removable partial denture**. A **bilateral** partial denture replaces the teeth and structures on both sides of the arch, whereas a **unilateral** partial denture replaces teeth and structure on only one side. Although construction of the partial denture resembles that of the complete denture, the partial has more components. Some of these components are illustrated in Figure 12-2, Chapter 12, Prosthodontics.

framework: the skeleton of the partial to which acrylic material and artificial teeth will be applied.

abutment: the remaining natural tooth or implanted device that supports and stabilizes the prosthesis.

connector: metal framework that unites the left and right sides of the partial appliance. Major connectors may be in the form of a bar, plate, or strap. A connector is termed **palatal** in the maxillary prosthesis and **lingual** in the mandibular prosthesis. Minor connectors may unite the framework with the saddles.

saddle: mesh extension of the framework that rests upon the alveolar ridge; the mesh will be covered with pink acrylic material to resemble oral tissue.

stress breaker: a device placed in stress-bearing areas to assist with occlusal forces.

retainer: a clasp or removable partial denture attachment that is applied to an abutment tooth to provide retention; may be clasp-type or an intracoronal retainer and fabricated as a cast, wrought-wire, or combination of the two. The two styles of clasps are:

1. **bar:** originates at the prosthesis base or connector border and extends upward toward the tooth undercut.
2. **circumferential** (ser-**kum**-fer-**EN**-shal = *around*): a clasp that encircles a tooth more than 180 degrees with one terminal end in the undercut of the tooth crown.

rest: metal projector or clasp extension that fits into the prepared area or restoration of the abutting tooth. Rests supply support and stabilization and are described according to their surface position, such as occlusal rests or lingual rests.

FIXED PROSTHODONTIC DENTAL LABORATORY PROCEDURES

A dental prosthesis that is prepared and cemented into or onto the teeth is called a fixed prosthesis. Examples of fixed prostheses are inlays, onlays, veneers, various crowns, and fixed bridges. These prostheses are cast and prepared in the dental laboratory from impressions or patterns supplied by the dentist. Some common terms and illustrations used to describe fixed prosthodontic items were introduced in Chapter 12, Prosthodontics.

inlay: cast restoration that sits inside of the tooth cusps and is constructed to fit in the tooth preparation of the proximal walls and a portion of the occlusal surface.

onlay: cast restoration that covers one or more of the tooth cusps and is constructed to fit the tooth preparation of the proximal walls and most or all of the occlusal surface.

three-quarter crown: cast restoration that is applied to a tooth prepared on all surfaces except the facial surface.

full crown: cast restoration that covers the entire visible, anatomical tooth.

porcelain fused to metal crown (PFM): full cast crown restoration that has a porcelain (ceramic) veneer applied to the prepared surfaces; PFM gives an esthetic, natural appearance to the metal casting.

veneer: a thin, tooth-colored shell that is applied to the prepared facial surface of a tooth.

porcelain jacket crown (PJC): thin metal and ceramic veneered crown for an anterior tooth.

post and core crown (PCC): crown for use in an endodontically treated tooth with significant loss of tooth structure. The crown has an internal post to fit into the pulp chamber and the prepared core to give full coverage and strength.

temporary crown: acrylic, aluminum, or composite crown constructed and provisionally cemented on for protection while construction of the permanent crown is completed.

fixed bridge: prosthesis that replaces one or more missing teeth; usually involves adjoining teeth (abutment) to space, and therefore is termed *crown and bridge prosthesis.*

cantilever (KAN-tih-lee-ver) bridge: prosthesis in which only one side of the device is attached to the retainer or abutment tooth.

Maryland bridge: conservative, prepared resin-retained prosthesis using a bonding procedure to hold to adjacent teeth: may be used in either anterior or posterior area.

Prosthesis Fabrication

Fabrication of the dental prosthesis is completed in the dental laboratory. The construction process of these dental devices also has specialized terminology.

occlusal records: measurements of jaw relationships and articulation of teeth; measurements are obtained with impressions and/or articulation devices.

facebow: measurement device used to record the occlusal position (see Figure 19-5). A waxed-lined bitefork is placed in the mouth for a bite registration, and calipers from the facebow are inserted into the patient's ears for axis relation. The nosepiece is placed on the nasal bridge and noted. After the device is removed, all measurements are repeated on the articulator to simulate the patient's occlusal record.

die: exact stone replica of the tooth preparation that is receiving the prosthesis; usually made of dental stone and may be electroplated for extra strength.

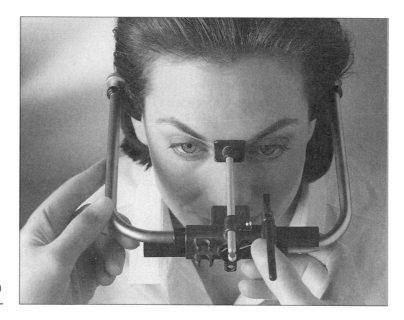

FIGURE 19-5
Facebow for recording measurements. (Courtesy of Kavo Dental Corporation)

FIGURE 19-6
Preparation of a gold inlay:
(A) wax pattern with sprue pin attached;
(B) sprue pin inserted into sprue base while investment material is being poured;
(C) pattern in inverted inlay casting ring after wax pattern has been melted away;
(D) casted gold inlay in casting ring before removing and polishing;
(E) completed gold inlay in the prepared tooth.

dowel **(DOWL) pin:** tapered brass post that is placed into the die when the stone is poured; used as handle of the die during waxing and carving of the pattern.

wax pattern: exact wax replica of the prosthesis to be completed; prepared by melting wax upon the die and carving it to proportion. The pattern is invested (encased) in a gypsum product, then melted out to leave a form or shape for the casting of the alloy reproduction (see Figure 19-6A).

separating medium: material placed upon the die before the wax is melted onto it to enable separation when completed. A thicker medium may be applied to provide **die relief,** a space in the prosthesis to accommodate the cement process.

sprue (SPROO) pin: a small, plastic pin or wax channel area attached to a wax pattern to provide space in the investment for the entry of melted metal in the casting procedure (see Figure 19-6B).

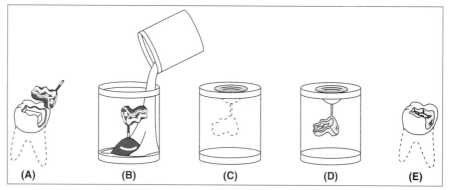

(A)   (B)   (C)   (D)   (E)

sprue base: a brass disc with rounded, pyramid top. It is used to hold the sprue pin that is attached to a wax pattern. The base receives the bottom of the casting ring and, when all assembled, it is filled with investment material, (see Figure 19-6B).

casting ring: small ring, 1-⅜″ by 1-¼″, that is used to hold the invested pattern during the investing of the gypsum material and the casting of the melted metal (see Figure 19-6B, C, and D).

liner: ring-lining material placed inside casting ring to allow for the investment expansion.

investment: gypsum, silica, and reducing agent material prepared to maintain the shape of the wax pattern during casting; may be mixed and placed into the ring with a vacuum machine or by hand.

wax elimination: burning or heating out of wax pattern from hardened investment material, leaving a void in the shape of the wax pattern. Wax elimination is completed in the lab furnace.

casting: procedure in which melted alloy is forced centrifugally from the crucible into the casting ring to fill the void in the shape of melted-out wax pattern. It is completed with a casting machine, either electrically heated and forced, or by manually melting the alloy and force-casting or throwing through a spring-action release.

blowtorch: compressed air heating device to melt the alloy for casting; produces a flame with four heating zones exiting from the nozzle.

Zone 1: junction area when gases meet; unproductive.
Zone 2: combustion area, oxidizing, slightly green; not to be used.
Zone 3: reducing area, bluish, hottest part of flame; the desirable use zone.
Zone 4: oxidizing area, where flame meets air; coolest part of the flame.

pickling solution: solution used to remove surface film from the cast restoration.

Finishing and Polishing Procedures

The finishing and polishing procedure refines the cast restoration. It may be completed with a sandblasting device or by using handpiece drills and bits along with polishing material and rag wheels on a dental lathe. The completed casting may be returned to the dentist for permanent cementation or used in a fixed appliance with other pieces.

Uniting Prothesis Units. After the construction of each independent part or unit of the appliance is complete, the units are united to form one piece of bridgework. The process of uniting parts or units together to form a single prosthesis has special terms associated with it.

soldering: joining of two metals by the fusion of an intermediate alloy that may be silver or gold.

flux (FLUKS = *flow*): an agent used to protect the alloy from oxidation during the heating process; may be a powder with a low fusing melting point that forms a molten state over the area to be soldered.

anti-flux: material, usually graphite, that is applied to retard the forward advance of the melted solder.

welding: the direct joining of two metals by a fusion process.

porcelain fused to metal: a process of bonding porcelain material to a metal sub-base, then firing it to hardness.

▌ MISCELLANEOUS DENTAL LABORATORY PROCEDURES

Besides the construction of dentures, castings, and prostheses, the dental technician may perform other procedures, such as denture reline, repair of dentures, denture duplications, replacement of broken teeth in dentures, fabrication of mouth guards, bleaching trays, biteplanes, orthodontic retainers and appliances, study models, and basic laboratory services required by the dental profession. Some dental laboratories perform all services, and others limit their services to specified procedures or materials.

▌ REVIEW EXERCISES

MATCHING

Match the following word elements with their meanings

1. _____ smile line

2. _____ adhesive

3. _____ PJC

4. _____ facebow

5. _____ flux

6. _____ liner

7. _____ casting ring

a. machine that imitates jaw and TMJ movements

b. denture placed in mouth at time of extraction surgery

c. sticky material applied to trays to hold impression

d. amount of tooth space viewed while patient is smiling

e. restoration for proximal and most of occlusal surfaces

f. thin metal and ceramic veneered crown for anterior

g. measurement device to take and record occlusal positions

8. _____ onlay

9. _____ wax pattern

10. _____ PFM

11. _____ immediate denture

12. _____ separating medium

13. _____ overdentures

14. _____ occlusal rims

15. _____ articulator

h. attached denture that is seated on bony ridge and gingiva

i. exact reproduction of prosthesis to be constructed

j. ring lining material to allow for casting expansion

k. ring used to hold investment pattern for prosthesis

l. material used to prevent oxidation of alloy during heating

m. ceramic material fused to metal process

n. material placed upon die surface prior to placement of wax

o. wax block placed upon baseplate to hold denture teeth

DEFINITIONS

Using the selection given for each sentence, choose the best term to complete the definition.

1. The stabilizing extension of the denture that extends over the present posterior anatomy is the:
   a. spacer
   b. flange
   c. base
   d. liner

2. The process of melting, shaping, and forming of the wax rims is called:
   a. pickling
   b. soldering
   c. welding
   d. festooning

3. The space height of the teeth while in occlusion is the:
   a. vertical dimension
   b. centric relationship
   c. retrusive aim
   d. protrusive aim

4. A grinding device used to shape diagnostic casts or study models is a:
   a. dental lathe
   b. vacuum press
   c. model trimmer
   d. casting machine

5. A full arch dental prosthesis that replaces the dentition is a/an:
   a. jacket crown
   b. denture
   c. implant
   d. full crown

6. The direct joining of two metals by a fusion heat process is called:
   a. vacuum pressing
   b. pickling
   c. soldering
   d. welding

7. The joining of two metals by the fusion of an intermediate or joining alloy is termed:
   a. vacuum pressing
   b. pickling
   c. soldering
   d. welding

8. A material, usually graphite, used to retard the advance of melted solder is:
   a. gold
   b. silver
   c. anti-flux
   d. flux

9. A process to fuse ceramic material to a metal subbase is called:
   a. PMF
   b. PJC
   c. PCM
   d. PFM

10. A solution used to remove surface film from a cast restoration is:
    a. pickling
    b. varnish
    c. liner
    d. acid etchant

11. A brass disk with elevated center to hold a sprued wax pattern for casting is a:
    a. casting ring
    b. sprue base
    c. sprue pin
    d. dowel

12. A cemented prosthesis that replaces one or more missing teeth, usually involving other abutting teeth is a:
    a. Maryland bridge
    b. cantilever bridge
    c. full crown
    d. fixed bridge

13. A conservative resin retained prosthesis for a small area with a missing tooth is a:
    a. Maryland bridge
    b. cantilever bridge
    c. full crown
    d. fixed bridge

14. A cast restoration applied to a tooth prepared on all surfaces except the facial view is a:
    a. porcelain jacket crown
    b. full crown
    c. three-quarter crown
    d. post and core crown

15. A crown used for an endodontically treated tooth with significant surface loss is a:
    a. porcelain jacket crown
    b. full crown
    c. three-quarter crown
    d. post and core crown

16. The position of the mandible as far anterior as possible while in occlusion is called:
    a. lateral excrusion
    b. cuspid eminence
    c. retrusion
    d. protrusion

17. The position of the mandible as far posterior as possible while in occlusion is termed:
    a. lateral excrusion
    b. cuspid eminence
    c. retrusion
    d. protrusion

18. The side-to-side sliding position of the mandible while in occlusion is called:
    a. lateral excrusion
    b. cuspid eminence
    c. extrusion
    d. protrusion

19. An indent or hole cut into the spacer to prevent the tray from being place too deeply is a:
    a. stop
    b. separator
    c. liner
    d. setup

20. Muscle trimming, the shaping of the impression material during the fabrication process is also called:
    a. casting
    b. molding
    c. festooning
    d. pickling

BUILDING SKILLS

Locate and define the prefix, root-combining form, and suffix (if present) in the following words:

1. **crematist**
   prefix   _____
   root/combining form   _____
   suffix   _____

2. **protrusion**
   prefix   _____
   root/combining form   _____
   suffix   _____

3. **denturist**
   prefix   _____
   root/combining form   _____
   suffix   _____

4. **festooning**
   prefix   _____
   root/combining form   _____
   suffix   _____

5. **excursion**
   prefix   _____
   root/combining form   _____
   suffix   _____

FILL-INS

Write the correct word in the blank space to complete each statement.

1. A/An _____is an air, water, or oil device used to heat prepared materials to 350 degrees F, or 200 degrees C.

2. The prescription to the laboratory to complete lab procedures is called a/an _____.

3. A/An_____ is a device placed in stress bearing area to assist with stress forces.

4. A metal projection or clasp extension that fits into prepared areas or restoration that is used for support or stabilization is a/an _____.

5. A/An _____ is a mesh extension of a prosthesis that rests upon the alveolar ridge.

6. The skeleton of a prosthesis is called the _____.

7. A/an _____is a thin, tooth-colored shell that is applied to the prepared facial surface of a tooth.

8. The remaining natural tooth or implanted device used to support a prosthesis is a/an _____.

9. A/an _____is an exact replica of a prepared tooth receiving a prosthesis.

10. A small pin attached to a wax pattern that permits the flow of molted metal in a casting is a/an _____pin.

11. A/an _____pin is a tapered brass post inserted into the die during the setup procedure.

12. The metal framework that unites the right and left sides of the prosthesis is called a/an_____.

13. _____ wax is supplied in thin sheets and used for construction of the denture base.

14. A blue stick wax used to make wax patterns is called _____ wax.

15. Wax blocks placed upon the baseplate wax and used to hold the teeth for the denture are called _____.

16. A/An _____ is the posterior part of the denture extending from side to side and provides the denture suction.

17. The exact replica of the prosthesis to be cast is a/an _____.

18. _____ is the procedure whereby melted alloy is forced from the crucible into the casting ring.

19. The agent used to protect the alloy from oxidation during the heating process is

_____.

20. The _____ is the vertical length of the cuspid placement in a denture.

WORD USE
Read the following sentences and define the bold-faced words.

1. The receptionist checks the amount of **working days** before making the next appointment for Mr. Smith's prosthesis.

_____

2. During the wax setup appointment, the dentist checks the **lateral excursion** of the patient's bite.

_____

3. The **ceramist** is very particular about the color and shaping of the porcelain fused to metal crown.

_____

4. The dentist advised Mr. Thomas that the tooth in question is a good candidate for a gold **onlay**.

_____

5. The hygienist gave instructions for the patient's home care of the newly received **prosthesis**.

_____

AUDIO LIST

This list contains selected new, important or difficult terms from this chapter. You may use the list to review these terms and to practice pronouncing them correctly. When you work with the audio for this chapter, listen to the word, repeat it, and then place a checkmark in the box. Proceed to the next boxed word and repeat the process.

❑ articulator (ar-**TICK**-you-lay-tore)
❑ cantilever (**KAN**-tih-lee-ver)
❑ ceramist (sir-**AM**-ist)
❑ circumferential (ser-kum-fer-**EN**-shal)
❑ dowel (**DOWL**)
❑ festoon (fes-**TUNE**)

❑ flux (**FLUKS**)
❑ protrusion (pro-**TRUE**-zhun)
❑ retrusion (ree-**TRUE**-zhun)
❑ solder (**SOD**-er)
❑ sprue (**SPROO**)

CHAPTER 20

Business Procedures

OBJECTIVES

Upon completion of this chapter the reader should be able to identify and understand terms related to:

1. **Office communication procedures.** Discuss the various avenues of communication, including oral and written methods.

2. **Appointment control.** Explain the different types of appointments and related scheduling terms.

3. **Patient records and filing procedures.** Identify the assorted terms used in patient recording and the methods or systems of filing and organization.

4. **Business correspondence.** List and identify the different types of correspondence used in the dental facility, including the major divisions of the business letter.

5. **Dental insurance terms.** Discuss the various types of dental insurance plans and related dental insurance terms.

6. **Financial disbursement and banking.** Define the types of financial disbursements used in the dental facility and list common banking terms.

7. **Inventory control.** Discuss the methods used in inventory control and the terms that relate to purchasing and inventory of supplies.

8. **Legal and ethical terms.** List and identify the major legal and ethical terms encountered in the dental practice.

OFFICE COMMUNICATION PROCEDURES

Whether a dental facility is a large clinic or a small office operation, the terms used to transact the business aspect of the practice are the same. Appointments must be made, letters written, and records maintained. Communication by oral (telephone) and written (mail) means is an essential part of the business aspect of dentistry.

Oral Communication

Oral communication involves a conversation between two or more persons either face-to-face or by phone. In the dental facility, much communication with others is by telephone. Often this is the first contact a patient will have with the dental facility.

incoming calls: phone calls received by the dental facility.

> appointment: call to request an appointment or information about an appointment matter.
> personal: call from a personal friend, colleague, family member, and the like.
> inquiry: call requesting information, such as a question about a statement or the result of a test.
> emergency: call requesting immediate attention for treatment or care.
> professional: call regarding specific care or concern in patient matters.

outgoing calls: calls made from the dental facility.

> confirmation: call to confirm an upcoming appointment.
> ordering: call to supplier or store to place an order.
> inquiry: call to request information regarding matter such as availability of a product.
> collection: call to arrange payment for an outstanding statement.

answering machine: device used to record incoming messages when no one is available to answer the phone, including automatic routing for certain calls, mailbox recording for specific personnel, and voice mail for the office.

answering service: professional service that will answer phone calls and take messages, forward messages, and advise callers of working hours and availability.

conference call: telephone service in which more than two persons at different locations may converse on the phone in the same conversation.

Written Communications

Many office communications are written, by use of traditional mail, e-mail, and by faxing messages.

first-class mail: letters, postcards, statements, business reply, and larger marked envelopes.

second-class mail: periodicals, magazines, newspapers.

third-class mail: catalogs, circulars, books, printed material weighing less than one pound.

fourth-class mail: printed matter and parcels weighing more than a pound; also called parcel post.

certified mail: postal fee service that records mail delivery by dating, numbering, and recording mailed pieces. The sender may track the progress of the mail using the receipt number.

C.O.D. mail: stands for "cash on delivery" fee service, in which postal employee collects money at time of delivery.

express mail: fast, 24 hour delivery of mail.

priority mail: mail delivery within two to three days.

insured mail: postal fee service insures item sent, for a set price declared by sender.

registered mail: postal fee service to record and protect mail to delivery site; post office supplies proof (card) that the material has been received; generally used for important papers.

restricted delivery: mail delivered to only the person specified.

special delivery: swift delivery of mail by the post office when received at local station; fee for service.

special handling: delivery of third and fourth class mail at fastest method but not special delivery.

e-mail (electronic mail): communication by means of computer.

fax (facsimile): communication by telephone line connection.

ground package service: parcels or packages containing dental cases, returns, items to be repaired, and so forth may be sent by Fed-Ex, UPS, or USPS. Pickup service can be arranged.

online postal services: include stamp purchase, calculation of postage, printing of labels, proof of delivery, and tracking of postal matters.

incoming mail: mail that has been delivered to the dental facility.

> invoice: printed from supplier regarding order or orders received by a facility; may or may not be a demand for payment.
>
> statement: request for payment for services, products, or material received by a facility.
>
> miscellaneous: may include lab reports, general information or correspondence, meeting information, samples, or advertisements.
>
> packages: may be from dental laboratories, suppliers, or sample products.
>
> personal: mail meant for a specific individual; not general business communication.
>
> payment: envelopes containing checks as payment for statement or treatment received.

outgoing mail: mail that is sent from the facility. May be sent as first class, special delivery, priority, registered, or certified.

zip code: specific numbers assigned by postal office to designated areas of the country.

▌ APPOINTMENT CONTROL

The appointment book is the center or hub of the dental practice. Proper scheduling helps the practice to run smoothly. Improper scheduling or deviation from the usual routine can be a source of frustration and increase the workload, as well as stress among the staff.

appointment: period of time set aside for a scheduled patient.

appointment card: printed reminder of patient's next appointment day and time.

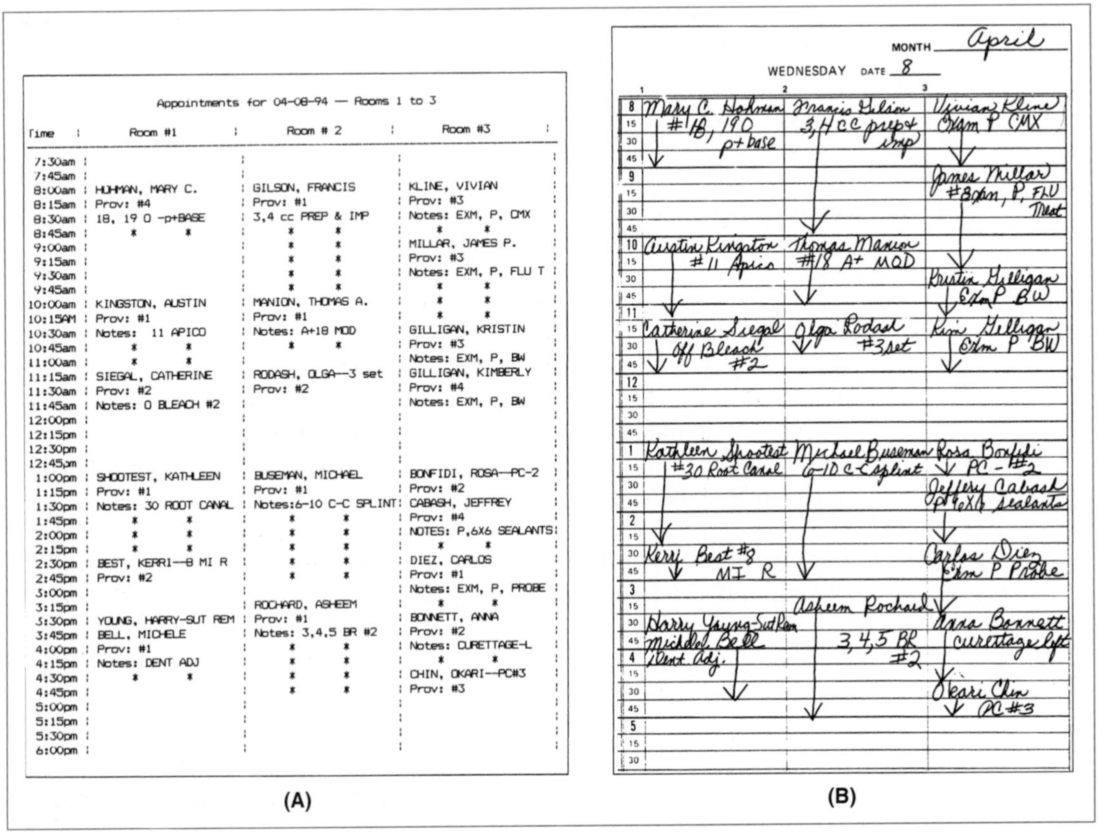

FIGURE 20-1

Examples of appointment control.
(A) Computer-generated
(B) Completed in an appointment book

Note: Both views show the same patients and procedures.

appointment entry: recording patient's name, procedure, phone number, and other required data into computer program or schedule book for a specific time and day. (See Figure 20-1 for two methods.)

buffer period: open unit or block of time that is maintained on schedule page; used for emergencies or to make up time when running behind schedule.

call list: list of patients willing to be summoned at first available opening or when cancellations occur.

daily schedule: copy of schedule of patients and procedures for the day. Copies are placed in strategic places for easy reference.

dovetail scheduling: process in which appointment times are scheduled into the day's procedures at a "down" period of another appointment. For example, suture removal for one patient may be scheduled during the waiting period of anesthesia onset of another patient.

matrix: pattern of work periods available for appointment scheduling. Nonworking hours, meetings, holidays, or any times the practice will not be in service are marked off the schedule.

recall list: system of monitoring patients' return to dental facility. Patients are listed in month of the desired service and called or notified at that time to make an appointment.

unit: section of an hour; may be 10, 15, or 20 minutes. Each procedure is allotted a specific amount of units for scheduling purposes.

PATIENT RECORDS AND FILING PROCEDURES

Patient records are legal recordings of treatment and care received. These records comprise a variety of different forms and items. When preparing and working with these various forms of patients' records, neatness and accuracy should be maintained.

patient information chart: questionnaire filled out by the patient, giving necessary data for office records. Usually divided into general or personal, medical, insurance, and financial information queries. Also called *patient registration form.*

clinical chart: printed chart showing anatomical drawings and diagnostic results of clinical observations; also may record procedures, fees charged, and payments received.

consent form: printed form signed by patient or guardian of a minor giving permission for treatment.

health history form: printed questionnaire regarding patient's present and past health history, medications taken, allergies, and other health matters.

insurance information form: printed questionnaire regarding insurance policy, numbers, type, and any other data supplied on the insurance card.

patient file envelope: large file envelope used to gather and hold together all the patient records in one central location.

Care of Patient Records

Patient records are legal documents. Generally, records and relative materials are placed in a central location. To avoid confusion and to maintain a system of easy retrieval, the records are filed or arranged in an order.

Filing Materials

An assortment of filing materials is needed to maintain dental records.

file cabinet: horizontal or vertical drawer cabinets that holds files; also, open-faced cabinets with clear access to records and more visible color-coding, and space-saving rotary files that rotate records for retrieval access.

file folder: thick envelope or tabbed folder used to contain patient records and notes or other grouping of items. Tab positions may be arranged with three divisions (left, middle, right) or four divisions, called cuts.

file guide: heavy cardboard sheet with letters or numbers on tabs; used to divide file drawer into sections.

out card: bright-colored card that is placed where a file is removed to ensure proper placement when the file is returned; may also have entry table to indicate location of the file that was removed.

Filing Systems

A routine or system helps to quickly place and locate items to be filed. The different documents and items require different filing systems.

alphabetical: filing material according to the order in the alphabet. This is the most common method of filing.

chronological: filing material according to date of occurrence; this method may be used for recall appointment or inventory scheduling and other time-related procedures.

geographical: filing material according to location, such as street, town, state. This method may be used in large cities or practices with branch offices.

numerical: assigning material a number and filing according to number sequence. This method may be used for procedures or study models. The system requires a numerical access book, listing numbers with names.

subject: filing material according to subject matter, such as utility bills, or products.

color coding: using color folders or tabs to indicate status, department, or any other separation desired.

Filing Methods

A standard method of filing is used when placing or retrieving an item during filing. Complying with this standard makes it easier to use and work with files in any setting.

coding: identifying the file alignment with marks, numbers, or color changes to aid in rapid placement and retrieval.

indexing: the process of identifying the position for placement of an item into the file system. Indexing requires breaking down names or titles into units and identifying the arrangement order of the units.

releasing: the process of identifying the readiness of an item to be placed into a file system. Each facility determines its individual method.

retrieving: the process of obtaining a file, using the procedural method of locating, removing, and returning the file for that file system.

purging: systematic process of reviewing and removing outdated or inactive files.

sorting: the process of arranging of files in preparation for indexing or classifying. This step simplifies the placement effort.

transferring: the process of moving a file folder from one file system to another— for example, from the active file to the inactive file station.

▌ BUSINESS CORRESPONDENCE

Correspondence from a dental facility represents the practice and establishes the image of the office. Attention should be given to all materials that are sent out.

letters: written correspondence between two or more parties. The content of the letter may be of assorted subjects such as: insurance reviews, referrals, thank-you's, inquiries regarding supplies or statements, case studies, news announcement, birthday regards, recalls, and other items.

postcards: small, heavy-paper cards that carry a message on one side and name and address of the person receiving the card on the other. Used for recalls, birthday greetings, and announcements.

memos: written correspondence that is less formal than letters and is a frequent means of communication within a practice or group setting. Date and message sender, along with referenced subject matter, appear at the top, followed by comments.

Parts of the Business Letter

The business letter is composed in a structured manner common throughout the commercial world and requires adherence to the letter standards The parts or divisions of a letter are shown in Figure 20-2.

dateline: on letterhead, independent line stating date of correspondence. If letterhead paper is not used, the address of the sender is inserted above the dateline.
inside address: name, title, street, and city with state and zip code address of person who will receive the correspondence.
salutation: greeting (Dear Sir or Madam).
body of letter: paragraphs that state the nature of the correspondence.
complimentary close: ending line, such as "Sincerely yours."
signature line: printed name of the person who is sending and signing the letter.
title line: title of person who is sending letter, placed immediately below the printed signature line.
reference initials: initials of person sending the letter (in upper case letters) and initials of person preparing the letter (in lower case letter). Initials are separated by a slash or colon. Some offices include only the initials of the preparer and the sender's signature.
enclosure line: line that indicates material enclosed with letter; multiple enclosures are so marked (e.g., Enclosures:3).

Styles of Business Letters

Letters may be composed in different styles. The style chosen is a matter of choice. Two standard letter styles are the block style and the modified block style, both shown in Figure 20-2.

1. block letter style. All parts of the letter (with the possible exception of preprinted letterhead) are placed on the left margin. Paragraphs are not indented.
2. modified letter style. All divisions of the letter, with exception of the dateline, complimentary close, and signature line are placed on the left margin. Paragraphs may or may not be indented.

DENTAL INSURANCE TERMS

Dental insurance is a cooperative arrangement of three parties involved in the dental care of a patient.

1. The patient—the subscriber or insured person.
2. The provider, or dentist
3. The insurance company, the carrier.

(A) Block Style

Sender's Street Address
Sender's City, State, ZIP   **(Return Address)**
Date of Letter

Receiver's Name and Title
Receiver's Street Address   **(Inside Address)**
Receiver's City, State, ZIP

Dear Name: **(Salutation)**

xxxxxxxxxx BODY OF LETTER – FIRST PARAGRAPH xxxxxxxxxx
xxxxxxxxxxxxxxxxxxxxxxxxxxxxxxxxxxxxxxxxxxxxxxxxxxxxxxxxxxxxxxx
xxxxxxxxxxxxxxxxxxxxxxxxxxxxxxxxxxxxxxxxxxxxxxxxxxxxxxxxxxxxxxx
xxxxxxxxxx.

xxxxxxxxxx BODY OF LETTER – SECOND PARAGRAPH xxxxxxxxxx
xxxxxxxxxxxxxxxxxxxxxxxxxxxxxxxxxxxxxxxxxxxxxxxxxxxxxxxxxxxxxxx
xxxxxxxxxxxxxxxxxxxxxxxxxxxxxxxxxxxxxxxxxxxxxxxxxxxxxxxxxxxxxxx
xxxxxxxxxx.

xxxxxxxxxx BODY OF LETTER – THIRD PARAGRAPH xxxxxxxxxx
xxxxxxxxxxxxxxxxxxxxxxxxxxxxxxxxxxxxxxxxxxxxxxxxxxxxxxxxxxxxxxx
xxxxxxxxxxxxxxxxxxxxxxxxxxxxxxxxxxxxxxxxxxxxxxxxxxxxxxxxxxxxxxx
xxxxxxxxxx.

Sincerely,   **(Closing)**

Signature Line

Enclosure Line

Reference Line

          (Return Address)   Sender's Street Address
                                         Sender's City, State, ZIP
                                         Date of Letter

Receiver's Name and Title
Receiver's Street Address   **(Inside Address)**
Receiver's City, State, ZIP

Dear Name: **(Salutation)**

   xxxxxxxx BODY OF LETTER – FIRST PARAGRAPH xxxxxxxxxx
xxxxxxxxxxxxxxxxxxxxxxxxxxxxxxxxxxxxxxxxxxxxxxxxxxxxxxxxxxxxxxx
xxxxxxxxxxxxxxxxxxxxxxxxxxxxxxxxxxxxxxxxxxxxxxxxxxxxxxxxxxxxxxx
xxxxxxxxxx.

   xxxxxx BODY OF LETTER – SECOND PARAGRAPH xxxxxxxxx
xxxxxxxxxxxxxxxxxxxxxxxxxxxxxxxxxxxxxxxxxxxxxxxxxxxxxxxxxxxxxxx
xxxxxxxxxxxxxxxxxxxxxxxxxxxxxxxxxxxxxxxxxxxxxxxxxxxxxxxxxxxxxxx
xxxxxxxxxx.

   xxxxxxx BODY OF LETTER – THIRD PARAGRAPH xxxxxxxxxx
xxxxxxxxxxxxxxxxxxxxxxxxxxxxxxxxxxxxxxxxxxxxxxxxxxxxxxxxxxxxxxx
xxxxxxxxxxxxxxxxxxxxxxxxxxxxxxxxxxxxxxxxxxxxxxxxxxxxxxxxxxxxxxx
xxxxxxxxxx.

         (Closing)   Sincerely,

                                Signature Line

Enclosure Line

Reference Line

FIGURE 20-2
The parts and
different styles of
a business letter.

(B) Modified Block Style

The financial arrangements and benefits in insurance coverage differ from one plan to another, from company to company, and from program to program. Various types of benefit plans are offered.

Prepaid Insurance Plans

Prepaid dental insurance plans are those in which the subscriber pays a specific amount (premium) of money for covered services. The subscriber has a choice of dental providers and services and pays for any service that the plan does not fully cover. The payment plans from the insurance companies are determined in a specific manner, based on several factors.

usual, customary, reasonable fee (UCR): The benefits are percentages of the UCR, determined through survey and research of local dentists' fees. Example: 80% coverage of three surface amalgam restoration would be 80 percent of the regional UCR fee for that procedure.

table of allowance: The insurance company policy establishes a specific amount for a specific service. The patient is responsible for any difference in fees between the cost of the service and the table of allowance fee.

fixed fee: A fixed schedule of fees for specific services determines the amount of benefits received. The provider agrees to accept this amount as full cost. Fixed fees are usually federally mandated (for example, Medicaid).

Capitation

A capitation dental insurance plan involves subscribers who are members of groups or organizations that enter into a contract for dental services. There are three principal types of capitation plans.

1. Health maintenance organization (HMO): The provider and the patient must belong to the plan that offers specific services to members and a stipulated payment allotment to the provider regardless of the number of procedures completed. Also called *closed panel dentistry*.
2. Preferred provider organizations (PPO): The employer, group, or organization contracts with the provider for lower-than-usual rates on dental services. The group or organization in return publicizes and encourages members to avail themselves of this program. The provider receives more patients and increased clientele in exchange for discounted fees.
3. Exclusive provider organization (EPO): The EPO is similar to the PPO program with the exception that the subscriber is offered service from only dentists who are members of the provider network.

Government Insurance Programs

The federal and state governments provide some health care, including dental services, to qualified persons. Occasionally some procedures, such as oral surgery, may be covered. The government offers four main health plans:

1. **Workers' compensation:** Covers employees injured at the working site or in fulfillment of their occupation.
2. **Medicaid:** Low-income and qualified persons receive medical treatment or care, with prior authorization, except in emergencies, in which case treatment is provided without waiting for approval.
3. **Medicare:** Health care for patients over age 65 who have registered for care. Medicaid is available in four parts:

   Part A: hospital care.
   Part B: physician care.
   Part C: Medicare-Advantage—provides extra health care coverage with additional patient premium costs.
   Part D: covers some pharmacy costs.

   Restorative and most dental care is not covered by Medicare, with the exception of some hospital surgical care and some prescription needs.
4. **Civilian Health and Medical Program of the Uniformed Services:** CHAMPUS provides care for dependents of military personnel, usually received in military or public health facilities.

Terms Used in Dental Insurance

When working with dental claims and insurance matters, knowledge of related terms is necessary.

approved services: all services covered by dental plan.

assignment of insurance benefits: policyholder's authorization to pay allowable claim benefits to the care provider (dentist). If not signed, the benefits will be sent to the policyholder.

authorization to release information: permission from patient or patient's guardian to release patient record data and treatment record to a specified party.

beneficiary: person entitled to receive the policy's payment of claim.

benefit: amount paid by insurance company to the policyholder or specified provider of care.

birthday rule: standards to determine primary insurance policy when two or more policies are involved, as with children of parents who each have a different policy or company. Primary policy is determined by earliest birthday of the two policyholders in the calendar year. If birthdates are same, the oldest policy is considered the primary policy.

calendar year: one year beginning with January 1 and extending to December 31.

carrier: insurance company or institution that does the insuring.

certificate of eligibility: official card identifying the individual covered by a company or group.

claim: a listing of rendered services, fees charged, and dates of service that is sent to insurer.

claim form: preprinted or computer-programmed form that contains information about the insurer, provider, services, and fees to be submitted for benefit payment.

coordination of benefits: plan by different insurance companies in which both pay on the claim. The primary company makes the first payment, and any remaining claim balance is sent to the secondary company. Both payments together may not exceed 100% payment of fees.

contract year: period of time for which a contract is written that may not begin on January 1; the year lasts from the date of issuance to the following anniversary date; also called *policy year.*

copayment: A specific amount or percentage of each claim for which the policyholder pays, per the plan agreement.

customary fee: average fee range for procedures completed by care providers in a given area or geographical section.

deductible: specified amount to be paid by the policyholder in an allotted time (calendar year or policy year), which must be paid before benefits from insurance company begin.

Individual deductible: requires each member to meet a specific amount per year before payments begin.

Family deductible: requires a group total amount from the entire family to meet requirements.

dependent: person who is carried as a member of the policy other than the holder; may be a spouse, a child, or an elder parent relying on the policyholder's financial assistance.

dual coverage: a patient's having two dental policies at the same time; may be individual or family policy.

effective date: date on which the contract becomes in force and benefits begin.

exclusion: dental service or procedure not listed under benefit plan.

fee schedule: listing of payable amounts for specific procedures performed; also called *Schedule of Benefits.*

fiscal year: any 12-month period set by the agency or company for accounting scheduling; many banks and government agencies start the year on July 1 and end June 31.

group policy: insurance policy covering a specific group or business group; only members of that group or business may belong to that plan. Companies have a multitude of policies.

insured: policyholder; the one who pays the premiums or enters into the contract.

maximum benefits: largest possible amount of payment permitted during a specified time, such as within a calendar year or a policy year or the life of the policy.

participating provider: health care giver who belongs to a specific organization's care plan and agrees to accept benefits for allowed care procedures. The insured will not be charged except policy-stated copayment fees, uncovered services, or deductibles.

pre-authorization: Request sent to insurance company to determine if the policy covers specified procedures or treatments and the amount of payment that will be received; also called *predetermination*; usually sent on claim form and marked "Pre-Treatment Estimate." After approval and completion of services, the form is resubmitted as a statement of actual services by the dentist.

premium: amount of payment required of policyholder to keep the policy in force; may be required monthly, quarterly, or yearly.

procedural code: code system constructed to provide a specific number to each treatment or procedure performed; used to file claims and determine benefits.

provider: the party who renders professional services; each provider has an identification number.

reasonable fee: amount determined by insurance company from survey of providers in area or region.

release of information statement: statement or form signed by patient or patient's guardian to authorize confidential information to be sent to a third party.

schedule of benefits: allotted benefits for specific procedures, same as fee schedule.

signature on file: area or space on initial registration form indicating continuing permission for payment and release of information; saves signature for each claim submission.

subscriber: insured person, the policyholder.

superbill: preprinted form listing procedure numbers and services rendered to patient.

third party: organization or person who makes payment but who is not part of provider–patient contract.

usual fee: average fee charged by provider for specific service.

FINANCIAL DISBURSEMENT AND BANKING

Each dental practice or facility will incur expenses necessary for its operation. The recording of the expenditures is an important aspect of the duties of the office manager or "front desk" receptionist. There is a vocabulary of important terms relative to the disbursement and record keeping of monies handled by any business, including a dental practice.

account: record of transactions, charges, fees paid, and any adjustments. May be individual or family account. An *aged* account is one which has been outstanding for a specified period of time, such as 30, 60, 90, or 120 days.

bookkeeping: structured method of maintaining records of financial transactions.

charge slip: paper form used to show the procedure performed, fees charged, and need for follow-up appointment. The slip travels with a patient throughout treatment and to the front office for posting.

collection: request for payment of aged account; may be attempted with a phone call, letter, or with assistance of a collection agency.

day sheet: daily record of appointments, services, and business activities of the day; also called *daily journal sheet*; or it may be the basis for a daily pegboard bookkeeping system.

ledger card: a record keeping sheet of services, charges, and payments for a person or a family.

pegboard bookkeeping: a system for recording financial activities of the dental practice day. All forms are strategically layered over each other, allowing a written entry to be recorded on several documents; also called a *one-write system*.

statement: form sent to an individual or a responsible party requesting payment for services.

Disbursements

Disbursements are monies leaving the facility. These payments are made using the practice's checking account, which provides a legal record of the transaction for bookkeeping and tax purposes. Some disbursements are fixed, and some are variable. Fixed expenses are those that occur regularly, such as utilities and rent. Variable expenses occur with use, such as supplies.

Checks

A check is a written order to the bank for a draft or transfer of funds. It is payable to the person or business named on the check. The different types of checks are:

cancelled: a check that represents a completed transaction and is returned to the account holder.

cashier's: a check written on the bank's account and signed by bank treasurer or official. The purchaser determines the name of payee, supplies the money for the check, and pays a fee for the procedure.

certified: a check that has been endorsed by the bank to be valid. The bank removes and holds the amount of check from the account to assure that the transaction is covered. The bank charges a fee for this service.

traveler's: a check in which the bank sells agency checks in specified amounts ($10, $20, $50, etc.) The purchaser signs the face of the check once at the time of purchase and again at the time of use. A fee is charged for this service, but traveler's checks are usually accepted more readily than personal checks when a person is traveling.

voucher: a check with an attached stub indicating payment information, such as a payroll check with hours worked, gross and net pay, deductions, and yearly totals. The stub is removed when the check is cashed.

money order: similar to a check, as it is a written order, but may be issued by stores or business establishments and post offices. The purchaser denotes the amount and the name of the person to be placed on the check. The purchaser pays the issuer the money for the amount of the money order, plus an additional fee for service.

Miscellaneous Payment Terms

Other form of payment and terms that may be used when working with checks and disbursements include:

electronic transfer of funds: paperless method of transferring monies. The payee may call or contact the banking institution, provide identification, and place an order to transfer funds to another account or business.

automatic payment: arrangement by payee authorizing specified parties to automatically deduct specific funds to cover fixed or other monthly charges such as utilities. The funds are withdrawn and the transaction is noted on the monthly statement.

credit card transaction: using a credit card to cover an expense. A monthly statement is sent, and payee submits a payment.

Miscellaneous Banking Terms

The following are miscellaneous terms related to banking transactions.

deposit slip: a form for recording submitted cash and checks, included with monies deposited to the business account. A deposit may be made in person at the bank, through the mail, or placed in a night deposit vault after banking hours.

endorsement: payee's signature placed on the back of the check to show that the payee has cashed the check. The three types of endorsements are:

blank endorsement: signature of the payee only; may be cashed by anyone.

restricted endorsement: signature of the payee following a restriction line such as, "For deposit only." It can be deposited only in the payee's account.

third-party endorsement: signature of the payee following instructions to pay the check amount to a third person, such as "Pay to order of Delta Dental Supply Co." This type of endorsement is also called *endorsement in full* and is difficult to cash.

petty cash: a fund set up in an office to pay for incidental office purchases in cash. A record of expenditures is kept and the fund is replenished when needed.

reconciliation: determination if checkbook balance agrees with the bank balance; done monthly when the statement and canceled check records are returned to the office. Any deposits or checks that were written and not yet received or recorded by the bank at the statement date are called "outstanding."

non-sufficient funds (NSF): designation for a check written for more money than is present in the account; commonly called "a bounced check" The bank charges the check-writer a fee for returning the check and the person receiving the check also may charge the payor an extra fee.

stop payment: payee order to the bank not to honor or cash a specific check. If processed before the check has cleared the bank, a fee is charged to the payee.

▌INVENTORY CONTROL

To run an efficient dental practice, the office must maintain the proper supply of materials and functioning equipment. One of the duties of the receptionist or office manager is to see that all supplies and materials are on hand, up-to-date, and in good working order. The best way to accomplish this task is to maintain an accurate inventory list that is updated when making purchases and repairs.

back order: an item that was not included in an order and will be shipped at a later date.

capitol supply: items of major cost that are used on an ongoing basis, such as dental chair, autoclave, or radiograph developer.

expendable supply: items that are used up or consumed during procedures, such as cements, tissues, and gloves.

invoice: listing of materials or items included in an order; may also include demand for payment.

nonexpendable supply: items that are used more than once but are not of major cost, such as dental instruments.

purchase order: printed request for materials or equipment that is used mainly in large institutions; may require authorization before being processed.

reorder point: minimum quantity or amount of an item that is necessary to have on hand before another order is necessary.

lead time: amount of time between the reorder of a supply and its arrival.

inventory **or** order control card: printed card listing major supply, reorder point, and information regarding source, price, and quantity needed.

shelf life: expected amount of time a material can be retained before it loses its effectiveness or before a product's expiration date.

▎ LEGAL AND ETHICAL TERMS

All dental professionals should be aware of the ethical and legal aspects associated with providing treatment and care. Each State Board of Dental Examiners regulates the dental practice and those performing the services. Federal laws control the distribution of drugs, and local zoning or municipal statues also affect practices. Dental professionals should understand the terminology regarding ethical and legal relationships involved with patient care.

abandonment: lack of follow-through by the provider in the care of an established patient.

abuse: any care or relationship that harms, pains, or causes mental anguish to another.

breach of confidentiality: unauthorized release of confidential data, either spoken or written.

confidentiality: respect for the privacy of another's status, data, or condition.

consent: patient's agreement to treatment; may be written, oral, or implied. A parent or guardian gives consent for a minor.

contract: an agreement between two or more parties for the performance of services or care.

defamation: a false statement causing damage to a person's reputation or resulting in ridicule.

defendant: accused or person named in a lawsuit.

deposition: testimony given under oath regarding specific event or occurrence.

ethics: rules and standards of conduct set forth by the profession.

felony: a serious crime, with stricter penalties than a misdemeanor or petty crime.

fraud: deliberate misrepresentation of facts or information.

incompetent: not mentally able; one who lack skills or abilities.

judgement: final decision by the court.

liability: bearer of responsibility for the course of action.

licensure: certification of a candidate's ability and knowledge in a chosen profession.

litigation: lawsuit.

malpractice: failure to provide proper care and treatment; indication of a lack of proper skill or ability, such as failing to remove a broken-off root tip in oral surgery.

negligence: failure to provide reasonable skill, care, and judgment: for example, improper sterilization of instruments.

plaintiff: injured person or guardian in a lawsuit; the party who initiates or files a lawsuit.

res ipsa loguitor (in Latin, "the deed speaks for itself"): the cause.

respondeat superior (in Latin, "the master answers"): responsibility of the employer for actions of the employees.

statute: law.

statute of limitations: period of time following the event during which a lawsuit or legal action may be instituted.

subpoena: legal summons requiring a person to report to a trial or to provide testimony.

testimony: statement, given under oath, regarding details of an event or occurrence.

REVIEW EXERCISES

MATCHING

Match the following word elements with their meanings.

1. _____unit

2. _____indexing

3. _____beneficiary

4. _____carrier

5. _____consent form

6. _____back order

7. _____modified block letter

8. _____ethics

9. _____call list

10. _____invoice

11. _____check

12. _____block letter

13. _____exclusion

14. _____account

15. _____title line

a. position or station of the person sending a letter

b. list of patients who are willing to accept last-minute appointment

c. services or procedures not listed in the benefit plan

d. insurance company or institution doing the insuring

e. written draft or demand of payment from bank account

f. record of services, transactions, charges, fees paid

g. form in which some letter parts are not placed next to left margin

h. section of an hour, used for scheduling appointment purposes

i. person entitled to receive payment from claim

j. part of supply order to be shipped at later date

k. aligning position for file placement using names, dates, etc.

l. list of items and costs shipped in order

m. form in which all letter parts are placed at the left margin

n. code of conduct set by a profession

o. form signed by patient/guardian giving permission for care

DEFINITIONS

Using the selection given for each sentence, choose the best term to complete the definition.

1. The scheduled time set aside for treatment of a specific patient is a/an:
   a. index
   b. matrix
   c. appointment
   d. procedure block

2. Mail that is composed mostly of magazines and printed matter is:
   a. first class mail
   b. second class mail
   c. third class mail
   d. parcel post

3. Time set aside during schedule day to allow for emergency or makeup periods is:
   a. initial time
   b. recall
   c. matrix
   d. buffer

4. Filing a utility bill receipt under "Utility" is an example of which filing system?
   a. alphabetical
   b. chronological
   c. numerical
   d. subject

5. A printed item to remind a patient of a scheduled return visit is a/an:
   a. statement
   b. appointment card
   c. index card
   d. account card

6. A fund of money used to pay for small items purchased for office needs is called:
   a. petty cash
   b. recount money
   c. voucher check
   d. draft

7. The process of arranging items for filing, using names, dates, numbers, or subject is called:
   a. sorting
   b. coding
   c. transferring
   d. retrieving

8. Which telephone call setup permits more than two parties at different locations to speak?
   a. station call
   b. cellular call
   c. conference call
   d. long-distance call

9. A serious or major crime, such as arson or murder, is a:
   a. misdemeanor
   b. petty crime
   c. tort
   d. felony

10. Which of the following selections is considered a part of the return address division of a letter?
    a. title line
    b. dateline
    c. closing line
    d. signature line
    e. none of these

11. Special and immediate processing and delivery of a letter is marked:
    a. first class
    b. special delivery
    c. registered
    d. priority

12. Purposeful misrepresentation of facts or knowledge is a case of:
    a. fraud
    b. libel
    c. slander
    d. felony

13. A requirement for the family or individual to pay the first $100 is known as:
    a. primary carrier
    b. coordination of benefits
    c. split-fee
    d. deductible

14. In three-party payment plans, the health care giver is termed the:
    a. provider
    b. insurer
    c. subscriber
    d. individual

15. Marking off holidays and setting up a new appointment book is the making of a/an:
    a. cross-file
    b. index
    c. matrix
    d. appointment schedule

16. An autoclave is considered which type of expense?
    a. disposable
    b. capital
    c. nonexpendable
    d. expendable

17. Keeping record information secret and private is an act of:
    a. negligence
    b. screening
    c. legality
    d. confidentiality

18. A law or legal regulation set forth by the legislature is a:
    a. restriction
    b. tort
    c. statue
    d. license

19. What kind of check is signed at time of purchase and at time of use?
    a. voucher
    b. traveler check
    c. certified
    d. cashier check

20. A check written on a person's account that is guaranteed by the bank is a:
    a. voucher
    b. traveler's check
    c. certified
    d. cashier's check

BUILDING SKILLS

Locate and define the prefix, root/combining form, and suffix (if present) in the following words.

1. **malpractice**
   prefix   _____
   root/combining form   _____
   suffix   _____

2. **reconciliation**
   prefix   _____
   root/combining form   _____
   suffix   _____

3. **chronological**
   prefix   _____
   root/combining form   _____
   suffix   _____

4. **incompetent**
   prefix   _____
   root/combining form   _____
   suffix   _____

5. **bookkeeping**
   prefix   _____
   root/combining form   _____
   suffix   _____

FILL-INS

Write the correct word in the blank space to complete each statement.

1. A telephone call placed by the assistant from the facility is a/an _____ call.

2. _____ mail has a rapid 24-hour delivery.

3. A rendering of a patient's account that is sent monthly to the patient is a/an _____.

4. A six-month check up appointment is termed a/an _____ appointment.

5. Personal correspondence and business letters are considered _____ class mail.

6. A service or procedure covered by the insurer is a/an _____ service.

7. A private letter to the doctor would be considered _____ mail.

8. _____ is the dividing of a name or item in preparation for filing.

9. A/An _____ form is permission from a patient/guardian for care.

10. A/An _____ is placed in the file drawer to indicate the spot for replacement.

11. Numbered radiographs may be filed in a/an _____ file system.

12. The greeting "Dear Sir" is the _____ _____ part of the letter.

13. The time span from the start of the policy to a year later is called the _____ year.

14. A/An _____ is typically used by institutions to place orders for supplies.

15. An endorsed check assigned to another is called a/an _____ endorsement.

16. A/An _____ is the recorded testimony of an event or occurrence.

17. The act of harming a person bodily or mentally is called _____.

18. A/An _____ is a legal finding of a court.

19. A patient's partial payment on an insured service is called _____.

20. A/An _____ is an interdepartmental or facility correspondence.

WORD USE

Read the following sentences and define the bold-faced words.

1. Our office has a policy of making **confirmation** calls the day before the appointment.

   _____

2. Mr. Walker requested to be placed on the **call list.**

   _____

3. The receptionist explained to Mrs. Keefer that her maximum insurance coverage for the **calendar year** was less than the estimated treatment plan.

   _____

4. Mr. Siegel signed the **consent form** for his son's tooth extraction.

   _____

5. The receptionist requested the new patient to bring his **certificate of eligibility** so she could make a copy of it.

   _____

Appendix A: Word Elements

PREFIXES

A

a	without, away from
ab	away from, absent, negative
ad	toward, in the direction of
albus	white
ambi	both, both sides
an	without
ante	before, forward
anti	against, counteracting
auto	self

B

bi	two, twice
bio	life
brachy	short
brady	slow
bucca	cheek, buccal

C

cent	hundred
circum	around
co, com	together
con	with
contra	against, opposed
cut/o	skin
cyano/o	blue

D

de	from, lack
demi	half
dent	tooth, teeth
derma	skin
di	twice, double
dia	complete, through
dipl/o	double
dis	negative, absence of
dors	back
dys	pain, difficulty

E

e	out of, from
ec	out, out from
ecto	external, outside
edem	swelling
end/o	within, inside
epi	over, upper
ex	outside, away from
exo	out
extra	beyond, outside

F

faci	face
fore	in front of, before

G

gene	origin, start
gyne	woman

H

hem	blood
hemi	half
homo	same
hydra	water
hyper	above, excessive, more than
hypo	low, deficient, less than

I

im	into/position
in	not, into
infra	beneath, under, below
inter	between, among
intra	within, inside

L

leuco	white

M

macro	large
mal	bad
med	middle
mega	large, grand
melan/o	black
mes, mes/o	middle
micro	small
mid	middle
mono	one, single
multi	many
myxa	mucus, slime

N

neo	new
non	no, not

O

ob	against

ortho

ortho	straight
os	bone, mouth

P

pan	all
para	beside, abnormal
per	through
peri	around
poly	many
post	behind, after
pre	before, in front of
primi	first
pro	forward
pseudo	false

Q

quad/quat	four

R

re	back, again
retro	after, behind, back of

S

semi	half, partial
sub	under, less
super	over, above
supra	above, excessive
sym	with, together
syn	together, union

T

tachy	fast, rapid
trans	across, through
tri	three

U–X

ultra	excess, beyond
un	not
uni	one
vaso	vessel
ventro	body front
xanth	yellow

▌ROOT WORDS/COMBINING FORMS

A

abdomin/o	abdomen
acr/o	extremities
aden/o	gland
adren/o	adrenal gland
angi/o	vessel
ankyl/o	looped, crooked, stationary
anter/o	before, in front of
apic/o	apex
arteri/o	artery
arthr/o	joint
audi/o	sound
aut/o	self

B

bifid/o	split, cleft in two parts
blepharo	eyelid
brachi/o	arm
bronch/o	bronchial tubes
brux/o	gland, chew
bucc/o	cheek

C

carcin/o	cancer
cardi/o	heart
cari/o	decay, rot
caud/o	tail
cement/o	cementum
cephal/o	head
cerebr/o	cerebrum
cervic/o	neck
cheil/o	lip
chol/e	gall, bile
cholecyst	gallbladder
chondr/o	cartilage
cocc/i, cocc/o	round, spherical bacteria
col/o	colon, large intestine
coll/i	neck
coron/o	crown
cost/o	rib
crani/o	skull

cutane/o	skin
cyst/o	fluid-filled sac, bag, bladder
cyt/o	cell

D

dacry/o	tear duct
dactyl/o	fingers, toes
decidu	falling off, shed
dent/i, dent/o	tooth
derm/o	skin
dextr/o	right
dipl/o	double
duct/o	lead, carry
duoden/o	duodenum

E

edemat/o	swelling
edentul/o	toothless
electr/o	electric
emet/o	vomit
encephal/o	brain
enter/o	intestine
erythr/o	red
esophag/o	esophagus
esthesi/o	feeling
excis/o	cutting out

F

faci/o	facial
fasci/o	fibrous, band
fiss/o	crack
flu/o	flow
foramin/o	opening
foss/o	shallow depression
freno	connecting band

G

gangli/o	nerve plexus
gastr/o	stomach
genit/o	birth, reproductive organs

geront/o	old age
gingiv/o	gum
glen/o	socket, pit
gloss/o	tongue
glott/i/o	back of tongue
gluc/o	sugar
gynec/o	woman, female

H

halo/o, halit/o	breath
hemo, hemat/o	blood
hepat/o	liver
hered/o, heredit/o	inherited
hist/o	tissue
hom/o	same
hydr/o	water
hyster/o	uterus

I

ile/o	ileum
immun/o	immune, protected
incis/o	cutting into
infer/o	under, below
iri/o	iris

J

jejun/o	jejunum (intestine)
jugul/o	throat

K

kerat/o	cornea, hard, horny

L

labi/o	lips
lacrim/o	tears, lacrimal duct
lact/o	milk
lapar/o	abdomen
laryng/o	larynx
later/o	side
leuk/o	white
lingu/o	tongue
lip/o	fat
lith/o	stone, calculus
lymph/o	lymph

M

mamm/o	breast
mastic/o,	
masticat/o	chew
maxill/o	maxilla, upper jaw
melan/o	black
men/o	menstruation
mesi/o	middle
muc/o, mucos/o	mucus
muscul/o	muscle
my/o	muscle
myel/o	spinal cord, bone marrow

N

nar/i	nose, nostrils
necr/o	death
nephr/o	kidney
neur/o	nerve

O

occlud/o	shut, close up
ocul/o	eye
odont/o	tooth
onc/o	tumor
oophor/o	ovary
opthalm/o	eye
orchis/o	testes
oste/o	bone
ot/o	ear
ovario	ovary
ovi/o	egg

P

palat/o	palate, roof of mouth
part/o	birth, labor
path/o	disease
ped/o	child, foot
phag/o	swallow
pharyng/o	pharynx, throat
phas/o	speech
phleb/o	vein
phob/o	fear, dread
pleur/o	pleura of the lungs
pneum/o	lung, air
pod/o	foot

proct/o	rectum
psych/o	mind, soul
pulm/o	lung
pyel/o	kidney
py/o	pus

Q

quadr/o	four

R

rect/o	rectum
ren/o	kidney
rhin/o	nose

S

salping/o	oviduct, tube
scler/o	hardening, sclera (white of the eye)
scoli/o	twisted
semin/i	seed
sept/o	poison, infection
sinistr/o	left
somat/o	body
splen/o	spleen
spondyl/o	spine
squam/o	scaly
stat/i	standstill, stop
sten/o	contracted, narrow
stern/o	sternum

stomat/o	mouth
stric/o	narrowing
syring/o	fistula, tube

T

tars/o	ankle
tax/o	order, arrangement
tend/o	tendon, stretch out
tens/o	stretch, strain
therm/o	heat
thromb/o	clot
thorac/o	chest
thym/o	thymus
thyr/o	thyroid
tox/o	poison
trache/o	windpipe, trachea

U–Z

ur/o	urine, urinary
urethr/o	urethra
urin/o	urine
uter/o	uterine
vas/o	vessel
ven/o	vein
vesic/o	bladder, sac
viscer/o	viscera, internal organ
xer/o	dryness
zygoma/o	yoke, cheekbone

SUFFIXES

A

ac	pertaining to, relating to
al	pertaining to, relating to
algesia	suffering, pain
algia	pertaining to pain
ar	pertaining to
ase	enzyme

C

cele	swelling, hernia

cente	puncture
centesis	surgical puncture to remove fluid
cide	kill
cise	cut
coccus	round, spherical bacteria
crine	secrete
cyte	cell

D

dema	swelling

desis	surgical fixation
dynia	pain

E

ectasis	dilation
ectomy	surgical removal of
ectopy	displacement
emesis	vomiting
emia	blood condition
ent	agent
esthesia	sensation

F

ferous	producing
form	shape, resembling
fuge	driving away, pushing

G

genic	originated
gram	picture, record
graph	picture, record
graphy	recording a picture or record

I

ia	pertaining to
iasis	in the presence of, abnormal condition
ic	pertaining to
ical	pertaining to
id	condition
ile	pertaining to
ion	state, condition
itis	inflammation
ism	state of, condition
ium	small, little
ize	take away, remove

L

lith	stone
logist	specialist
logy	study of
lysis	destruction

M

malacia	abnormal softening
megaly	large, enlargement

N

necrosis	death of tissue

O

oid	resembling
ology	study of
oma	tumor
orrhagi	hemorrhage
orrhaphy	suture
orrhea	flow
osis	condition of
ostomy	creating a surgical opening
otomy	cutting into
ous	pertaining to

P

para	bring forth
parous	giving birth, bearing
pathy	disease
penia	few
pexy	fixation
phage	ingest, swallow
phasia	speech, speak
phobia	fear
plakia	plate, thin flat layer
plasty	surgical repair
plegia	paralysis
pnea	breathing
ptosis	organ drooping, drooping
ptysis	spitting

R

rrhage	abnormal flow, excessive flow
rrhaphy	stitch, suture
rrhea	flow, discharge
rrhexis	rupture

S

sarcoma	tumor, cancer

scopy	scan, visual exam	*trophy*	nourishment, growth
sis	state of	*tropia*	turn
spasm	involuntary muscle move, twitch		
		U	
stalsis	constriction, contraction	*um*	pertaining to
stasis	constant level	*uria*	urine, urination
stenosis	stricture, abnormal narrowing		
		Y	
T		*y*	act, result of an act
tic	pertaining to		
tome	cutting instrument		

Appendix B: Answers to Word Exercise—Chapter 1

Exercise 1–1

1. two	6. half/two
2. none/without	7. one
3. three	8. first
4. one	9. half/two
5. many	10. four

Exercise 1–2

1. b 2. c 3. a 4. e 5. d 6. e

Exercise 1–3

1. large	4. small/tiny
2. over/excess	5. all around
3. under/below	6. extreme/beyond

Exercise 1–4

1. ad	5. ex/o	9. supra
2. exto	6. peri	10. ab
3. endo	7. post	11. in
4. infra	8. trans	12. retro

Exercise 1–5

1. f	3. i	5. j	7. b	9. h
2. g	4. d	6. a	8. e	10. c

Exercise 1–6

1. mandible	4. dens
2. glossa	5. gingiva
3. occlude	6. cheilo
7. mesial	9. distal
8. frenum	10. stoma

Exercise 1–7

1. al	5. ary	9. form
2. ior	6. ic or tic	10. ar
3. gram	7. ac	11. graph
4. oid	8. ous	12. eal

Exercise 1–8

1. ic—acidic	5. tion—mastication
2. ion—incision	6. tic—neucrotic
3. ia—bacteria	7. pathy—myopathy
4. oma—lipoma	8. cule—molecule

Exercise 1–9

Students may select own answers.

Exercise 1–10

1. plasty	5. rrhea	9. phobia
2. algia	6. ize	10. opsy
3. scope	7. ectomy	
4. algia	8. ate	

Exercise 1–11

1. indices	5. calculi	9. vertebrae
2. ganglia	6. irides	10. carcinomas
3. bacteria	7. biopsies	
4. fungi	8. prostheses	

Glossary

abandonment—lack of provider follow-through for the care of an established patient.

ABC—A = open airway; B = respiration; C = external compression to heart.

abducens (AB-due-senz)—sixth cranial nerve.

abfraction (ab-FRACK-shun)—loss of tooth surface in the cervical area, caused by tooth grinding and compression forces.

abrasion (ah-BRAY-zhun)—an injury in which skin is scraped away; wearing away of a tooth surface from abnormal causes.

abscess (AB-sess)—collection of pus.

absorption (ab-SORP-shun)—transfer of drug substance from the administration site by body fluids.

abutment (ah-BUT-ment)—natural tooth or teeth prepared to hold a bridge retainer in position.

accessory (ack-SESS-ore-ee)—auxillary; XI cranial nerve assisting with spinal movements.

acetaminophen (ah-seat-ah-MIN-oh-fen)—drug used as an aspirin replacement in children.

acid etchant—material to prepare cavity margins for retention of the bonding and restorative materials.

acidity (ah-SID-ih-tee)—condition of being sour; makes litmus paper red.

acquired pellicle (PEL-ah-kol)—little skin; thin covering on teeth, plaque.

acrylic (ah-KRIL-ick)—synthetic resin material used in fabrication of appliances.

activator (ACK-tih-vay-tor)—substance that reacts with the initiator to start polymerization.

acute (ah-cute)—sharp or severe.

acute radiation exposure—radiation resulting from a massive, short-term, ionizing dose, such as in an accidental exposure or explosion of radiation material.

addiction (ah-DICK-shun)—compulsive, uncontrollable dependence on a drug.

adenoid (ADD-eh-noyd)—lymphatic tissue found in the nasopharynx area.

adhesive (ad-HEE-siv)—sticky or adhering material or substance.

adjacent (ah-JAY-sent)—nearby or adjoining.

adjunctive orthodontics—procedures necessary to correct or restore function.

adrenocorticosteroids (ah-dren-oh-kor-tih-koh-STARE-oyds)—byproducts from the adrenal cortex.

adverse effect—response to a drug that is not desired (too intense, weak, toxic, etc.).

aerobes—microorganisms that cannot survive without oxygen; may be facultative (adaptable) or obligate (strict).

aerobic (air-OH-bick)—requiring oxygen to live; bacteria that need oxygen to live.

ala-tragus line—imaginary line from the ala (wing) of the nose to the ear meatus (center of ear).

alginate (**AL**-jih-nate)—seaweed, agar-based elastic impression material.

allergic reaction—sensitivity to an antigen present within the body, resulting in various symptoms.

allergy—specific response to a drug; also called hypersensitivity.

allograft (**AL**-oh-graft)—human bone graft from a person other than the patient.

alloy (**AL**-oy)—a mixture of metals.

alternating pulse sound—alternate weak and strong pulsations.

alveolar (al-**VEE**-oh-lar)—pertaining to the alveolus.

alveolectomy (al-vee-oh-**LECK**-toe-mee)—surgical removal of alveolar bone crests.

alveolitis (al-**vee**-oh-**LIE**-tis)—infection or inflammation of the alveolar bone; a dry socket.

alveolus (al-**VEE**-oh-lus)—bone growth on border of maxilla and mandible.

alveoplastomy (al-vee-oh-**PLASS**-toe-me)—surgical reshaping or contouring of alveolar bone.

amalgam (ah-**MAL**-gum)—soft alloy mass containing mercury, which hardens into restoration.

amalgamation (ah-mal-gah-**MAY**-shun)—blending or pulverizing of an alloy with mercury.

amalgam carrier—hand instrument used to carry plastic (moveable) amalgam to a restorative site.

AMBU bag—bag placed over the nose and mouth of the victim to force air into the lungs.

ameloblasts (ah-**MEAL**-oh-blasts)—enamel-forming cells; encourage cell growth for enamel tissue.

amelogenesis imperfecta (ah-**meal**-oh-**JEN**-ih-sis im-purr-**FECK**-tah)—incomplete or improper development of enamel tissue.

amoxicillin (ah-mox-ih-**SILL**-in)—antibiotic drug (examples: Amosil, Larotid).

ampicillin (am-pih-**SILL**-in)—antibiotic type of drug (examples: Polucillin, Omnipen).

anaerobic (an-**AH**-roh-bick)—bacteria that do not need oxygen for survival.

analgesia (an-al-**JEE**-zee-ah)—without pain; feeling of a lack of pain.

analgesic (an-al-**JEE**-zick)—drug that relieves pain.

anaphylactic (an-ah-fil-**ACK**-tick)—shock arising from reaction to a body allergen.

anaphylaxis (an-ah-fil-**ACK**-sis)—allergic reaction to drug or food.

aneroid (**AN**-er-oyd)—dial-type blood pressure device using air pressure readings.

anesthesia (an-ess-**THEE**-zee-ah)—without sensation. Topical anesthesia: in a specific place, the surface. Local anesthesia: limited to one place. Block anesthesia: produces a regional loss of sensation. General anesthesia: involves loss of consciousness.

aneurysm (**AN**-you-rizm)—dilation of a blood vessel due to wall weakness, possible rupture.

angina pectoris (an-**JYE**-nah **PECK**-tore-iss)—pain or pressure around the heart.

angle of the mandible—area from where ramus ascends on the lower border of the mandible.

ankyloglossia (ang-key-loh-**GLOSS**-ee-ah)—shortness of the lingual frenum; "tongue-tied."

ankylosis (ang-kill-**OH**-sis)—stiff joint; tooth fixation, retention of a deciduous tooth.

anode (**ANN**-ode)—positive pole in x-ray tube that serves as the target for the electron force.

anodontia (an-oh-**DON**-she-ah)—absence of teeth; partial or total loss of teeth.

anomalies (ah-**NOM**-ah-leez)—out of the normal range, development, or general rule.

anopsia (an-**OP**-see-ah)—blindness.

anosmia (an-**OZ**-me-ah)—loss of sense of smell.

antagonism (an-**TAG**-oh-nizm)—opposite or contrary action of a drug.

antagonist (an-**TAG**-oh-nist)—opposing tooth; tooth that occludes or counteracts.

antecubital fossa—interior depression of the elbow; blood pressure site.

anterior (an-**TEE**-ree-or)—before or in front of; front of mouth from canine to canine.

anti-anxiety drug—drug used to produce sedation.

antibody (**AN**-tie-bah-dee)—protein material to destroy an antigen; part of the immune system.

anticoagulants (an-tie-koh-**AGG**-you-lants)—drugs used to delay or prevent the clotting of blood.

antiflux—material, usually graphite, applied to retard the forward advance of melted solder.

anti-fungal drug—agent used to destroy or hamper the growth or multiplication of fungus.

antigens (**AN**-tih-jens)—foreign substance introduced into or produced by the body.

antihistamines (an-tie-**HISS**-tah-meens)—drugs that counteract the effects of histamines in the body.

antihyperlipids (an-tie-high-per-**LIP**-ids)—drugs that decrease or prevent high blood lipid plasma.

antihypertensives (an-tie-**high**-per-**TEN**-sivs)—drugs used to lower or decrease high tension.

antimicrobial (**an**-tih-my-**CROW**-bee-ahl)—substance that kills or destroys microbes.

antipyretic (an-tih-**PYE**-ret-ick)—drug used to reduce a fever.

antiseptic (an-tih-**SEP**-tick)—usually a diluted disinfectant that helps to inhibit growth of microbes.

aorta (ay-**ORE**-tah)—main trunk artery that exits from the heart.

aperture (**AP**-er-chur)—opening or port in the lead collimator disk that regulates the size of the beam.

apex (**AY**-pecks)—root end of tooth.

apexification (ay-**pecks**-ih-fih-**KAY**-shun)—treatment of a nonvital tooth to stimulate closure.

apexogenesis (ay-pecks-oh-**JEN**-ih-sis)—treatment of vital pulp to continue natural development.

aphthous ulcer (**AF**-thuss UHL-sir)—small ulcer; also called a canker sore.

apical (**AY**-pih-kahl)—pertaining to the apex of the tooth.

apicoectomy (ay-pih-koh-**ECK**-toh-mee)—surgical amputation of the apex of the root.

aplasia (ah-**PLAY**-zee-ah)—failure of an organ or body part to develop.

apnea (**APP**-nee-ah)—cessation of breathing, usually temporary.

apposition (ap-oh-**ZIH**-shun)—addition of parts; fourth stage of tooth development.

arch—curved or bow-like; one half of the mouth, either maxillary or mandibular.

archwire—horseshoe-shaped orthodontic wire; when tied, it helps to shape the arch.

armamentarium (**ar**-mah-men-**TARE**-ee-um)—layout of dental equipment and material.

arrested caries—decay showing no progressive tendencies.

arrhythmia (ah-**RITH**-mee-ah)—absence of rhythm of the heart; irregular heartbeat.

arteriosclerosis (ar-**teer**-ee-oh-skleh-**ROH**-siss)—small artery closing; may be caused by plaque.

artery (**ARE**-ter-ee)—vessel that carries blood from the heart to tissues of the body.

arthrotomy (ar-**THRAH**-toh-mee)—cutting into a joint; surgical joint repair.

articular eminence (ar-**TICK**-you-lar **EM**-ih-nense)—forms anterior boundary of the glenoid fossa and helps to maintain the mandible in position.

articulate (ar-**TICK**-you-late)—coming together in a pattern or design.

articulating (are-**TICK**-you-lay-ting) **paper**—color paper strip for testing the level of occlusion.

articulation (ar-**tick**-you-**LAY**-shun)—movement of teeth of the lower jaw in an up-and-down, tooth position relationship.

articulator (ar-**TICK**-you-lay-tore)—mechanical device that simulates jaw joint actions.

artificial acquired immunity—immunity to a disease, obtained from inoculation or vaccination.

asculate (awe-**SKUL**-ate)—to listen to movement.

asepsis (ay-**SEP**-sis)—condition of being germ-free.

aseptic (ay-**SEP**-tick)—without disease; a condition without pathogens.

asphyxiation (ass-**fick**-see-**AY**-shun)—not breathing; result of oxygen imbalance.

aspirating tips—tip ends placed into suction tubes; used to remove mouth moisture.

asthma (**AZ**-mah)—shortness of breath accompanied by wheezing sounds, caused by swollen or spastic bronchial tubes or mucous membranes.

astringent (ah-**STRIN**-jent)—agent that has a binding effect or constricts.

asymmetric (ay-**SIM-ET**-rick)—lack of balance of size and shape on opposite sides.

atherosclerosis (ath-er-oh-skleh-**ROH**-sis)—narrowed arteries caused by buildup of plaque.

atrioventricular (ay-tree-oh-ven-**TRICK**-you-lar)—a valve situated between the atrium and the ventricle.

atrium (**AY**-tree-um)—upper chamber of the heart, one on each side.

attenuated (at-**TEN**-you-ate-ed)—diluted or reduced virulence of a pathogenic microbe.

attrition (ah-**TRISH**-un)—chafing or abrasion of tooth; final stage of tooth development.

auditory meatus (mee-**AY**-tus)—large opening in temporal bone for passage of the auditory nerve.

auditory ossicles (**AHS**-ih-kuls)—small bones in the ear; not considered part of the face or skull.

augmentation (awg-men-**TAY**-shun)—buildup of gingival and bone tissue in collapsed area, resulting from tooth extraction.

aura (**AW**-rah)—awareness of oncoming physical or mental disorder.

aural (**ORE**-ahl)—pertaining to the ear; site for taking temperature.

autoclave (**AW**-toh-klave)—apparatus for total sterilization by means of pressurized steam.

autogenous (awe-toh-**JEE**-nus)—in transplantation, moving a tooth from one area to another area in the same cavity.

autograft—bone graft from another site in the same patient.

auxillary springs—stainless steel attachments used to apply force for directional pull.

avulsion (ah-**VULL**-shun)—pulling away from; tearing or knocking out of tooth or body part.

axial (**AX**-ee-al) **surface**—long-length surface of a tooth; axis (**ACK**-sis).

axillary (**ACK**-sih-lair-ee)—under the armpit; site for taking armpit temperature.

bacteria (back-teer-ee-ah)—one-celled microorganisms lacking chlorophyll (singular, bacterium).

bacteriacide (back-**TEER**-ee-ah-side)—agent that kills or destroys bacteria.

bacteriostatic (back-teer-ee-oh-**STAT**-ick)—inhibitor or retarder of bacterial growth.

band—orthodontic circle made of stainless steel to be cemented on to tooth surface.

band and loop—type of space maintainer used to hold tooth area open.

band pusher—orthodontic instrument used to push bands onto teeth; also termed band driver.

band-removing pliers—orthodontic instrument used to remove orthodontic bands.

bar—solid-line construction, usually made of metal, uniting one side of an appliance to the other side, such as a palatial bar (maxillary) and a lingual (mandibular) bar.

barbiturates (bar-**BIT**-you-ret)—anti-anxiety drugs (examples: Surital, Nembutal, Seconal).

barrier control—an obstacle or impediment; rubber dam that prevents saliva and germs from infecting a site.

barrier technique—a method to avoid contamination by applying material between germs and object.

basal cell carcinoma—malignant epithelial cell growth.

base—barrier against chemical and thermal irritation to pulp.

baseplate wax—supplied in sheets; used in denture construction and bite registration.

Bell's palsy (**PAUL**-zee)—sudden but temporary unilateral facial paralysis from unknown cause.

benign (bee-**NINE**)—not malignant.

benzocaive—(**BEN**-zoe-kave)—anesthetic drug; usually topical.

benzodiazepines (ben-zoe-dye-**AZ**-eh-peens)—anti-anxiety drugs (examples: Librium, Valium).

bevel (**BEV**-el)—slanted edge; a technique to prepare tooth surface for a prosthetic device.

bicuspidization (bye-cuss-pih-dih-**ZAY**-shun)—a surgical division of a tooth with both sides retained.

bifurcation (bye-fer-**KAY**-shun)—branching into two parts, such as lower molar roots.

binary (**BYE**-nar-ee)—an alloy made up of two different metals.

biodegradable (bye-oh-dee-**GRADE**-ah-bull)—metabolic material for breakdown of protein matter.

biofilm—bacterial cells adhering to moist surfaces in a protective slime or covering.

biohazard container—receptacle to hold discarded biohazardous trash and items.

biomechanical (bye-oh-meh-**KAN**-ih-kuhl)—RCT procedure using biological (chemical) and mechanical (twisting) means.

biopsy (**BYE**-op-see)—a tissue sample for microscopic study.

bisecting angle technique—a method in which the central x-ray beam is directed perpendicularly at an imaginary line that is bisecting the angle between the film placement and tooth surface.

biteblock—a device used to hold radiation film in the mouth for exposure to radiation film.

biteloop/tab—loop that encircles periapical film, used by patient to hold film in mouth.

biteplane—acrylic appliance constructed to correct simple crossbites.

bite registration—impression of teeth in a biting, occlusal position to help position study models.

bitestick—wooden stick used to push appliances on the teeth; may "seat" appliances.

bitewing film exposure—x-ray of crowns of the maxillary and mandibular teeth while in occlusion.

bitewing survey—x-ray scan of teeth and their interproximal areas (BWX).

bitewing window—area or designated space in x-ray mount for placement of processed fill.

blood pressure—indication of the pulsating force of blood circulating through the blood vessels; a vital sign.

bonding agent—used to unite some restorative agents to tooth surface and underlying materials.

bone file—larger hand instrument with serrated edges, used to smooth larger areas of bone.

bone graft—transplanting bone to restore bone loss resulting from periodontal disease.

boxing pour method—use of a wax strip around impression seated in an impression tray to make a box to receive mixed gypsum for a study model.

boxing wax—supplied in strips; used to box or wrap around an impression prior to pouring.

bracket (**BRACK**-et)—holding device used to support and stabilize archwires in place.

bradycardia (bray-dee-**KAR**-dee-ah)—slow pulse rate, under 60 beats per minute.

breach of confidentiality—relating personal and confidential matters to others.

bridge—prosthesis used to replace one or more missing teeth.

broach—a thin, barbed, sharp-ended instrument inserted to remove pulpal tissue.

bruxism (**BRUCK**-sizm)—grinding of teeth, especially during sleep or from bad habits.

buccal (**BUCK**-uhl)—pertaining to the cheek; surface of the posterior tooth touching the cheek.

buccal tube—orthodontic device cemented onto the tooth and fitted to hold archwire in place.

buccinator (**BUCK**-sin-ay-tore)—principal cheek muscle; gives name to the buccal surface.

burnish (**BUR**-nish)—to smooth or rub out.

burnisher—hand instrument with rounded head of various shapes, used to smooth out surfaces.

button—orthodontic device added to bands to help support or supply additional directional force.

calcification (kal-sih-fih-**KAY**-shun)—deposit of lime salts; hardening in the fifth stage of tooth development.

calculus (**KAL**-kyou-luss)—deposit of hard mineral salts on tooth surfaces.

canaliculi (kan-ah-**LICK**-you-lie)—small channels or canals, may be present in the cementum.

candidiasis (kan-dih-**DYE**-ah-sis)—infection of the mouth; thrush.

cantilever (**KAN**-tih-lee-ver) **bridge**—prosthesis in which only one side of the device is attached.

capillaries (**KAP**-ih-lair-eez)—tiny blood vessels that transport blood from veins to arteries.

carcinoma (kar-sih-**NO**-mah)—tumor of connective-tissue origin.

cardiogenic (kar-dee-oh-**JEN**-ick)—shock arising from improper heart action.

cardiopulmonary resuscitation—act of providing air and heartbeat to a victim.

caries (**CARE**-eez)—tooth decay.

cariogenic (**CARE**-ee-oh-**JEN**-ick)—start of decay, causes of decay.

carious lesion (care-ee-us **LEE**-zhun)—decay area.

carotid (care-**OT**-id)—large artery arising from the aorta to branch into the internal and external carotids.

carpule (**CAR**-pule)—glass vial container for anesthetic solution, also called cartridge.

casting—metal reproduction of a wax pattern.

casting ring—small ring, 1⅜ inches by 1¼ inches, used to hold the invested pattern during casting.

casting wax—square sheet of various thicknesses; used for construction of patterns for cast.

catalyst (**CAT**-ah-list)—substance that speeds up a chemical reaction.

cathode (**KATH**-ode)—negative pole in an x-ray tube that serves as electron source.

cellulitis (sell-you-**LYE**-tiss)—inflammation of cellular or connective tissue.

cement—thicker dental material that helps to maintain or lute items together.

cementation (see-men-**TAY**-shun)—bonding or uniting two or more items.

cementoblasts (see-**MEN**-toh-blasts)—cementum-forming cells; encourage growth of cementum cells.

cementoclasts (see-**MEN**-toh-klasts)—germ cells that destroys tooth cementum.

cementoenamel junction—tooth area where cement and enamel tissues meet.

cementum (see-**MEN**-tum)—tissue covering the root of a tooth.

centric (**SEN**-trick) **relationship**—occlusal relationship of the teeth occurring when biting on rear teeth; a seated mouth closure.

cephalometric (seff-ah-loh-**MEH**-trick)—pertaining to the head; in x-ray, a cephalometric film is a view of the entire head.

cephalometric film—large-sized radiographic film for exposure of head.

cephalostat (**SEF**-ah-loh-stat)—a pin used to stabilize a patient's head in position during x-ray exposure.

ceramist (sir-**AM**-ist)—an expert in construction of dental ceramic appliances.

cerebrovascular (sare-ee-broh-**VAS**-kyou-lar) **accident**—stroke; result of insufficient blood supply to the brain.

cervical (**SIR**-vih-kul)—pertaining to the neck.

cervical line—cementoenamel junction.

cervical traction—orthodontic appliance worn on the head; attaches to a facebow and applies external force to the bands.

cervix (**SIR**-vicks)—neck of tooth.

chamfer (**SHAM**-fur)—tapered margin at tooth crevix; a preparation for crown replacement.

cheilosis (kee-**LOH**-sis)—inflammation of the lips, particularly at the corners.

chelator (**KEY**-lay-tor)—chemical ion softener used to soften dentin walls during an RCT.

chemical vapor sterilization—total sterilization by means of chemical vapor under pressure.

cherubism (**CHAIR**-you-bizm)—enlargement of the cheek tissue; may be a family trait.

Cheyne-Stokes respiratory sound—respirations gradually increasing in volume until climax and then subside and cease for a short time, then starting again.

chronic (**KRON**-ick)—not acute; drawn out, lasting.

chronic radiation exposure—accumulated radiation effects from continual or frequent exposures.

cingulum (**SIN**-gyou-lum)—smooth, convex, or rounded bump on lingual of maxillary anteriors.

circumferential (ser-kum-fer-**EN**-shal)—clasp that encircles a tooth more than 180 degrees with one terminal end in the undercut of the tooth crown.

circumvallate (sir-kum-**VAL**-ate)—largest, V-shaped papilla found on tongue's dorsal aspect.

clasp—extension of a partial appliance that grasps the adjoining teeth to provide support.

cleft lip—tissue fissure or incomplete junction of maxillary lip tissues.

cleft palate—congenital fissure in the roof of the mouth with an opening into the nasal cavity; can be unilateral (one-sided), bilateral (two-sided), complete, or incomplete.

cleft tongue—bifid tongue, usually split at the tip.

cleoid/discoid (**KLEE**-oyd/**DISK**-oyd)—double-ended instrument used for excavating or carving.

clonic (**KLON**-ick)—alternating contraction and relaxation of muscles.

closed-bite registration—registration taken while teeth are in occlusion.

coagulant (koh-**AG**-you-lant)—agent that causes blood to congeal, clot.

collimator (**KAHL**-ih-may-tore)—device used to regulate the exit beam from an x-ray tube.

commensal (koh-**MEN**-sahl)—organism living in or on another without harming its host; oral flora.

commissure (**KOM**-ih-shur)—corner of the mouth where the lips meet.

complex cavity—decay involving more than two surfaces of a tooth.

composite (cahm-**PAH**-zit)—resin material used for tooth-colored replacement.

compound—nonelastic impression material used in edentulous impressions.

compound cavity—decay involving two surfaces of a tooth.

compression—force upon the chest to provide pressure on the heart to imitate the heartbeat.

conchae (**KONG**-kee)—small bones in interior of the nose.

concussion (kun-**CUSH**-un)—shaken violently, such as a tooth injured in an accident or sports.

condensation (**kon**-den-**SAY**-shun)—act of compressing or plugging soft material into a mass.

conduction anesthesia—nerve block anesthesia given at the base of mandible in the condyle neck.

condylar inclination (**KAHN**-dih-lar **in**-klih-**NAY**-shun)—angular movement of the mandible depending upon placement and function of condyle of mandible.

condyle (**KON**-dial)—posterior process of the mandible; part of the temporomandibular joint TMJ.

condyloid (**KON**-dih-loyd)—posterior growth on ramus of the mandible.

cone cutting—placement error in x-ray exposure, resulting in incomplete film exposure.

congenital (kahn-**JEN**-ih-tahl)—occurring or present at birth; one factor in malocclusion.

connector (kahn-**ECK**-tore)—device used to unite or attach two or more parts together.

conscious sedation—calming of nervous anxiety without loss of consciousness.

contact area—surface point where two teeth meet, side by side.

contact infection—direct passage of disease through intimate relationship; transmitted through saliva, blood, or mucus.

contrast—variations in shade from black to white.

convenience form—stage of tooth preparation when tooth material is cut to provide needed access.

coping (**KOH**-ping)—thin covering placed over remaining tooth surface.

core buildup—use of synthetic material to enlarge tooth core area to provide support for a crown.

coronal (kor-**OH**-nal)—suture at junction of frontal and parietal bones.

coronoid (**KOR**-oh-noyd)—anterior growth on ramus of mandible.

corrective orthodontics—procedures taken to reduce or eliminate malocclusion.

cortical plate—outer bone layer growth of alveolar bone.

cotton forceps—tweezer-like pinchers used to transport materials to or from the mouth.

cranium (**KRAY**-nee-um)—portion of the skull that encloses the brain.

crepitus (**KREP**-ih-tus)—grinding, joint abrasion.

cribriform (**KRIB**-rih-form) **plate**—thin lining of alveolar socket; also called lamina dura.

cricothyrotomy (kry-koh-**thigh**-**ROT**-oh-me)—incision or cut into thyroid and cricoid cartilage.

crown—top part of the tooth; portion of tooth covered by enamel.

crossbite—midsagittal alignment between central incisors not in agreement.

Crozat appliance—removable orthodontic appliance with molar clasp.

cumulative effect—long-term outcome; refers here to radiation effects resulting from multiple exposures.

cure process—hardening of material through an auto (chemical) or a light-activated method.

curettage (**CURE**-eh-tahj)—scraping of a cavity; during an apicoectomy, when the alveolar crest is shaped or in a prophylaxis, a scraping of cementum found in a periodontal pocket.

curette (**KYOU**-rett)—round-tipped blade instrument with a longer extended neck and two cutting edges.

cusp (kusp)—elevation or mound on the biting surface of a tooth.

cuspid (**KUSS**-pid)—third tooth posterior of the midline; also called canine, eye tooth.

cuspid eminence—vertical length or height of cuspid placement in denture construction.

cusp of Carabelli—extra cusp present on lingual surface of maxillary first molar.

cuspidor (**KUSS**-pih-dore)—basin area at chairside where patients may empty their mouths.

cuticle (**KYOU**-tih-kul)—tissue layer covering tooth surface; also called Nasmyth's membrane.

cyanosis (sigh-ah-**NO**-sis)—blue condition; discoloration of the face from lack of oxygen.

cyst (SIST)—abnormal, closely walled sac present in or around tissues.

debridement (deh-**BREED**-ment)—removal of damaged tissue or foreign matter.

deciduous (deh-**SID**-you-us)—primary teeth; first set of teeth.

defibrillation (dee-fib-rih-**LAY**-shun)—reversal of cardiac standstill.

deficit (**DEF**-ih-sit)—lower pulse rate at wrist site than at heart site; also called "heart flutter."

definition—sharpness and clarity of the outline of the image on the radiograph.

degenerative (**DEE**-jen-er-ah-tiv)—disease resulting from natural aging, such as arthritis.

deglutition (dee-gloo-**TISH**-un)—the act of swallowing.

dens in dente (**DENZ** in **DEN**-tay)—tooth in tooth; usually found on linguals of maxillary laterals.

density—film blackening resulting from percentage of radiation transmitted through the film.

dental dam (rubber dam)—thin sheet of rubber used as a mask to isolate a work area.

dental dam forcep (rubber dam forcep)—device used to spread open and transport the dam clamp.

dental dam frame (rubber dam frame)—device used to hold or maintain the dam material in place.

dental dam ligature (rubber dam ligature)—floss or thread strings; small pieces of dam material or a device used to tie or hold down the clamp and dam material.

dental dam punch (rubber dam punch)—device used to place measured holes in dam material.

dental lamina (**LAM**-ih-nah)—membrane band containing organs of future teeth.

dental sac (sack)—pocket covering; derived from the mesoderm, it makes up the tooth covering.

dentated (**DEN**-tay-ted)—bur with extra cutting teeth in a crosscut pattern.

denticle (**DEN**-ti-kul)—small tooth growth, also known as pulp stone.

dentifrice (**DEN**-tih-friss)—tooth powder or paste used to clean teeth.

dentigerous (den-**TIJ**-er-us)—cystic sac containing a tooth or tooth bud.

dentin (**DEN**-tin)—main tissue of the tooth, present in the root and the crown; surrounds the pulp.

dentinogenesis imperfecta (den-tin-oh-**JEN**-eh-sis im-per-**FECK**-tuh)—inadequate formation of the tooth, resulting in weakened teeth.

dentition (den-**TISH**-un)—tooth arrangement; set of teeth.

denture (**DEN**-chur)—removable appliance to replace an entire arch of missing teeth. A partial denture is an appliance that replaces a few missing teeth in an arch.

denture base—acrylic part of a denture prosthesis that substitutes for gingival tissue.

denturist (**DEN**-ture-ist)—independent specialist in the construction of dentures; may practice only in states where recognized and licensed.

desiccant (**DES**-ih-kant)—chemical to dry the prep area, remove matter.

desquamative (des-**KWAM**-ah-tiv)—shedding or scaling off; tissue loss.

detail—point-to-point delineation or view of tiny structures in a radiographic image.

developing—process used to produce the latent image on a radiographic film.

diabetic coma—loss of consciousness resulting from severe untreated or unregulated diabetes.

diagnosis (die-agg-**NO**-sis)—term denoting the name of a disease.

diamond rotary instrument—bur instrument with diamond surface for rapid or gross tooth removal.

diaphragm (**DYE**-ah-fram)—layer over disk end of stethoscope; enlarges, amplifies pulse sounds.

diastema (dye-ah-**STEE**-mah)—an opening or gap between two teeth.

diastolic (dye-ah-**STAHL**-ick)—pressure or force of blood circulating through blood vessels while at rest.

die—reproduction of a prepared tooth.

differentiation (dif-er-en-she-**AY**-shun)—growth stage causing changes in bud shape, makeup.

digital sensor exposure—radiographic exposure of a sensor rod placed in the oral cavity, transmitted to a computer monitor for viewing and recording.

diplopia (die-**PLOH**-pee-ah)—double vision.

direct bond (DB)—the technique of cementing brackets directly onto the tooth surface.

direct dentin stimulation—scratching of dentin tissue to obtain a pain reaction; a method of locating and diagnosing pulpal conditions.

disclosing dye—food-coloring material that is placed in the mouth to dye matter and plaque.

disease—pathological change in body or body functions.

disinfectant (**dis**-inn-**FECK**-tant)—chemical that kills many microbes, but not spore-forming bacteria.

disinfection (**dis**-inn-**FECK**-shun)—application of chemicals to kill, reduce, or eliminate germs.

dissipate (**DISS**-ih-pate)—to scatter, spread out; to let heat escape.

distal (**DIS**-tal)—pertaining to the far or away side; side farthest from the midline of the face.

distal end cutter—an orthodontic cutting instrument used to cut, hold archwire in a buccal tube.

distocclusion (dis-toh-**KLOO**-zhun)—Class II malocclusion; lower teeth in a retruded position.

distribution—process of dividing and circulating an absorbed drug to the desired site.

diuretics (dye-you-**RET**-ick)—drugs to increase secretion of urine.

dorsal (**DOOR**-sal)—back, pertaining to the rear.

dosimeter (doh-**SIH**-meh-ter)—device to measure the amount of stray or secondary x-ray exposure.

double pour method in study models—after filling in impression area with gypsum, mixing another gypsum batch and placing the first pour onto another mixed pile of gypsum.

dowel (**DOWL**)—tapered brass post placed into a die to use as a handle during construction.

droplet infection—infection from pathogens released from the mouth or nose of infected person.

drug interaction—effect resulting from combination of two or more drugs at one time.

dry heat sterilization—sterilization by means of a dry heat oven; hot air bake.

duct—narrow vessel or opening that allows secretions from glands to enter the body.

ductility (duck-**TILL**-ih-tee)—ability to be drawn or hammered into a fine wire without breaking.

duplication of films—process of making a copy of a radiographic film.

duration—lasting effect of a drug.

dysphagia (dis-**FAY**-jee-ah)—difficulty swallowing.

dyspnea (**DISP**-nee-ah)—out of breath; difficult or labored breathing.

ectoderm (**ECK**-toh-derm)—outer layer of development.

ectopic (eck-**TAH**-pick)—out of place; one factor in malocclusion.

edema (eh-**DEE**-mah)—swelling.

edentulous (ee-**DENT**-you-luss)—without teeth.

efficacy (**EFF**-ih-kah-see)—intensity of a drug.

elasticity (ee-las-**TISS**-ih-tee)—ability of a material to be stretched and resume its original shape.

elastics—bands with an elastic ability to apply pressure by attachment to opposing brackets.

elastomeric (**ee**-las-toh-**MARE**-ick)—having properties similar to rubber.

electroplate (ee-**LECK**-troh-plate)—thin metal covering applied to a surface through electrolysis.

elixir (ee-**LICK**-sir)—sweetened, aromatic, hydroalcoholic solution.

elongation (ee-lon-**GAY**-shun)—radiographic placement error resulting in an extended length of the tooth image; ability of a metal to stretch before permanent deformation begins.

embolism (**EM**-boh-lizm)—floating clot lodging in an artery.

embrasure (em-**BRAY**-zure)—V-shaped tooth gap between contact area and gingival crest.

eminence (**EM**-inence)—high place, projection, or prominence.

emulsion—mixture of two liquids that are not mutually soluble.

enamel (ee-**NAM**-el)—outer covering of the crown of a tooth.

enamel hypoplasia (**high**-poh-**PLAY**-zee-ah)—underdevelopment of enamel tissue.

enamoplasty (ee-**NAM**-oh-plas-tee)—selective reduction of enamel tissue to reduce fissures and pits.

endemic (en-**DEM**-ick)—disease occurring within the same population or locality.

endocardium (en-doh-**KAR**-dee-um)—inner layer of the heart, lining the four heart chambers.

endodontia (en-doh-**DAHN**-she-ah)—branch of dentistry concerned with diagnosis, treatment, and prevention of diseases of dental pulp and surrounding tissues.

endodontic (en-doh-**DAHN**-tick)—pertaining to the area within a tooth, pulp tissue.

endodontist (en-doh-**DAHN**-tist)—dentist specializing in the treatment of diseased pulp.

endogenous (en-**DAH**-jeh-nuss)—arising from within the cell or organism; illness from within.

endosseous (en-**DOE**-see-us)—within the alveolar bone, such as an implant into the bone.

endosteal (en-**DOSS**-tee-al)—implant placement with the bone.

endotoxins (en-doh-**TOCKS**-inz)—poisons within or internal.

enflurane (**EN**-floh-rane)—volatile general anesthetic liquid.

enteral (**EN**-ter-al)—taken into the gastrointestinal system.

enteric-coated drug (en-**TARE**-ick)—specially coated pill that prevents release and absorption of its contents until reaching the gastrointestinal tract.

enzymes (**EN**-zimes)—body-produced chemicals that break down food.

epicardium (ep-ih-**KAR**-dee-um)—the outer serous layer of the heart.

epidemic (ep-ih-**DEM**-ick)—among people; widespread, occurring in many places.

epilepsy (**EP**-ih-lep-see)—seizure; disease with recurrent attacks of disturbed brain functioning.

epistaxis (ep-ih-**STACK**-sis)—nosebleed.

epithelium (ep-ith-**EE**-lee-um)—tissue lining or layer.

epulis (ep-**YOU**-liss)—gumboil; fibrous tumor of oral tissue.

erosion (ee-**ROE**-zhun)—gnawed away; destruction of tooth tissue caused by disease, chemicals.

eruption (ee-**RUP**-shun)—breaking out of teeth; growth stage in which tooth enters oral cavity.

erythema (air-ith-**EE**-mah)—skin redness; may be result of allergy.

esthetic (ehs-**THET**-ick)—pertaining to beauty; act of making something appealing.

etching (**ET**-ching)—application of acid to tooth tissues to prepare for adhesion.

ethmoid (eth-**MOYD**)—spongy bone forming part of the anterior nasal fossa of the skull.

etiology (ee-tee-**AHL**-oh-jee)—cause of a disease or beginning of the illness.

excavator (**ECKS**-kah-vay-tore)—hand instrument used to remove decayed matter from prep site.

excretion (ecks-**KREE**-shun)—process of eliminating waste products from the body.

excursion (ecks-**KER**-zhun)—lateral movement of the mandible.

exfoliate (ecks-**FOH**-lee-ate)—to shed teeth.

exfoliation (ecks-**FOH**-lee-**AY**-shun)—shedding or falling off.

exodontia (**ecks**-oh-**DAHN**-shah)—extraction of teeth.

exogenous (ecks-**AH**-jeh-nuss)—produced outside, disease occurring from causes outside the body.

exolever (**ECKS**-oh-lee-ver)—device used in oral surgery to raise and elevate a tooth or root tip.

exothermic (ecks-oh-**THER**-mick)—giving off heat, as in some chemical union reactions.

exostosis (ecks-ahs-**TOH**-sis)—bony outgrowth.

expander (ecks-**PAN**-der)—device used to expand or enlarge the maxillary jaw.

expectorate (ex-**PECK**-toe-rate)—to spit or empty the mouth.

expiration (ecks-purr-**AY**-shun)—expulsion of air from the lungs.

explorer—sharp pick-end instrument of various shapes and angles, used to detect small caries.

exposure time—duration of the interval that the electric current will pass through the x-ray tube.

expros—instrument with combination ends, one an explorer and the other a periodontal probe end.

extirpation (ecks-ter-**PAY**-shun)—rooting out; removal of nerve and pulp in RCT.

extraction (ecks-**TRACK**-shun)—surgical removal of a tooth or teeth.

extraoral film—radiographic film that is placed and exposed outside of the oral cavity.

extrinsic (ecks-**TRIN**-sick)—outer; stains on outside of the tooth.

extruded (ecks-**TRUE**-ded)—pushed out of normal position.

extruder (ecks-**TRUE**-dur)—device to measure and blend two materials into a homogenous mixture.

extrusion (ecks-**TROO**-zhun)—orthodontic movement of tooth out of the alveolus.

exudate (**ECKS**-you-dayt)—passing out of pus.

facebow—stainless steel orthodontic archbow device to attach to intraoral buccal tubes, headgear.

facial (**FAY**-shal)—pertaining to the surface of the cheek and lips (face).

facultative anaerobes—bacteria that grow best without oxygen but do not require its absence.

fauces (**FOH**-seez)—constricted opening leading from mouth and oral pharynx, composed of tissue pillars; area where tonsils are located.

febrile (**FEEB**-ril)—pulse sound; normal pulse rate becoming weak and feeble upon illness or prostration.

Federation Dentaire Internationale—a method of tooth identification in which each quadrant has a specific starting number to designate that area.

festoon (fes-**TUNE**)—to trim and finish off.

fiber—thread-like film/element; also called Tome's dentinal fibril.

fibroblasts (**FIE**-broh-blasts)—fiber-forming cells that encourage growth of the periodontium.

fibroma (fie-**BROH**-mah)—benign tumor of connective tissue.

filament (**FILL**-ah-ment)—tungsten coil in the cathode focusing cup to generate the electrons.

file—a thin, rough serrated instrument used in RCT.

filiform (**FIL**-ih-form)—smallest, hair-like papillae covering the tongue's entire dorsal aspect.

filler—substance added to a mixture to alter or modify its purpose.

film-holding instrument—device used to hold radiographic film in place during exposure.

film-safe container—lead-lined container used to hold x-ray film before or after exposure.

film speed—comparison rate of exposure time the film requires for proper exposure.

filter—aluminum disk placed between the collimeter attachment and the exit spot to screen x-rays.

finger sweep—placing a finger into the mouth to locate and wipe out airway obstruction.

fissure (**FISH**-er)—groove or natural depression; slit or break.

fistula (**FISS**-tyou-lah)—pathway for escape of pus; opening in tissue for pus drainage.

fixing—chemical process of making a radiographic image permanent.

flagella (flah-**JELL**-ah)—small whip-like hairs providing movement for some bacteria.

flange (flanj)—projecting rim or lower edge of a prosthesis.

floss—string or thread composed of silk, nylon, Teflon, or synthetic materials used to eliminate plaque buildup.

floss holder—device used to hold floss; useful for patients with limited use of hands.

fluoride—decay-preventive natural element that strengthens teeth tissues.

fluorosis (floor-**OH**-sis)—reaction to overfluoridation; also called mottled teeth.

flux (flucks)—agent employed to protect alloy from oxidation during the heating process.

focal spot—target or area where the x-ray beam is projected.

fog—clouded, darkened, or blemished x-ray film results; caused by multiple factors.

foliate (**FOH**-lee-ate)—tissue bits located on the posterior lateral borders of the tongue.

fomes (**FOH**-mez)—inanimate objects that absorb and transmit infection, such as a doorknob; plural, **fomites** (**FOH**-mights).

fontanel (fon-tah-**NELL**)—literally, "little fountain"; baby's "soft spot" on the skull.

foramen (foh-**RAY**-men)—an opening or hole in the bone for passage of nerves and vessels.

forceps (**FOUR**-seps)—plier-like instrument used to remove teeth.

forensic (for-**EN**-sick) **dentist**—dentist who discovers and uses pathological evidence.

foreshortening—radiographic placement error resulting in shortened tooth image on film surface.

fossa (**FAH**-sah)—shallow, rounded, irregular depression or concavity on lingual surface of anterior teeth and on occlusal surface of posterior teeth.

fracture—a breakage; in a tooth, root, crown, or all may be fractured.

framework—metal skeleton or spine onto which a removable prosthesis is constructed.

frenectomy (freh-**NECK**-toh-me)—excision of the frenum and its attached periosteum.

frenetomy (freh-**NET**-oh-me)—incision and suturing of the frenum to the periosteum.

frenum (**FREE**-num)—tissue fold attachment that connects two parts; plural, frena.

frequency of pulse sound—pulse count.

friction grip (FG) bur—smooth-ended bur that slips into an FG handpiece and is held by friction grip.

frontal (**FRON**-tal)—the anterior area bone that makes up the forehead.

full-mouth survey (FMX)—multiple exposures of radiographs resulting in a view of entire area.

fungus (**FUNG**-us)—division of chlorophyll-lacking plants that include slimes and molds.

furcation (fur-**KAY**-shun)—branching off; area where the tooth roots branch apart.

furrow (**FER**-oh)—shallow, concave groove located on either the crown or the root.

fusion (**FEW**-zhun)—joining together; union of tooth buds resulting in large crown or tooth.

galvanic (gal-**VAN**-ick) **shock**—electrical charge emitted from reaction and meeting of two dissimilar metals.

Gasserian ganglion (**GAS-AIR**-ee-an **GANG**-glee-un)—nerve bundle or union center of trigeminal nerve branches.

gastric distension—condition resulting from air forced into the abdomen instead of the lungs.

Gates-Glidden drill—latch-type bur with flame-shaped tip; used to open and access during RCT.

generic (jeh-**NARE**-ick)—drug name conferred by the U.S. Adopted Name Council.

genioplasty (**JEE**-nee-oh-**plas**-tee)—plastic surgery of the chin or cheek.

germicide (**JER**-miss-eyed)—substance that destroys germs.

germination (jerm-ih-**NAY**-shun)—single tooth germ separating to form two crowns on one root.

gingiva (**JIN**-jih-vah)—mucous tissue that surrounds the teeth; attached gingiva is firm, bound.

gingival crest—lip edge of free gingiva; also called gingival margin.

gingival margin trimmer—bladed hand instrument with cutting edge to adapt to tooth margin.

gingivectomy (jin-jih-**VECK**-toh-me)—surgical excision of unattached gingival tissue.

gingivitis (jin-jih-**VIE**-tis)—inflammation of gingival tissues.

gingivoplastomy (jin-jih-voh-**PLAS**-toh-me)— surgical recontour of the gingival tissues.

glenoid fossa (**GLEE**-noyd **FAH**-sah)— depression in the temporal bone; location of the condyle.

glossa (**GLOSS**-ah)—tongue.

glossitis (glah-**SIGH**-tiss)—inflammation of the tongue.

glossopalatine (glahs-oh-**PAL**-ah-tine) **arch**— anterior tissue pillar in throat; tonsil location.

glossopharyngeal (**gloss**-oh-fair-en-**JEE**-al)— ninth cranial nerve.

glucose (**GLUE**-kohs)—a blood sugar.

gnarled (**NARLD**) **enamel**—enamel rods twisting and curving within the enamel tissue.

gold foil—thin sheet of gold used for restorations.

gomphosis (gahm-**FOH**-sis)—the holding and anchoring action of a tooth in its socket.

grand mal seizure—noticeable epileptic attack.

granuloma (gran-you-**LOH**-mah)—granular tumor or growth, usually in the root area.

groove—a rut, furrow, or channel; may be a developmental or surface groove.

gutta-percha point—endodontic canal point made of a rubber-like, thermoplastic material.

gypsum—calcium sulfate product of various grits, speeds, strengths, and colors; used for models.

halothane (**HAL**-oh-thane)—volatile general anesthetic liquid.

hamulus (**HAM**-you-luss)—hook-like end of bone that serves as a site for muscle attachment.

handpiece—motor-driven drill; available in different speeds, shapes, and types.

hardness—ability of a material to withstand penetration.

hatchet—hand instrument with hatchet-like edge, used to break away decayed tooth tissue.

Hawley appliance—removable, orthodontic appliance worn to maintain space after correction.

headgear—orthodontic appliance worn on the head to support and apply forces to an internal appliance.

Health maintenance organization (HMO)— plan offering specific services to its members and a stipulated payment allotment to the provider.

Heimlich maneuver—abdominal thrusts to force air to expel or to dislodge an obstruction in the airway.

hemangioma (he-**man**-jee-**OH**-mah)—tumor of dilated blood vessels.

hematoma (hee-mah-**TOE**-mah)—blood swelling or bruise.

hemiplegia (hem-ih-**PLEE**-jee-ah)—paralysis on only one side of the body.

hemisection (**HEM**-ih-seck-shun)—cutting a tissue or organ in half.

hemorrhage (**HEM**-or-ahj)—blood burst; excessive bleeding.

hemostat (**HE**-moh-stat)—device or drug used to arrest the flow of blood.

hemostatic (he-moh-**STAT**-ick)—a chemical that causes cessation of blood flow.

herpes (**HER**-peez)—a viral disease; cold sore.

herringbone effect—exposure error resulting in an image of the lead washer upon an x-ray.

heterodont (**HET**-er-oh-dahnt)—teeth of various shapes.

heterogenous (het-er-**AH**-jen-us)—transplant of a tooth from one species to another.

high-volume evacuator (HVE)—suction device with hand instrument tip, used to suction mouth.

histodifferentiation (his-toh-dif-er-en-she-**AY**-shun)—branching into different parts.

hoe—smaller bladed hand instrument with an angled cutting tip resembling a garden hoe.

holding solution—disinfectant solution with a biodegradeable chemical; used to soak items.

homogenous (hoh-**MAH**-jeh-nus)—same or alike; uniform mixture.

homogeneous transplantation—transferring and inserting a tooth from one patient to another.

horizontal angulation—placing the central x-ray beam is perpendicular to the film.

horizontal window—placement in an x-ray mount, usually for posterior tooth exposures.

How or Howe pliers—orthodontic pliers used to make archwire adjustment.

Hutchinson incisors—rounded, small teeth caused by maternal syphilis during tooth formation in the fetus.

hydrocolloid (high-droh-**KAHL**-oyd)—an agar impression material able to change forms.

hydrophilic (high-droh-**FIL**-ick)—ability to attract and hold water.

hydrophobia (high-droh-**FOH**-bee-ah)—fear of water; giving or shedding water.

hygroscopic (high-groh-**SKAH**-pick) **expansion**—submersion into or addition of water to material prior to the initial set.

hyoid (**HIGH**-oyd)—small bone in neck area, called "Adam's apple."

hypercementosis (**high**-per-**see**-men-**TOH**-sis)—overgrowth of cementum from stress or trauma.

hyperdontia (high-per-**DAHN**-she-ah)—excess number of teeth, supernumerary teeth.

hyperemia (high-per-**EE**-mee-ah)—increase in blood or lymph because of irritation.

hyperextension—condition in which the tooth arises out of its socket.

hyperglossal (**high**-per-**GLOSS**-al)—twelfth cranial nerve.

hyperglycemia (high-per-glye-**SEE**-me-ah)—condition where there is an excessive amount of blood sugar.

hyperkinetic (**high**-per-kin-**NET**-ick)—low pain tolerance ability; over sensitive or superactive response to pain.

hyperplasia (high-per-**PLAY**-zee-ah)—excessive tissue; swollen gingiva.

hyperplastic (**high**-per-**PLAS**-tick)—excessive tissue growth.

hypersensitivity (**high**-per-**sen**-sih-**TIV**-ih-tee)—abnormal sensitivity, reaction to pain or stimuli.

hyperthermia (high-pur-**THER**-mee-ah)—body temperature over 104°F (40°C).

hypertrophy (**HIGH**-per-troe-fee)—increase in size; puffy gingiva.

hyperventilation (**high**-per-vent-tih-**LAY**-shun)—increased inspiration resulting in carbon dioxide decrease.

hypo (hyposulfite)—in film processing, the chemical that removes the silver grains from the exposed x-ray film.

hypocalcification (**HIGH**-poh-kal-sih-fih-**KAY**-shun)—underbonding or incomplete calcification, resulting in weak, susceptible teeth.

hypodontia (**high**-poh-**DAHN**-she-ah)—congenital missing of teeth, lack of teeth.

hypoglycemia (**high**-poh-glye-**SEE**-me-ah)—condition where blood sugar is abnormally low.

hypokinetic (**high**-poh-kih-**NET**-ick)—high pain tolerance ability; under sensitive or underactive response to pain.

hypoplasia (**high**-poh-**PLAY**-zee-ah)—underdevelopment of tissue; lack of enamel covering.

hypothermia (high-poh-**THER**-me-ah)—body temperature under 95°F (35°C).

hypoxia (high-**POCK**-see-ah)—lack of oxygen, as in tension.

ibuprofen (eye-byou-**PROH**-fenn)—anti-inflammatory medication, such as *Advil* and *Motrin*.

idiosyncrasy (id-ee-oh-**SIN**-krah-see)—effect from unusual and abnormal drug response.

imbibition (**im**-bih-**BISH**-sun)—taking on of moisture or fluid absorption.

immediate denture—denture that is placed into the mouth at the time of teeth extraction.

immunity (im-**YOU**-nih-tee)—resistance to organisms because of previous exposure.

immunocompromised (**im**-you-no-**KAHM**-proh-mizd)—having a weakened immune system, resulting from drugs, disease, malnutrition, etc.

immunoglobulin (**im**-you-no-**GLOB**-you-lin)—plasma-made proteins that can act as antibodies.

impaction—a covering or interference with normal growth; may be bone, tissue, or both.

implant—device that is inserted into the alveolar bone to anchor a prosthetic device; also, a drug planted under skin surface for sustained slow release.

implantation (im-plan-**TAY**-shun)—placing an implant into bone or tissue.

impregnated (im-**PREG**-nay-ted)—saturated or filled with a solution or substance.

impression tray—device used to hold material that records an impression.

in utero (in **YOU**-ter-oh)—during pregnancy.

incipient (inn-**SIP**-ee-ent) **caries**—beginning decay of tooth tissue.

incisal (in-**SIGH**-zel)—cutting edge of anterior teeth.

incisive (in-**SIGH**-siv) **suture**—located in anterior area of premaxilla and palatine processes.

incisive papilla—tissue growth situated in anterior of the palate behind the maxillary centrals.

incisor (in-**SIGH**-zore)—cutting, anterior tooth.

incontinence (in-**CON**-tin-ense)—loss of bladder control.

increment (**IN**-kreh-ment)—an increase or add in small amounts.

incus (**IN**-kus)—ossicle of the middle ear; "anvil."

index (**IN**-decks)—measurement of conditions or standards; plural, indices.

indicator—in sterilization, tape showing that sterile conditions have been met.

indirect infection—infection caused by improper handling of materials or contamination of items leading to infection.

infarction (in-**FARK**-shun)—decreased blood supply causing necrosis of the heart.

inferior conchae (**KONG**-kee)—lowest of three scroll-like bones on both sides of the nasal cavity.

infiltration (in-fill-**TRAY**-shun)—injecting anesthetic into the gingival and alveolar.

infraorbital (in-frah-**OR**-bih-tahl)—growth process from the zygomatic bone articulating with the maxilla to form the lower side of the eye orbit.

ingestion (in-**JEST**-shun)—taking a substance into the gastrointestinal tract.

inguinal (**IN**-guee-nahl)—pertaining to the abdomen or groin.

inhalation (in-hah-**LAY**-shun)—breathing vapor or gas into the lungs.

inhibitor (in-**HIH**-bih-tore)—substance that prevents polymerization.

initial set—period of time when the material assumes the shape but remains pliable.

initiation (ih-**nish**-ee-**AY**-shun)—first stage of tooth development.

initiator (ih-**NISH**-ee-ay-tore)—agent capable of starting the polymerization process.

injection (in-**JECT**-shun)—forced placement into the body or vessel, tissue, or cavity.

inlay (**IN**-lay)—a solid, casted restoration made in the shape of a prep and cemented into place.

inlay wax—hard, blue stick wax melted onto a die and carved to become a wax pattern.

inoculation (inn-ock-you-**LAY**-shun)—injection of serum or toxin into the body to produce immunity.

inscription—the part of a prescription giving the drug name, dose form, and amount of drug.

inspiration (in-spur-**AY**-shun)—breathing in.

instrumentation (in-strew-men-**TAY**-shun)—use of instruments.

insulation (in-sue-**LAY**-shun)—setting apart; preventing the transfer of heat.

insulin (**IN**-sue-lin)—hormone released by the pancreas.

insulin shock—condition resulting from overdose of insulin, which results in lower blood sugar levels.

intensifying screen—fluorescent-treated cassette screen to reduce patient's exposure to radiation.

interceptive orthodontics—procedures to lessen the severity of existing malfunctions.

interdental aids—appliances or devices that assist in cleansing teeth.

interferon (in-ter-**FEAR**-ahn)—proteins produced by cells exposed to viruses; they aid immunity.

interleukins (in-ter-**LOO**-kins)—chemicals produced by the white blood cells that elicit responses.

interpulpal (inn-ter-**PUHL**-puhl) **injection**—anesthetic injection that is directly injected into the pulpal area.

intolerance (inn-**TAHL**-er-anse)—effect from the inability to endure or the incapacity for a drug.

intradermal (in-trah-**DER**-mal)—implanted under the skin for sustained slow release.

intraligamentary (in-trah-ligg-ah-**MEN**-tah-ree)—injection of anesthetic into the peridental ligament.

intramuscular (in-trah-**MUSS**-kyou-lahr)—injection given within the muscle; parenterally administered.

intraosseous (in-trah-**OSS**-ee-us)—anesthetic material is injected into the bone.

intraperitoneal (in-trah-**pare**-ih-toh-**NEE**-ahl)—within the peritoneal cavity.

intrapulpal (in-trah-**PUL**-puhl)—anesthetic injection given within the pulp.

intrathecal (in-trah-**THEE**-kal)—within the spinal cavity.

intravenous (in-trah-**VEE**-nus)—injection within a vessel.

intrinsic (in-**TRIN**-sick)—stain from within the tooth.

intrusion (in-**TROO**-zhun)—tooth movement into the alveolus during orthodontic treatment.

invert (in-**VERT**)—to turn toward or reverse material; turning in the edges of a dental dam.

inverted pour method for study models—inverting filled impression material over a gypsum pile.

investment—gypsum used to surround and hold denture or appliance form until pouring or casting.

irrigation—use of liquid material or substances to wash or bathe an area.

ischemia (iss-**KEE**-me-ah)—holding back blood.

isoflurane (eye-soh-**FLUR**-ane)—volatile general anesthetic liquid.

isolation (eye-so-**LAY**-shun)—separation or detachment from others or other areas.

jugular (JUG-you-lar)—large vein that carries blood from the brain back to the heart.

juvenile diabetes—onset of diabetes condition in someone under 15 years of age.

Kaposi's sarcoma—skin disease or growth caused by a virus.

keratinized (KARE-ah-tin-ized)—hard tissue; also called masticatory mucosa.

ketone (KEE-tone)—acidic substance resulting from metabolism.

kilovolt (KILL-oh-volt) **power**—1000 volt unit in radiation (kVp).

labia (LAY-bee-ah)—lips (Latin); singular, labium.

labial (LAY-bee-al)—pertaining to the lips; anterior surface of anterior teeth.

lacuna (lah-**KYOU**-nah)—small open space in the cementum.

lacrimal (LACK-rih-mal)—two bones at inner side of orbital cavity.

lambdoid (LAM-doyd)—suture located between the parietal and upper border of occipital bone.

lamellae (lah-**MEL**-ah)—developmental imperfections of the enamel, extending to the dentin.

lamina dura (LAM-ih-nah **DUR**-ah)—membrane covering or lining tooth area.

laminate (LAM-ih-nate)—thin plate or layer, the applying of a thin layer to another object.

latch-type bur—rotary bur that fits into a right or contra-angled handpiece.

lateral (LAT-er-ahl)—side; position on the side; second tooth from midline.

lateral excessive/deficient—too much bone in one direction and not enough in another.

lateral excursion (ecks-**KERR**-zhun)—measurement with side-to-side movement of the mandible.

lead apron/thyrocervical collar—radiation protection drope.

Lentulo spiral drill—thin, endodontic, latch-type rotary instrument used to spin-spread calcium hydroxide or cement into the canal.

lesion (LEE-zhun)—injury or wound.

leukocytes (LOO-koh-sites)—white blood cells.

leukoplakia (loo-koh-**PLAY**-key-ah)—precancerous white patches on oral tissues.

ligature (LIG-ah-chur)—bound or tied; material used to tie or hold down.

line angle—junction of two tooth surfaces, such as the mesial and incisal surfaces.

liner—a thin coat of material that provides a barrier against chemical leakage into tooth structure; a ring lining placed inside the casting ring to allow for investment expansion.

lingual (LIN-gwal)—surface of tooth or area touching the tongue.

lobe—well-defined part of an organ that develops during tooth formation.

lozenge (LAH-zunj)—solid mass of drug, flavored for holding in the mouth and dissolving slowly.

Luer-loc syringe—barrel instrument with piston force plunger to force or inject fluids.

luting (LOO-ting)—holding together; binding two items.

luxation (luck-**SAY**-shun)—movement; a loose tooth may be moved or loosened before extraction.

lymph (**LIMF**)—body alkaline fluid found in the lymphatic vessels.

lymphangioma (lim-**fan**-jee-**OH**-mah)—tumor made up of lymphatic tissue.

lymph nodes—mass of lymph cells forming units of lymphatic tissue.

lymphocytes (**LIM**-foh-sites)—lymph cells that assist body defenses by attracting antigens.

lymphokines (**LIM**-foh-keens)—active lymph cells that attract antigens.

lymphoma (lim-**FOH**-mah)—new tissue growth within the lymphatic system.

macrodontia (**mack**-roh-**DAHN**-she-ah)—abnormally large teeth.

macrogenia (mack-roh-**JEE**-nee-ah)—large or excessive chin.

macroglossia (**mack**-roh-**GLOSS**-ee-ah)—large tongue.

macrophages (**MACK**-roh-fayges)—large cells that ingest dead cells and tissues.

magnum foramen (**MAG**-num **FORE**-ah-men)—large opening in the occipital bone for passage of spinal cord.

malady (**MAL**-ah-dee)—disease or disorder.

malar (**MAY**-lar)—zygomatic bone; cheekbone.

malignant (mah-**LIG**-nant)—harmful or growing worse; usually refers to cancer.

malleability (**mal**-ee-ah-**BILL**-ih-tee)—capability of material to withstand deformation without fracture while undergoing maximum compression stress.

mallet (**MAL**-ett)—surgical hammer.

malleus (**MAL**-ee-us)—largest of the three ossicles of the ear; mallet-shaped bone.

malocclusion (**mal**-oh-**KLOO**-zhun)—irregular or improper occlusion.

mamelon (**MAM**-eh-lon)—bumps or scalloped edges on newly erupted incisor teeth.

mandible (**MAN**-dih-bull)—strong, horseshoe-shaped bone forming the lower jaw.

mandibular (man-**DIB**-you-lahr)—pertaining to the mandible or lower jaw.

mandibular notch—small notch or depression in jaw edge located on mandible's lower border.

mandrel (**MAN**-drell)—rotary instrument that holds abrasive or treated wheels and disks.

manipulation (mah-nip-you-**LAY**-shun)—the skillful operation or handling and use.

marginal—pertaining to the margin, portion of gingiva that is unattached to underlying tissues.

Maryland bridge—bridge that is cemented to adjacent teeth.

masseter (mass-**EE**-ter)—principal muscle of mastication that closes the mouth.

mastication (mass-tih-**KAY**-shun)—the act of chewing.

mastoid (**MASS**-toyd)—natural growth on temporal bone behind the ear, used for muscle attachment.

matrix (**MAY**-tricks)—artificial wall material; may be metal or celluloid.

matrix holder—device to hold matrix band in place during use.

matrix wedge—small V-shaped wedge made of wood or plastic to support matrix band and shape.

maxilla (**MACK**-sih-lah)—upper jaw.

maxillary (**MACK**-sih-lair-ee)—left and right bones that form the upper jaw.

maxillofacial (mack-sill-oh-**FAY**-shal) **surgeon**—a specialist who provides surgical care for the teeth, jaws, and related areas.

maximum permissible dose (MPD)—maximum x-ray exposure permissible for an occupationally exposed person.

meatus (mee-**AY**-tus)—opening in temporal bone for auditory nerves and vessels.

medicament (meh-**DICK**-ah-ment)—medicine or remedy; agent used for treatment.

melanoma (mel-ah-**NO**-mah)—malignant, pigmented mole or tumor.

meniscus (men-**IS**-kus)—articular disc located between the TMJ bones.

mental (**MEN**-tal)—pertaining to the chin.

mentalis (men-**TAL**-iss)—chin muscle that moves the chin tissue and raises the lower lip.

mesenchyme (**MEZ**-en-kime)—connective tissue cells forming the mesoderm cells.

mesial (**ME**-zee-al)—to the middle; side surface closest to the middle of the face.

mesioclusion (me-zee-oh-**KLOO-**zhun)—Class III malocclusion; condition of protruding lower jaw.

mesoderm (MESS-oh-derm)—middle layer of growth; development germ of middle cells.

metabolic (met-ah-**BAHL-**ick) **shock**—shock arising from diseases, diabetes.

metabolism (meh-**TAB-**oh-lizm)—the sum of all physical and chemical changes taking place in the body.

metals—an assortment of dental materials; base materials are common, and more precious metals are termed **noble metals.**

metallic oxide paste—two-paste impression system of zinc oxide eugenol (ZOE) base.

metastasize (meh-**TASS-**tah-size)—move; movement of cancer throughout the body.

microdontia (my-kroh-**DAHN-**shee-ah)—abnormally or unusually small teeth.

microgenia (my-kroh-**JEE-**nee-ah)—small or undersized chin.

micrognathia (my-kroh-**NAY-**thee-ah)—abnormally small jaw, undersized mandible.

microphages (MY-kroh-fayges)—cells that ingest smaller matter, such as bacteria.

micropump—implanted device for a sustained, timed release of a drug.

midline—imaginary vertical line bisecting the head at the middle of the face; determines right and left.

milliampere (mA) (mill-ee-**AM-**peer) **control**—one-thousandth of an ampere (electric current).

mobility (moh-**BIL-**ih-tee)—capable of movement; a diagnostic test in RCT.

modifier—substance used to change the condition of a material.

molar (MOH-lar)—large grinding teeth located in posterior of the mouth.

molding—shaping an impression material over the edge of the tray for better adaption.

molten metal/glass bead sterilization—method used in endodontics to sterilize small tips.

morphodifferentiation (more-foh-diff-er-en-she-**AY-**shun)—tooth development stage of shape change.

mouth prop—device to maintain the mouth in an open position during surgery and dental procedures.

mucin (MYOU-sin)—slimy or sticky secretion that produces mucus.

mucocele (MYOU-koh-seal)—mucous cyst.

mucoperiosteum (myou-koh-**pear-**ee-**AHS-**tee-um)—mucous lining covering tissues in mouth.

mucogingival (myou-koh-**JIN-**jih-vahl)—site where the gingiva and mucous membrane unite.

mucogingival excision—procedure used to correct defects in shape, position, or amount of tooth's gingiva.

mucosa (myou-**KOH-**sah)—tissue lining an orifice.

mutation effect—abnormal growth or development resulting from radiation that causes a genetic change.

mylar (MY-lar)—heavy, cellophane-type material that provides matrix support for anterior areas.

mylohyoid (my-loh-**HIGH-**oyd) **ridge**—horizontal layered edge located on the mandible's lingual.

myocardial infarction (my-oh-**KAR-**dee-ah in-**FARK-**shun)—necrosis of the myocardium; heart attack.

myocardium (my-oh-**KAR-**dee-um)—middle cardiac muscular layer.

myotherapeutic (my-oh-thare-ah-**PYOU-**tick)—exercise or treatment to heal or correct misalignments.

naproxen (nah-**PROX-**en)—anti-inflammatory medication, such as *Naprosyn* or *Anaprox*.

nasal (NAY-zal)—left and right bones that form the arch or bridge of the nose.

nasion (NAY-zhun)—point where nasofrontal suture transverses skull midplane.

nasociliary (nay-zoh-**SIL-**ee-air-ee)—branch of the ophthalmic division of the trigeminal nerve.

nasocomial (nay-zoh-**KOH-**me-al)—pertaining to or beginning in a hospital.

nasopalatine (nay-zoh-**PAL-**ah-tine)—combined area of nose and palate, spot for tooth infiltration.

necrotic (neh-**KRAH-**tick)—dead or nonvital tissue or organ.

negative angulation—upward angle of the PID, x-ray beam in minus angulation.

negative reproduction—an impression opposite of the condition.

nematodes (**NEM**-ah-toads)—small parasitic worms, such as threadworm and roundworm.

neoplasm (**NEE**-oh-plazm)—new tissue, growth.

neurofibromatosis (**new**-roh-fie-**broh**-mah-**TOH**-sis)—tumor of the peripheral nerves.

neurogenic (**new**-roh-**JEN**-ick)—shock arising from nervous impulses.

neutroclusion (**new**-troh-**KLOO**-zhun)—Class I malocclusion; teeth are occluding in a normal manner but may have a misplaced or titled tooth.

nitroglycerin—medication for immediate relief of heart problems, angina pectoris.

noble metals—precious metals used in prostheses: gold, palladium, platinum.

nosocomial (**noh**-soh-**KOH**-me-al)—disease arising in health-care settings, such as staph.

objective symptom—evidence observed by someone other than victim; also called a sign.

oblique line—slanted, bony growth line on facial side of mandible.

obturation (ahb-too-**RAY**-shun)—to close or stop up; a procedural step in RCT.

occipital (ock-**SIP**-ih-tahl)—large bone in lower back of head forming the skull base.

occlude (oh-**KLUDE**)—jaw closing.

occlusal (oh-**KLOO**-zahl)—chewing surface of posterior teeth.

occlusal film packet—radiographic film used intra- or extraorally for exposure of larger areas.

occlusal guard—custom-formed acrylic night guard to prevent tooth grinding.

occlusal records—measurements of jaw relationships and articulation of teeth.

occlusal rims—wax blocks placed on contoured baseplate wax in preparation for dentures.

oculomotor (ock-you-loh-**MOE**-tor)—third cranial nerve.

odontalgia (oh-dahn-**TAHL**-jee-ah)—toothache, pain in a tooth.

odontoblasts (oh-**DAHN**-toh-blasts)—dentin-forming cell.

odontoclasts (oh-**DAHN**-toh-klasts)—cells that break down hard tooth surface, causing resorption.

odontogenesis (oh-**dahn**-toh-**JEN**-eh-sis)—pertaining to tooth production.

odontology (oh-dahn-**TAHL**-oh-jee)—study of teeth characteristics, shapes, sizes, and care.

odontoma (oh-dahn-**TOH**-mah)—tumor of a tooth or a dental tissue.

olfactory (ol-**FACK**-toh-ree)—first cranial nerve.

onlay (**ON**-lay)—cast restoration to fit preparation of proximal walls and most of occlusal surface.

open bite—condition occurring when the anterior teeth do not have contact with each other.

operatory (**AH**-purr-ah-tore-ee)—dental room with chair, unit, and items needed for performing dental treatments.

operatory light—chairside light used to illuminate patient's oral cavity.

ophthalmic (off-**THAL**-mick)—sensory nerve branch of the trigeminal nerve.

opioid (**OH**-pee-oyd)—narcotic drugs.

opportunistic (ah-pore-too-**NISS**-tick)—a disease or infection occurring when body resistance is low.

opposing arch—the arch opposite the working arch; upper or lower jaw; impression may be taken on arch opposite of worksite.

oral pathologist—dentist who specializes in the nature, diagnosis, and control of dental diseases.

oral shield—vestibule device placed between the teeth and lip to train, correct, and maintain function.

orbicularis oris (ore-bick-you-**LAIR**-iss **OR**-iss)—circular muscle around the mouth; "kissing muscle."

oris—inferius oris is the lower lip; superior oris is the upper lip.

orthodontia (ore-thoh-**DON**-shuh)—the specialty of prevention and correction of malocclusion.

orthodontist (ore-thoh-**DON**-tist)—dentist who straightens teeth or corrects malocclusion.

osseointegration (oss-ee-oh-inn-teh-**GRAY**-shun)—union of bone with implant device.

osseous surgery—surgery that involves alteration in bony support of the teeth.

osteoblasts (**AHS**-tee-oh-blasts)—bone-forming germ cells.

osteoclasts (**AHS**-tee-oh-klasts)—cells that destroys or causes absorption of the bone tissue.

osteomylitis (oss-tee-oh-my-**LYE**-tiss)—an infection of the bone and bone marrow.

osteopenia (ahs-tea-oh-**PEE**-nee-ah)—lack of bone tissue.

osteoplasty (**OSS**-tee-oh-**plas**-tee)—forming or recontouring bones.

osteotomy (oss-tee-**OT**-oh-me)—bone incision.

outline forms—tooth cuts used to prepare the size, shape, and placement of the restoration.

overdenture—prosthetic denture that is prepared to fit and be secured upon posts.

overjet—condition in which the anterior teeth overbite or improperly extend over the lower incisors.

overlapping—positioning error in an x-ray resulting in an overlapping shadow of adjacent tooth cusps.

palate (**PAL**-utt)—roof of the mouth; composed of soft and hard palate.

palatine (**PAL**-ah-tine)—relating to the palate area.

palliative (**PAL**-ee-ah-tiv)—relieving or alleviating pain.

Palmer numbering system—method for identifying teeth, using numbers and letters.

palpation (pal-**PAY**-shun)—application of finger pressure to a questionable area; a diagnostic test.

pandemic (pan-**DEM**-ick)—a disease in epidemic stages and occurring in many places.

panoramic (pan-oh-**RAM**-ick) **radiograph**—special radiograph that exhibits the entire dentition area on one film.

papilla (pah-**PILL**-ah)—tissue growths or buds; plural, papillae (pah-**PIH**-lie).

papillary—the part of the marginal gingiva that occupies the interproximal spaces.

papilloma (pap-ih-**LOH**-mah)—epithelial tumor of the skin or mucous membrane.

papoose board—wrapping device for restraining a child patient.

paresthesia (par-es-**THEE**-zee-ah)—abnormal feeling; may occur after anesthesia has worn off.

paralleling technique—method of exposing intraoral films at a parallel angle to the film surface.

parenteral (pare-**EN**-ter-ahl)—not entering the body through the gastrointestinal system, such as an injection or needle-stick.

parietal (pah-**RYE**-eh-tal)—bone that makes up the roof and side walls covering the brain.

parotid (pah-**ROT**-id)—largest salivary gland, located near the ear.

passive acquired immunity—immunity obtained from antibodies from another source, such as breast milk or injections.

passive natural immunity—immunity that passes from mother to fetus; congenital.

patch—a medicated adhesive strip applied to skin for timed release of a drug.

pathogenic (path-oh-**JEN**-ick)—disease-producing substance.

pathology (**PATH**-ahl-oh-jee)—study of disease.

pediatric (pee-dee-**AT**-rick)—concerning the child patient.

pedodontist (**PEE**-doh-**don**-tist)—dentist who cares for the teeth and oral tissues of children; also called a pediatric dentist.

pellicle (**PELL**-ih-kul)—adhering film on the surface of the teeth.

percussion (per-**KUSH**-un)—tapping on body tissue; a diagnostic test in RCT.

periapical (**pear**-ee-**APE**-ih-kahl)—area around the apex of a tooth.

periapical film—most commonly used radiographic film for intraoral exposure.

pericardium (pair-ih-**KAR**-dee-um)—sac encasing the heart.

pericementitis (**pear**-ih-seh-men-**TIE**-tiss)—inflammation and necrosis of the tooth alveoli.

pericoronitis (**pear**-ih-core-oh-**NIGH**-tiss)—inflammation around the crown of a tooth.

periodontal (**pear**-ee-oh-**DAHN**-tahl)—area around the tooth.

periodontal abscess—collection of pus in the periodontal tissue; also called pyorrhea.

periodontal flap surgery—surgical movement or treatment of the periosteum and pocket tissues.

periodontal ligaments—fiber bundles located around the tooth.

periodontal pocket—abnormal open space between the tooth and the gingival; caused by gum recession or loss of epithelial attachment.

periodontist (pear-ee-oh-**DAHN**-tist)—dentist who specializes in treatment of the periosteum.

periodontitis (**pear**-ee-oh-don-**TIE**-tiss)—inflammation of the gingiva and the supporting tissues.

periodontium (pear-ee-oh-**DANT**-um)—tissues surrounding the teeth.

periodontology (pear-ee-oh-dahn-**TAHL**-oh-jee)—treatment of diseases of tissues around teeth.

periodontosis (pear-ee-oh-don-**TOH**-sis)—inflammation of the gingival and periodontal ligaments, accompanied by destruction of the alveolar bone.

periosteal (pear-ee-**OSS**-tee-al)—pertaining to the area round the periosteum.

periosteotome (pear-ee-**OSS**-tee-oh-tome)—instrument used for cutting around the bone.

periosteum (pear-ee-**AH**-stee-um)—fibrous membrane lining on all oral mouth tissue surfaces.

periradicular (pear-ee-rah-**DICK**-you-lar)—around the root area; a cyst around the root apex.

petit mal (**PEH**-tee-mahl)—smaller brain seizures consisting of momentary unconsciousness.

phagocytes (**FAG**-oh-sites)—white blood cells that ingest and destroy antigens.

phantom (**FAN**-tum)—device used for practice in learning radiation-exposure techniques.

pharmacokinetics (**far**-mah-koh-kaih-**NEH**—ticks)—study of drugs and their actions on the body.

pharmacology (far-mah-**KAHL**-oh-jee)—the study of drugs and their effects.

pharyngopalatine (fare-in-goh-**PAL**-ah-tine)—a rear fauces between the pharynx and palate area.

philtrum (**FILL**-trum)—median groove on the external surface of the upper lip.

pickling solution—mixture used to remove surface film from a cast restoration.

pit—pinpoint depression located at the junction of developed grooves or at the groove ends.

plaque (**plack**)—buildup or plate; invisible film on tooth surface.

plasticizer (**PLAS**-tih-sigh-zer)—substance that causes a softening effect upon polymerization.

plexus (**PLECK**-sus)—network, grouping of vessels.

point angle—meeting of three surfaces of a tooth, such as the mesial, incisal, and labial.

polycarboxylate (pahl-ee-kar-**BOX**-ih-late)—permanent cementation for crowns, inlays, onlays, and bridges.

polyether (**PAHL**-ee-ee-thur)—elastic impression material.

polymerization (pahl-ee-mare-ih-**ZAY**-shun)—change of compound elements into another shape.

polysulfide (pohl-ee-**SUL**-fide)—also known as mercaptan, rubber base impression material.

polyvinylsiloxane (pahl-ee-vine-ih-sil-**OX**-ane)—rubber base impression material.

pontic (**PON**-tick)—artificial tooth part of a bridge that replaces the missing tooth area.

porcelain (**POOR**-sih-lin)—hard, ceramic ware used in shells, veneers, facings, artificial teeth.

porcelain jacket crown (PJC)—a thin metal and ceramic veneered crown for an anterior tooth.

porcelain fused to metal crown (PFM)—full metal crown with all surfaces covered with a porcelain veneer.

positive angulation—angle achieved by positioning the PID downward for a plus-radiation angle.

positive cast—reproduction of the patient's mouth.

post and core crown—crown used for endodontically treated tooth with significant tooth loss.

post dam—posterior edge of the maxillary denture that provides suction hold.

posterior (pahs-**TEE**-ree-or)—toward the rear; area of mouth back from the corner of the lips.

posterior nasal spine—located in the upper arch between the nasal bone and the superior maxilla.

post placement—insertion of a metal retention pin into the root canal or prepared area to provide stability to the restoration.

postural (**POSS**-chu-ral) **shock**—shock arising from sudden body position changes.

potency (**POH**-ten-see)—strength of a drug.

premolar (pree-**MOH**-lar)—a bicuspid tooth; teeth between the canine and molars.

prescription—written order for a drug.

preventive orthodontics—methods used to prevent or avoid future occurrences of malocclusion.

primary—first; first set of teeth, deciduous teeth or "baby teeth."

primary radiation—desired radiation beam during an x-ray exposure; radiation from the primary beam.

process—projection or outgrowth of bone or tissue.

prognosis (prahg-**NO**-sis)—prediction about the course of the disease.

prognastic (prahg-**NAS**-tick)—position with the mandible forward.

proliferation (pro-**lif**-er-**AY**-shun)—second growth stage of teeth; reproduction of new parts.

prophy (**PRO**-fee)—short term for prophylaxis; a professional tooth cleaning.

prophylactic (proh-fih-**LACK**-tick)—warding off disease, anti-infective.

prophylaxis (proh-fih-**LACK**-sis)—professional cleaning and polishing of teeth.

proprietary (proh-**PRY**-eh-tare-ee) **drug name**—registered U.S. patented name of a drug.

prosthesis (prahs-**THEE**-sis)—artificial appliance for missing body part; plural is prostheses.

prosthodontist (**prahs**-thoh-**DAHN**-tist)—dental specialist dealing with artificial tooth replacements.

protocol (**PROH**-toe-kall)—steps or method to follow.

protozoa (proh-toh-**ZOH**-ah)—small animal parasite or organism that must live upon another.

protrusion (proh-**TRUE**-zhun)—mandible thrust forward with lower jaw out.

protuberance (proh-**TOO**-ber-ans)—projection, such as the chin.

provider—one who renders professional services.

proximal—side wall of tooth that meets with or touches side wall of another tooth.

pseudomacrogenia (soo-doh-mack-roh-**JEE**-nee-ah)—excess of soft tissue presenting a look of abnormal size, such as "witch's chin."

psychogenic (sigh-koh-**JEN**-ick) **shock**—shock arising from mental origins.

pterygoid (**TER**-eh-goyd)—wing-shaped process; growth of sphenoid bone extending downward.

ptosis (**TOH**-sis)—drooping or sagging of an organ; may be termed "witch's chin."

public health dentist—specializes in dental diseases among the community or general population.

pulp—living tissue of the tooth; contains blood, lymph vessels, and nerve endings.

pulpalgia (puhl-**PAL**-jee-ah)—pain in the pulp or toothache from irritated pulp.

pulp canal—small trench area in center of root, containing the pulpal vessels.

pulp capping—placement of medication to sedate and treat an inflamed pulp.

pulp chamber—open area in center of tooth, found in the crown area; place for pulpal tissues.

pulp cyst (**sist**)—closed, fluid-filled sac in pulp tissues.

pulpectomy (puhl-**PECK**-toh-mee)—surgical removal of the pulp tissue from the tooth; also known as root canal treatment.

pulpitis (pul-**PIE**-tis)—pulp inflammation; also called toothache.

pulpotomy (puhl-**POT**-oh-me)—partial excision of the pulpal tissue.

pulp stone—small tooth growth in pulpal tissue; also called denticle.

pulp tester—electric stimulation device used to detect pulp conditions.

pulse—beating force of blood circulating through the arteries.

putrefaction (**pyou**-trih-**FACK**-shun)—decaying animal matter.

pyorrhea (**pie**-oh-**REE**-ah)—pus discharge from a periodontal pocket.

quadrant (**KWAH**-drant)—one-fourth of the mouth, half of the maxillary or mandibular arch.

quaternary (**KWAH**-ter-nare-ee)—an alloy composed of four metals.

quinary (**KWIN**-ar-ee)—an alloy composed of five different metals.

R (Roentgen)—the basic unit of x-ray exposure; the international unit is the coulomb per kilogram (C/kg).

rad (radiation absorbed dose)—international unit is gray (Gy), calculated as equal to 100 ergs (energy units) per gram of tissue.

radiant energy—energy that is given off from a central source.

radicular (rah-**DICK**-you-lar)—area near the tooth root; site of root tip cysts.

radiographic unit—x-ray device; may be single unit or have multiple heads with a single control board.

radiolucent (ray-dee-oh-**LOO**-sent)—radiograph that appears dark or the ability of a substance to permit passage of x-radiation for film exposure.

radiopaque (**RAY**-dee-oh-payk)—portion of the radiograph that appears light; the ability of a substance to resist radiation penetration resulting in light area on the film.

rales—respiration sounds heard on inhaling and expelling of air as noisy, bubbling sounds.

rampant caries—widespread or growing tooth decay.

ramus (**RAY**-mus)—ascending part of the mandible.

ranula (**RAN**-you-lah)—cystic tumor found on the underside of the tongue or in the sublingual ducts.

raphe (**RAH**-fay)—ridge or union between two halves.

reamer (**REE**-mer)—endodontic instrument used to scrape and enlarge the root canal.

rectal sedation—sedative administered by placement of drugs in the rectum.

recurrent caries—decay occurring under or near a previously repaired margin of a restoration.

reduction (ree-**DUCT**-shun)—lessening or reducing in size; preparation; or a restoration to normal position, as in a fracture.

refractory (ree-**FRACK**-tore-ee)—resistant to treatment; gingival disease that will not heal.

rem (roentgen equivalent measure)—unit of ionizing radiation needed to produce the same biological effect as one R of radiation; international unit is sievert (Sv).

remission (ree-**MISH**-un)—a lessening or abating of a disease or condition.

remnant radiation—radiation rays reaching the film target after passing through the patient.

replantation—replanting or replacing a tooth that has been avulsed.

replenisher solution—superconcentrated chemical solution added to tank to restore fluid level.

resin—plastic-type material used for dental appliances; may be self- or auto-cured when no other material is needed for the set, or it may require a curing light to cause the setup.

resistance—ability of a microorganism to be unaffected by a drug.

resistance form—preparation cuts to ensure that the restored natural tooth can withstand trauma.

resorption (ree-**SORP**-shun)—removal of hard tooth surface and degeneration of the root tissues.

respiration—inhaling or the taking in of oxygen and the exhaling of carbon dioxide; a vital sign.

respiratory (**RESS**-purr-ah-tore-ee) **shock**—shock arising from insufficient breathing.

rest—small extension of removable prosthesis made to fit or seat atop the adjoining teeth.

restoration—a repair that replaces an area; a renewing; tooth filling.

retainer (ree-**TAIN**-ur)—part of an appliance joining the abutting, natural tooth to the support.

retention form—stage of tooth preparation for the undercut of walls to provide a mechanical hold.

reticulation (reh-**tick**-you-**LAY**-shun)—cracked effect on radiograph caused by extreme temperature changes.

retraction cord—chemically treated string or cord put into the gingival sulcus to prepare the gingiva.

retractor (ree-**TRACK**-tor)—device used to hold back cheek or muscle tissue from surgical area.

retrograde (**REH**-troh-grade)—backward step; in RCT, the restoration of a tooth from the root apex to the crown, instead of from the crown to the root.

retromolar (ret-trow-**MOLE**-ar) **area**—located at the rear of the mouth distal to the molars.

retrusion (ree-**TRUE**-zhun)—measurement with the mandible drawn backward.

rheostat (ree-oh-**STAT**)—a foot petal or lever is used to regulate the speed of the handpiece.

rickettsia (rih-**KET**-see-ah)—microbes smaller than bacteria but larger than viruses.

ridge—linear elevation that receives its name from its area or location.

right angled bur (RA)—rotary bur that fits into right-angled handpiece.

right-angled handpiece—power-driven drill with head angled at 90°.

rinsing—in radiation, the water bath immersions between chemical dips and final water bath.

rod (enamel rod)—prism-like, slender bar that extends from dentinoenamel junction to outer surface of tooth.

rongeurs (**RON**-jeers)—cutting instrument, clipper; used to snip or nip off bone points.

root—bottom part of a tooth; may be single-, double-, or triple-rooted.

root amputation (**am**-pyou-**TAY**-shun)—surgical removal of a root.

root canal condenser/plugger—long-necked instrument used to condense the gutta-perch a material placed in the canal during RCT treatment.

root canal spreader—instrument used to spread cement that has been placed in the root canal.

root hemisection—cutting off a tissue or a root part.

root planing—removal of all detectable deposits and endotoxins on the root surfaces.

rotary instrument—instrument that is placed into the handpiece for operation; includes bur, mandrels, diamonds, points, and stones.

rotation—movement of tooth; turn on the tooth axis; orthodontic movement.

rugae (**RUE**-guy)—irregular folds on the surface of the palate; singular, ruga.

saddle—that part of a removable prosthesis that is astride or straddles the gingival crest.

safelight—device used for illumination in a processing darkroom.

saggital (**SAJ**-ih-tahl) **suture**—union line between two parietal bones on top of the skull.

saggital plane—in radiation, an imaginary vertical line bisecting the face.

salicylates (sah-**LIH**-sil-ates)—analgesic, antipyretic and anti-inflammatory drugs; example: aspirin.

saliva ejector tip—small tube-like device used to suction mouth fluids; may be bent and hooked into patient's mouth during procedures, or may be hand-held.

sanitation (san-ih-**TAY**-shun)—application of methods to promote favorable germ-free state.

saprophytes (**SAP**-roh-fights)—organisms living on dead or decaying organic matter.

sarcoma (sar-**KOH**-mah)—tumor of the flesh or tissues.

scaler—hand instrument with sharp blade used to scrape or fleck off calculus.

scalpel (**SKAL**-pell)—cutting instrument; may be one piece or have a handle and detachable blade.

scattered radiation—radiation that is deflected from its path.

scorbutic (skor-**BYOU**-tick)—lacking vitamin C.

sealant—clear or tinted acrylic substance painted on tooth surfaces to prevent decay.

seating—process of placing and fitting an appliance into the oral cavity.

secondary effect—indirect consequence from a drug action.

secondary radiation—radiation given off from matter other than the area that is primarily exposed.

sedation (see-**DAY**-shun)—induced state of relaxation.

selected removal—removal and restoration of occlusal irregularities to prevent decay.

semilunar valves—two heart valves—aortic and pulmonary.

sensitivity—ability of x-rays to penetrate and possibly ionize the body.

separating medium—material placed on a die before wax is melted on it, to ease separation.

separator—device used to prepare interproximal space between teeth to receive orthodontic bands.

septic (**SEP**-tick) **shock**—shock caused by excessive microbial infection.

sequestra (see-**KWESS**-trah)—small bone spicules working to the surface after surgery; singular, sequestrum.

serum (**SEE**-rum)—watery fluid produced by the body.

setting time—period when material becomes as hard as it will be.

shank—part of a rotary bur that fits into handpiece; may be plain or have a latch-notched end.

Sharpey's fibers—part of the periodontal ligaments that attach and hold the tooth.

shoulder (**SHOAL**-dur)—preparation of gingival margin edge to provide an appliance junction.

sialoadenitis (**sigh**-al-oh-**add**-en-**EYE**-tiss)—inflammation of a salivary gland.

side effect—reaction from a drug that is not the desired treatment outcome.

sigmoid notch—S-shaped curvature between condyle and coronoid processes.

silicone (sill-ih-**KONE**) **impression material**—putty base with a liquid accelerator, or as a two-paste system.

silver point—endodontic restorative point that is cemented into the prepared canal.

simple cavity—dental decay on only one surface of a tooth.

sinus (**SIGH**-nus)—air pocket or cavity in a bone that lightens the bone and warms the air.

slurry (**SLUR**-ee)—thin, watery mixture; plaster slurry placed in the mix to speed up the set.

smile line—amount of tooth space viewed while the patient is smiling.

solder (**SOD**-er)—process of uniting two metal objects by melting into a common alloy.

solubility (sahl-you-**BILL**-ih-tee)—ability to be dissolved.

somatic (soh-**MAT**-ick)—pertaining to the body.

space maintainer—device used to retain space resulting from premature loss of tooth.

spacer—substance, usually wax, placed on cast surface to allow impression material space.

spectrum—range of a drug's activity in the body.

sphenoid (**SFEE**-noyd)—skull bone between occipital and ethmoid bones.

sphenopalatine (sfee-no-**PAL**-ah-tine)—sensory nerve branch ending for maxillary anterior mucosal and palatine tissues.

spherical (**SFEAR**-ih-kul)—round, in the form of a sphere.

sphygmomanometer (sfig-moh-man-**AHM**-eh-ter)—instrument to determine blood pressure.

spindle (**SPIN**-dul)—end area of union of odontoblasts and enamel rod endings.

spoon excavator—instrument with spoon-like tip; used to scrape out decay and necrotic matter.

spore—bacteria that encapsulate in a protective covering when conditions are adverse.

spot welding—electrical process of melting two metals together at a joint.

spray-wipe-spray method—process of using a disinfectant substance to disinfect large areas.

sprue (**SPROO**) **base**—used to hold wax pattern on a sprue pin during the investment process.

sprue pin—small plastic pin placed in the wax pattern to hold wax during the investment process.

squamous (**SKWAY**-mus)—also known as the temporoparietal suture.

stapes (**STAY**-peez)—ossicle in the middle ear; "stirrup."

Stim-U-Dent—flat, small wooden picks used to stimulate gingival tissue.

stabilization (stay-bill-ih-**ZAY**-shun)—condition of being fixed, steady, or firm.

sterilization (stare-ill-ih-**ZAY**-shun)—process of destroying all forms of microorganisms.

sternum (**STIR**-num)—breastbone in the middle of the ribs.

stertorous (**STARE**-toe-rus)—respiration sounds—rattling, bubbling snoring—that obscure normal breaths.

stethoscope (**STETH**-oh-scope)—device employed to intensify body sounds.

Stev plate—maxillary orthodontic biteplane covering incisal edges of the anteriors.

sticky wax—hard, brittle wax stick that is melted and placed to hold dental units together.

stippling (**STIP**-ling)—natural spotting or pigmentation on gingiva.

stoma (**STOW**-mah)—mouth, small opening.

stomatic (sto-**MAT**-ick)—pertaining to the mouth.

stop—indent or hole cut into wax spacer to prevent the tray from being seated too deeply.

strabismus (strah-**BIZ**-muss)—a condition in which the eyes do not fix at the same point.

stray radiation—radiation other than the useful beam; also called leakage radiation.

stress and tension gauge—orthodontic instrument used to test tension and internal forces.

stress breaker—connector applied in stress-bearing location to provide safe breakage area.

stripes of Retzius (**RET**-zih-us)—brownish lines in enamel tissue.

study model—gypsum reproduction of a patient's teeth and oral tissues.

styloid (**STY**-loyd)—natural growth from temporal bone for attachment of some tongue muscles.

subcutaneous (sub-kyou-**TAY**-nee-us)—under the skin.

sublingual—under the tongue.

subluxation (**sub**-lucks-**AY**-shun)—partially loosened.

submandibular—under the mandible.

submucosal (sub-myou-**COH**-sal)—under the mucous membrane.

subperiosteal (**sub**-pear-ee-**AHS**-tee-uhl) **implant**—device placed under the peritoneum to provide a hold for attaching prosthesis.

subscription—part of the prescription containing instructions to the pharmacist.

succedaneous (suck-seh-**DAY**-nee-us)—permanent teeth that replace deciduous teeth.

sulcus (**SULL**-kus)—long depression between ridges and cusps; valley on the tooth surface.

supernumerary (soo-per-**NEW**-mer-air-ee)—extra; more than normal number of teeth.

superscription—part of the prescription that contains name, address, age, and the Rx symbol.

suppository—medicated form to be inserted into the rectum or vagina for timed release.

suppurative (**SUP**-you-rah-tiv)—producing pus.

supraorbital (**soo**-prah-**OR**-bih-tal)—frontal bone opening above orbit of the eye.

supraperiosteal (**soo**-prah-pear-ee-**OSS**-tee-ahl)—about or above the periosteum injection site.

surgical bur—rotary bur with a larger head to smooth or score a tooth for bisectioning.

suspension—liquid drug obtained by mixing with, but not dissolving in, another substance.

suture (**SOO**-chur)—a line where two or more bones unite; a surgical stitch.

symmetric (sim-**MEH**-trick)—balanced, evenly placed body parts.

symphysis (**SIM**-fih-sis)—center of the mandible, mental (chin), or chin protuberance (projection).

symptom (**SIM**-tum)—perceptible change in the body or body function.

syncope (**SIN**-koh-pee)—fainting.

syndrome (**SIN**-drome)—grouping of multiple signs or symptoms characterizing a disease.

synergism (**SIN**-er-jizm)—harmonious action of two drugs to produce a desired effect.

synovial (sin-**OH**-vee-al) **fluid**—lubricating fluid contained in joint.

systolic (sis-**TAH**-lick)—pressure of the circulating blood while under pulsation.

tachycardia (tack-ee-**KAR**-dee-ah)—pulse rates above 100 beats per minute.

target–film distance—in radiation, the distance between the film and the source of radiation.

target–object distance—distance between the anode target and the object to be radiographed.

temperature—balance of heat loss and production in the body.

template—a pattern or design to follow.

temporal (**TEM**-pore-al)—fan-shaped bone, one on each side of the skull.

temporary coverage—protection for prepared tooth while awaiting permanent coverage; also called provisional coverage.

temporary crown—acrylic or composite crown prepared in the impression and provisionally cemented onto the prep for protection until the permanent crown is ready.

temporomandibular (tem-poe-roe-man-**DIB**-you-lar)—pertaining to the temporal and mandible joint area.

temporoparietal (tem-poe-roe-pa-**RYE**-eh-tal)—suture between the temporal and parietal bones.

tensile (TEN-sill) **strength**—a material's capability of being stretched.

teratogenic (tare-ah-toh-**JEN**-ick)—effects of drug on a fetus.

ternary (TURN-ah-ree)—an alloy composed of three metals.

tertiary (TERR-shee-air-ee)—later stage, such as a growth of reparative dentin.

thrombocytes (THROM-boh-sites)—blood platelets.

Tic douloureux (tick-**DOO**-loo-roo)—degeneration or pressure on the trigeminal nerve, causing pain and contractions.

therapeutic (thair-ah-**PYOU**-tick)—healing agent or action.

thermal—a heat measurement, condition; or diagnostic test in RCT.

thermal conductivity—ability of material to transfer heat.

thermoplastic (therm-oh-**PLAS**-tick)—material that softens and changes shapes when heated.

thrombosis (throm-**BOH**-sis)—blood clot.

thrush—fungus infection of mouth and/or throat.

tincture (TINK-chur)—diluted alcoholic solution of a drug.

tinnitus (tin-**EYE**-tuss)—ringing in the ears.

TMJ—temporomandibular joint, union of the mandible and the temporal bones.

tonic (TAHN-ick)—continuous muscular tension producing rigidity or violent seizures.

tonsil (TAHN-sill)—lymphatic tissue mass found in the fauces.

tooth stabilization—wiring or splinting of teeth to prevent movement.

topical (TAH-pih-cull)—in a specific place, as in topical application of a solution.

torque (tork)—orthodontic movement of the root without movement of the crown.

torus (TORE-us)—rounded, bony elevation (in the maxillary, it is a torus palatinus; in the lower jaw area, it is torus mandibularis).

tracheotomy (tray-kee-**AH**-toh-me)—cutting into the trachea to allow air to enter.

traction devices—orthodontic devices hooked onto a facebow and worn on the head.

transcription—part of a prescription that gives direction to a patient.

transient ischemic attack (TIA)—local and temporary anemia resulting from circulation obstruction.

transillumination (trans-ill-oo-mih-**NAY**-shun)—passage of light through an object; a diagnostic test in RCT.

transosteal (trans-**AHS**-tee-al)—implant placed through the bone.

transplantation (TRANS-plan-**tay**-shun)—the transfer of an object from one area to another.

traumatized (TRAW-mah-tizd)—wounded or injured from an outside force.

Trendelenburg position—patient lying supine with feet placed higher than the head.

trifurcation (try-fer-**KAY**-shun)—branching or separating into three roots (maxillary molar).

trigeminal (try-**JEM**-in-al)—pertaining to the trigeminal nerve; fifth cranial nerve.

trismus (TRIZ-mus)—grating or tonic contracting of the jaws.

trituration (try-chur-**AY**-shun)—mixing of mercury with other alloy material to form an amalgam.

troche—soft, flavored medicinal mass of a drug, for holding in the mouth and dissolving.

trochlear (TRAH-klee-ur)—fourth cranial nerve.

truncated (TRUN-kay-ted)—cut part off, lop off; shortened burs.

tubercle (TOO-ber-kul)—small knob-like prominence on a tooth surface.

tubule (**TOO**-bule)—small *S*-shaped tube or channel extending from dentinoenamel wall to pulp chamber; also known as Tomes' dentinal tubule.

tuft—abnormal clump of rods; irregular grouping of undercalcified enamel.

tympanic (tim-**PAN**-ick)—pertaining to the eardrum.

ultrasonic cleaner—machine to cleanse instruments by cavitration (exploding of bubbles).

undercut—removal of tooth structure near the gingival edge to provide a seat or placement area.

unit—in prosthetics, a part or section of an appliance.

Universal charting method—procedure for numbering of teeth from 1–32.

universal precaution—treating each case as if a disease is present.

urticaria (ur-tih-**CARE**-ee-ah)—vascular skin reaction; hives.

utility wax—soft, adhesive wax in stick or sheet form; used in mounting or adapting trays.

uvula (**YOU**-view-lah)—small, fleshy growth in back of throat that descends from the posterior of the palate.

vaccination (**VACK**-sih-nay-shun)—inoculation of serum or toxin to produce immunity.

vaccine (**VAK**-seen)—solution of killed or weakened or dead microbes.

vacuum tube—x-radiation tube producer.

vagus (**VAY**-gus)—tenth cranial nerve.

varnish—copal or resin gum sealing mixture that is placed under a restoration.

vascular (**VAS**-kyou-lar)—pertaining to the small blood vessels.

vasoconstrictor (vas-oh-kahn-**STRIK**-tore)—vessel tightener, chemical added to anesthetic to constrict blood vessels.

vector (**VEK**-tore)—carrier that transmits disease.

vector borne—diseased person with a natural immunity, one in an incubation period lacking signs.

veneer (veh-**NEAR**)—thin, resin, tooth-shaped layer applied to tooth surface, or a thin coating.

ventricle (**VEN**-trih-kul)—two lower chambers of the heart, one on each side.

vermilion (ver-**MILL**-yon) **border**—area where the pink–red lip tissue meets the facial skin.

verruca vulgaris (ver-**OO**-kah vul-**GAIR**-iss)—oral warts.

vertical angulation—central x-ray beam moving in an up or down position.

vertical overbite—overlap of upper and lower central incisors while in occlusion.

vertical window—placement position in a radiograph mount used for anterior films.

vertigo (**VER**-tih-go)—dizziness.

vesicle (**VES**-ih-kuhl)—small blister.

vestibule (**VES**-tih-byul)—open gum area between teeth and cheek.

vestibulocochler (vest-**tib**-you-loh-**COCK**-lee-ar)—eighth cranial nerve.

vestibuloplasty (ves-**TIB**-you-loh-**plas**-tee)—surgical alteration of the gingival mucous membrane in mouth vestibule.

virulence (**VEER**-you-lence)—power or strong ability of a disease.

virus (**VYE**-rus)—class of parasitic, tiny organisms that cause a variety of diseases.

viscosity (**VISS**-**KAHS**-ih-tee)—sticky or gummy ability or condition.

vital signs—body indications of a patient's present health status.

vomer (**VOH**-mer)—bone forming lower and posterior part of the nasal septum.

wax elimination—burnout of wax pattern from investment material, leaving a void.

wax pattern—exact replica of the prosthesis to be constructed.

welding—direct joining of two metals by a fusion process.

working time—time period when it is possible to manipulate a material without adverse effects.

xenograft (**ZEE**-no-graft)—bone graft taken from another species, such as a cow or pig (experimental).

xerostomia (zee-roh-**STOH**-me-ah)—dry mouth.

xiphoid (**ZIF**-oyd)—process or bone at the lowest portion of the sternum (breastbone).

x-ray—radiant energy produced from a vacuum tube.

yield strength—maximum amount of stress a material can withstand without deformation.

zero angulation—position of x-ray source in a neutral angle, not up or down; zero degree angle.

zygomatic bone (zye-goh-**MAT**-ick)—facial bone on the underside of each eye that gives form and shape to the cheekbone.

zygomaticofacial (zye-goh-**MAT**-ee-coe-fay-shal) **foramen**—opening in bone for nerve passage.

Glossary of Acronyms

ALARA	as low as reasonably achievable
ADA	American Dental Association
	Americans with Disabilities Act
ADAA	American Dental Assistants Association
ADHA	American Dental Hygienists Association
AIDS	Acquired Immune Deficiency Syndrome
ANSI	American National Standard Institute
ANUG	acute necrotic ulcerative gingivitis
ARC	AIDS-related complex
BIS-GMA	polymer used in pit and fissure sealants
BPM	beats per minute
CAHP	contra angle handpiece
CDA	Certified Dental Assistant
CDCP	Centers for Disease Control and Prevention
CDPMA	Certified Dental Practice Management Assistant
CDT	Certified Dental Technician
CERP	Continuing Education Recognition Program
CHF	congestive heart failure
CNS	central nervous system
COA	Certified Orthodontic Assistant
COMSA	Certified Oral Maxillofacial Surgery Assistant
CPR	cardiopulmonary resuscitation
CVA	cerebrovascular accident
DANB	Dental Assisting National Board
DB	direct bonding
DDS	Doctor of Dental Surgery
DEA	Drug Enforcement Agency
DHCW	Dental Health Care Worker
DMD	Doctor of Medical Dentistry
DNA	deoxyribonucleic acid

DR	digital radiography
EBA	ortho-ethoxybenzoic acid
EFDA	Expanded Function Dental Auxiliary
ELISA	Enzyme-Linked Immunosorbent Assay (HIV antibody test)
ENAP	excisional/new attachment procedure
EPA	Environmental Protection Agency
FDA	Food and Drug Administration
FDC	Federal Drug and Cosmetic Act
FDI	Federation Dentaire Internationale
FFD	film focus distance
FG	friction grip
HAV	Hepatitis A virus
HBIG	Hepatitis B immune globulin (plasma antibody for hepatitis)
HBV	Hepatitis B virus
HCV	Hepatitis C virus
HCW	health care worker
HIV	Human Immunodeficiency Virus
HIV+	positive serotest for HIV antibody
HVE	high-volume evacuator
IOR	interocclusal registration (bite registration)
IPA	Independent Practice Association
MMWR	Morbidity and Mortality Weekly Report
MPD	maximum permissible dose
MSDS	manufacturer's safety data sheet
NADL	National Association of Dental Laboratories
NIOSH	National Institute for Occupational Safety and Health
OPIM	other potential infectious material
OSHA	Occupational Safety and Health Administration
PFI	plastic filling instrument
PFM	porcelain fused to metal
PID	position indicating device (radiology)
PIM	potential infectious material
PPE	personal protection equipment
PPO	preferred provider organization
RCT	root canal treatment
RDH	Registered Dental Hygienist
RPE	rapid palatal expander
SBDA	State Board of Dental Examiners
SDPA	State Dental Practice Act
SOP	standard operating procedure
TIA	transient ischemic attack
UCR	usual, customary, and reasonable (fees)
ZOE	zinc oxide eugenol

Index

IMPORTANT! READ CAREFULLY: This End User License Agreement ("Agreement") sets forth the conditions by which Thomson Delmar Learning, a division of Thomson Learning Inc. ("Thomson") will make electronic access to the Thomson Delmar Learning-owned licensed content and associated media, software, documentation, printed materials, and electronic documentation contained in this package and/or made available to you via this product (the "Licensed Content"), available to you (the "End User"). BY CLICKING THE "I ACCEPT" BUTTON AND/OR OPENING THIS PACKAGE, YOU ACKNOWLEDGE THAT YOU HAVE READ ALL OF THE TERMS AND CONDITIONS, AND THAT YOU AGREE TO BE BOUND BY ITS TERMS, CONDITIONS, AND ALL APPLICABLE LAWS AND REGULATIONS GOVERNING THE USE OF THE LICENSED CONTENT.

1.0 SCOPE OF LICENSE

1.1 *Licensed Content.* The Licensed Content may contain portions of modifiable content ("Modifiable Content") and content which may not be modified or otherwise altered by the End User ("Non-Modifiable Content"). For purposes of this Agreement, Modifiable Content and Non-Modifiable Content may be collectively referred to herein as the "Licensed Content." All Licensed Content shall be considered Non-Modifiable Content, unless such Licensed Content is presented to the End User in a modifiable format and it is clearly indicated that modification of the Licensed Content is permitted.

1.2 Subject to the End User's compliance with the terms and conditions of this Agreement, Thomson Delmar Learning hereby grants the End User, a nontransferable, nonexclusive, limited right to access and view a single copy of the Licensed Content on a single personal computer system for noncommercial, internal, personal use only. The End User shall not (i) reproduce, copy, modify (except in the case of Modifiable Content), distribute, display, transfer, sublicense, prepare derivative work(s) based on, sell, exchange, barter or transfer, rent, lease, loan, resell, or in any other manner exploit the Licensed Content; (ii) remove, obscure, or alter any notice of Thomson Delmar Learning's intellectual property rights present on or in the Licensed Content, including, but not limited to, copyright, trademark, and/or patent notices; or (iii) disassemble, decompile, translate, reverse engineer, or otherwise reduce the Licensed Content.

2.0 TERMINATION

2.1 Thomson Delmar Learning may at any time (without prejudice to its other rights or remedies) immediately terminate this Agreement and/or suspend access to some or all of the Licensed Content, in the event that the End User does not comply with any of the terms and conditions of this Agreement. In the event of such termination by Thomson Delmar Learning, the End User shall immediately return any and all copies of the Licensed Content to Thomson Delmar Learning.

3.0 PROPRIETARY RIGHTS

3.1 The End User acknowledges that Thomson Delmar Learning owns all rights, title and interest, including, but not limited to all copyright rights therein, in and to the Licensed Content, and that the End User shall not take any action inconsistent with such ownership. The Licensed Content is protected by U.S., Canadian and other applicable copyright laws and by international treaties, including the Berne Convention and the Universal Copyright Convention. Nothing contained in this Agreement shall be construed as granting the End User any ownership rights in or to the Licensed Content.

3.2 Thomson Delmar Learning reserves the right at any time to withdraw from the Licensed Content any item or part of an item for which it no longer retains the right to publish, or which it has reasonable grounds to believe infringes copyright or is defamatory, unlawful, or otherwise objectionable.

4.0 PROTECTION AND SECURITY

4.1 The End User shall use its best efforts and take all reasonable steps to safeguard its copy of the Licensed Content to ensure that no unauthorized reproduction, publication, disclosure, modification, or distribution of the Licensed Content, in whole or in part, is made. To the extent that the End User becomes aware of any such unauthorized use of the Licensed Content, the End User shall immediately notify Thomson Delmar Learning. Notification of such violations may be made by sending an e-mail to delmarhelp@thomson.com.

5.0 MISUSE OF THE LICENSED PRODUCT

5.1 In the event that the End User uses the Licensed Content in violation of this Agreement, Thomson Delmar Learning shall have the option of electing liquidated damages, which shall include all profits generated by the End User's use of the Licensed Content plus interest computed at the maximum rate permitted by law and all legal fees and other expenses incurred by Thomson Delmar Learning in enforcing its rights, plus penalties.

6.0 FEDERAL GOVERNMENT CLIENTS

6.1 Except as expressly authorized by Thomson Delmar Learning, Federal Government clients obtain only the rights specified in this Agreement and no other rights. The Government acknowledges that (i) all software and related documentation incorporated in the Licensed Content is existing commercial computer software within the meaning of FAR 27.405(b)(2); and (2) all other data delivered in whatever form, is limited rights data within the meaning of FAR 27.401. The restrictions in this section are acceptable as consistent with the Government's need for software and other data under this Agreement.

7.0 DISCLAIMER OF WARRANTIES AND LIABILITIES

7.1 Although Thomson Delmar Learning believes the Licensed Content to be reliable, Thomson Delmar Learning does not guarantee or warrant (i) any information or materials contained in or produced by the Licensed Content, (ii) the accuracy, completeness or reliability of the Licensed Content, or (iii) that the Licensed Content is free from errors or other material defects. THE LICENSED PRODUCT IS PROVIDED "AS IS," WITHOUT ANY WARRANTY OF ANY KIND AND THOMSON DELMAR LEARNING DISCLAIMS ANY AND ALL WARRANTIES, EXPRESSED OR IMPLIED, INCLUDING, WITHOUT LIMITATION, WARRANTIES OF MERCHANTABILITY OR FITNESS FOR A PARTICULAR PURPOSE. IN NO EVENT SHALL THOMSON DELMAR LEARNING BE LIABLE FOR: INDIRECT, SPECIAL, PUNITIVE OR CONSEQUENTIAL DAMAGES INCLUDING FOR LOST PROFITS, LOST DATA, OR OTHERWISE. IN NO EVENT SHALL THOMSON DELMAR LEARNING'S AGGREGATE LIABILITY HEREUNDER, WHETHER ARISING IN CONTRACT, TORT, STRICT LIABILITY OR OTHERWISE, EXCEED THE AMOUNT OF FEES PAID BY THE END USER HEREUNDER FOR THE LICENSE OF THE LICENSED CONTENT.

8.0 GENERAL

8.1 *Entire Agreement.* This Agreement shall constitute the entire Agreement between the Parties and supercedes all prior Agreements and understandings oral or written relating to the subject matter hereof.

8.2 *Enhancements/Modifications of Licensed Content.* From time to time, and in Thomson Delmar Learning's sole discretion, Thomson Delmar Learning may advise the End User of updates, upgrades, enhancements and/or improvements to the Licensed Content, and may permit the End User to access and use, subject to the terms and conditions of this Agreement, such modifications, upon payment of prices as may be established by Thomson Delmar Learning.

8.3 *No Export.* The End User shall use the Licensed Content solely in the United States and shall not transfer or export, directly or indirectly, the Licensed Content outside the United States.

8.4 *Severability.* If any provision of this Agreement is invalid, illegal, or unenforceable under any applicable statute or rule of law, the provision shall be deemed omitted to the extent that it is invalid, illegal, or unenforceable. In such a case, the remainder of the Agreement shall be construed in a manner as to give greatest effect to the original intention of the parties hereto.

8.5 *Waiver.* The waiver of any right or failure of either party to exercise in any respect any right provided in this Agreement in any instance shall not be deemed to be a waiver of such right in the future or a waiver of any other right under this Agreement.

8.6 *Choice of Law/Venue.* This Agreement shall be interpreted, construed, and governed by and in accordance with the laws of the State of New York, applicable to contracts executed and to be wholly preformed therein, without regard to its principles governing conflicts of law. Each party agrees that any proceeding arising out of or relating to this Agreement or the breach or threatened breach of this Agreement may be commenced and prosecuted in a court in the State and County of New York. Each party consents and submits to the nonexclusive personal jurisdiction of any court in the State and County of New York in respect of any such proceeding.

8.7 *Acknowledgment.* By opening this package and/or by accessing the Licensed Content on this Web site, THE END USER ACKNOWLEDGES THAT IT HAS READ THIS AGREEMENT, UNDERSTANDS IT, AND AGREES TO BE BOUND BY ITS TERMS AND CONDITIONS. IF YOU DO NOT ACCEPT THESE TERMS AND CONDITIONS, YOU MUST NOT ACCESS THE LICENSED CONTENT AND RETURN THE LICENSED PRODUCT TO DELMAR LEARNING (WITHIN 30 CALENDAR DAYS OF THE END USER'S PURCHASE) WITH PROOF OF PAYMENT ACCEPTABLE TO THOMSON DELMAR LEARNING, FOR A CREDIT OR A REFUND. Should the End User have any questions/comments regarding this Agreement, please contact Thomson Delmar Learning at delmarhelp@thomson.com.